WILLIAMS & LISSNER'S

BIOMECHANICS
OF
HUMAN
MOTION

THIRD EDITION

WILLIAMS & LISSNER'S

BIOMECHANICS OF HUMAN MOTION

THIRD EDITION

Barney F. LeVeau, PT, Ph.D.
Professor and Chairman, Department of Physical Therapy
University of Texas Southwestern Medical Center at Dallas
Southwestern Allied Health Sciences School
Dallas, Texas

W.B. SAUNDERS COMPANY
A Division of Harcourt Brace & Company
Philadelphia ■ London ■ Toronto ■ Montreal ■ Sydney ■ Tokyo

W.B. SAUNDERS COMPANY
A Division of
Harcourt Brace & Company

The Curtis Center
Independence Square West
Philadelphia, PA 19106

Library of Congress Cataloging-in-Publication Data

Williams, Marian
　　[Biomechanics of human motion]
　　Williams and Lissner's biomechanics of human motion /
Barney F. LeVeau.—3rd ed.
　　　　p.　cm.
　　Includes index.
　　ISBN 0-7216-5743-5
　　1. Human locomotion.　2. Human mechanics.　I.
Lissner, Herbert R.　II. LeVeau, Barney F. (Barney
Francis).　III. Title.　IV. Title: Biomechanics of human
motion.
　　QP303.W58　1991
　　612.7'6—dc20　　　　　　　　　　　　　　　91-21709
　　　　　　　　　　　　　　　　　　　　　　　　　CIP

Listed here is the latest translated edition of this book together with the language of the translation and the publisher.

French (*2nd edition*)—Decarie Editeur, Ville Mont-Royal, Quebec, Canada

Spanish (*2nd edition*)—Editorial Trillas, S.A. de C.V., Av. Rio Churubusco 385, Col. Pedro Maria Anaya, C.P. 03340, Mexico, D.F.

Editor:　Margaret M. Biblis
Designer:　Susan Blaker
Production Manager:　Peter Faber
Manuscript Editor:　David Prout
Illustration Coordinator:　Walt Verbitski
Indexer:　Roger Wall
Cover Designer:　Joan Wendt

Williams & Lissner's Biomechanics of Human Motion, 3/e.　　　　　ISBN 0-7216-5743-5

Last digit is the print number:　　9　8　7　6　5

*To my parents
who, although they had limited formal education,
provided opportunities and encouragement
for all of their children to obtain postgraduate degrees.*

PREFACE

The main purpose of the third edition of *Biomechanics of Human Motion* remains the same as for the original edition: that is, to suggest techniques for approaching biomechanical problems.

Several changes have been made in the current edition. A second color has been incorporated into many of the illustrations to enhance their clarity; an outline of chapter contents has been added at the beginning of each chapter to guide the student in locating specific topics; the units of measure have been changed from English to International System (SI) units, and a conversion table for these units is presented in Chapter 1; and discussions of nonbiological materials have been added. A major addition to the dynamics chapter (Chapter 7) addresses more thoroughly the equations of motion. A general discussion of applied biomechanical principles has been added to the applications chapter (Chapter 7), which has become the last chapter in this edition, and some of the repetitious examples have been deleted. The appendix has been changed by deleting the trigonometric tables, expanding the glossary, and adding answers to selected problems. Examples that relate to the fields of occupational therapy, prosthetics and orthotics, physical medicine, and orthopedics have been added, along with updated references.

By reading and practicing the examples in this book, the student may learn this material without the assistance of an instructor. The most difficult part of learning this material is that of visualizing the problem. The student reader must form a mental picture and draw the figure, or take an actual photograph to note the problem situation, including the acting forces and dimensions.

BARNEY F. LeVEAU, PT, PH.D.

ACKNOWLEDGMENTS

I would like to thank Michael Gross, Ph.D., from the University of North Carolina, and Sheik N. Imrhan, Ph.D., from The University of Texas at Arlington, for their useful critique of the new additions to Chapter 7, and Wang Te-Chih, from Beijing, People's Republic of China, for his suggestions for improvement of the Second Edition.

I would also like to thank Margaret M. Biblis, Editor, and Charles Keenan, Editorial Assistant, Health-Related Professions, W. B. Saunders Company; Martha W. Tanner, Development Editor; David Prout for editorial assistance; Mary Foster for secretarial assistance; and my wife and family for their patience.

CONTENTS

3

Strength of Materials 29

4

Composition and Resolution of Forces 60

5

Static Equilibrium 88

1

The Scope of Biomechanics

INTRODUCTION

The application of mechanical principles to the human body is as old as humanity itself. Only recently, however, have we seriously studied the implications of mechanics for the human body. Contini and Drillis (1954) briefly discussed the historical development of biomechanics up to the early 1950s. Since that time the study of biomechanics has grown rapidly. Increased awareness and interest have come from the fields of physical and occupational therapy, physical education, prosthetics and orthotics, sports medicine, orthopedics, and ergonomics (Rasch, 1958; Contini and Drillis, 1966; Fung et al., 1972; Miller and Nelson, 1973; Ghista, 1979; Radin et al., 1979; Ghista and Roaf, 1981a and 1981b; Chaffin and Andersson, 1984; Schmid-Schönbein et al., 1984; American Academy of Orthopedic Surgeons, 1985; Fess and Philips, 1987; Winter, 1987; Viano et al., 1989).

The purpose of this chapter is to give you only a brief idea of the breadth of biomechanics. The examples presented are discussed in more depth in the rest of the book. Many more examples exist. Biomechanics can be applied to many more areas than just those presented in this chapter.

Mechanics is the study of forces and their effects. The application of these mechanical principles to human and animal bodies in movement and at rest is biomechanics. Biomechanics is an attempt to combine engineering with anatomy and physiology. It covers a broad spectrum, from theoretical study to practical applications.

A full discussion of segmental forces in body movement should include not only biomechanical but also physiologic considerations of muscle length-tension relationships and controlling neuromotor mechanisms. Sensory feedback apparatus is a most important factor in adequate neuromuscular function. However, in this text we are concerned only with the mechanical aspects and will simply note in passing that these do not constitute the whole story.

The entire study of mechanics covers two basic areas: statics, the study of bodies remaining at rest or in equilibrium as a result of forces

1

acting upon them, and dynamics, the study of moving bodies. Dynamics, in turn, may be subdivided into kinematics and kinetics. Kinematics might be called "the science of motion" since it deals with the relationships that exist between displacements, velocities, and accelerations in translational or rotational motion. It does not concern itself with the forces involved, but only with the description of the movements themselves. Kinetics deals with moving bodies and the forces that act to produce the motion. For example, Eberhart and colleagues (1954) in their discussion of human locomotion dealt first with the kinematics of walking and described the displacements of the body segments in the three cardinal planes, covering flexion and extension of the thigh and leg, pelvic rotation, and so on. They considered next the kinetics of walking, analyzing the forces of the muscles as well as those of gravity and of floor reaction, all of which are necessary for propulsion of the body and control of segmental displacement. Dillman (1971) studied the kinematics and kinetics of the motion of the swinging leg during running, while Plangenhoef (1968) devised a method of studying dynamics using a computer. More recently, Isacson and associates (1986) studied three-dimensional kinematics of the lower limbs, and foot pressure studies have been reviewed by Lord and co-workers (1986). Hundreds of articles on locomotion alone have been published within the past three years. Hundreds of studies concerning statics and dynamics of other activities have been presented and published.

Some areas of study relevant to biomechanics include anatomy, growth, external loads, trauma, ergonomics, clinical applications, protective equipment, and body movement. Brief discussions of these topics relative to biomechanics follow.

ANATOMY

Biomechanical principles form the basis of musculoskeletal function. Muscles produce force that acts through the bony lever system to resist gravity or to create movement. (See Chapter 5.)

By observing the gross anatomy of the muscular system, we can see that muscles have different fiber arrangements. This internal structure of the muscle determines the relationship of the force that the muscle can produce and the distance over which the muscle can contract. The fusiform or longitudinal muscle fiber arrangement provides a small cross-sectional area and produces less force than other fiber forms. The attachments of a fusiform muscle, however, can span a greater distance. The pennate, or feather-shaped, muscles have the fiber attached at angles to the accompanying tendon. This fiber arrangement provides a greater cross-sectional area so that greater force may be produced. Since these fibers are at an angle to the tendon, not all of their force is directed through the tendon. Their excursion is less than a fusiform muscle. (See Chapters 3 and 4.)

The effect of muscle contraction also depends upon the muscle's attachments to the skeleton. The angle at which a muscle pulls upon the bony lever determines its rotatory and nonrotatory components of force. As the bony part moves through its range of motion, the rotatory and nonrotatory components change. For the effects of these components to be understood, analysis of these changes must be performed. The distance of the muscle attachment from the axis of the lever system determines the moment of force that can be produced. The instantaneous joint axis and the muscle insertion provide information to determine the lever arm length. (See Chapters 4 and 5).

When two or more muscles act on a bone, the final result depends upon the combined force developed by each muscle, their individual angles of pull, and their locations relative to the joint axis. As a muscle contracts it pulls at both attachments. The attachment that offers the least resistance will tend to move. The muscle may act as agonist, synergist, antagonist, or stabilizer. One muscle may act to produce the desired effect, but often several muscles contract to obtain the final result. Their magnitude, angle of pull, and position in relation to the joint and other muscles are important.

Ligaments, cartilage, and other soft tissues aid in joint control and are affected by body position and movement. Bones set up lever systems and provide pulley situations on which muscles and tendons may act.

GROWTH

Mechanical forces can provide a major effect on the growth of the body. Normal forces on the body allow it to grow in the typical manner. For example, the entire internal structure of bone is governed primarily by the loading history to which the bone was exposed (Carter et al., 1989). Abnormal forces, however, especially at times of rapid growth, can lead to abnormal growth patterns. The anomalies that result from these abnormal forces are called "deformations." Tissues respond to forces according to the type of loading, the duration of loading, and the direction of loading. The amount of tension, as opposed to compression, affects the response of chondrogenesis and osteogenesis. A prolonged loading affects the tissue differently than intermittent loading. The tissues respond to the direction of loading. If we can determine how a deformity has been or is being caused, we may be able to remove the deforming forces and apply forces that may reverse and correct the process. Night splints for the problem clubfoot and a Pavlic harness for a congenital dislocation of the hip are examples of the understanding of biomechanical principles applied to growth and development (LeVeau and Bernhardt, 1984; Graham, 1988). (See Chapter 3.)

EXTERNAL LOADS

The resistance offered to the forces of muscles, bones, and joints may come from the pull of gravity, water resistance, elasticity of materials, friction, stationary structures, or manual resistance. The angle of the line of application of the resistance, or load, and the distance of the load from the axis of the lever system determines the effectiveness of the load. Gravity, the most common load on the body, provides a line of force in a constant direction. Both the weight and position of the exercise resistance and of the body part are important when determining the effect of gravity. (See Chapters 2 and 5.)

Pulley systems are used to change the line of pull on the body. These may be set up to offer resistance or to aid in support or movement and may act in any direction. (See Chapter 4.)

The force of gravity may be reduced or neutralized by immersing the body, either totally or partially, in a tank of water. In this case, the gravitational force is balanced by the force of buoyancy, since the body is buoyed up by a force equal to the weight of the volume of water it displaces. Water also offers resistance, directly opposing a body part as that body part moves through it. Another method of reducing the effect of gravity is by suspension in slings, as advocated by Guthrie-Smith (1943). (See Chapter 2.)

A variety of elastic materials (such as springs, rubber bands, and balloons) can be used to provide resistance for muscular exercise. The line of resisting force lies along the length of the elastic material. (See Chapters 4 and 8.)

Many recently developed exercise devices make use of frictional resistance as load for the muscle contraction. Some exercise devices provide a line of force which is perpendicular to the bony lever throughout the range of motion. (See Chapters 5 and 8.) Stationary structures provide resistance for isometric contractions, whereas manual resistance can offer isometric resistance or can give a wide range of resisting loads. (See Chapter 8.)

TRAUMA

According to Radin (1980), of all the basic sciences, biomechanics has the clearest application to the understanding of injury and recovery of musculoskeletal problems. Generally, musculoskeletal injuries occur in a predictable manner (Gozna, 1982). Bony injury is dictated by five biomechanical factors: the type of load, the magnitude of load, the rate of loading, the material properties of the tissue, and the structural properties of the tissue (Gozna, 1982). Chapter 3 elaborates on the examples presented in the following paragraphs.

Forces may cause injury either directly or indirectly. A single force of large magnitude, such as a severe blow, may cause injury, or injury may result from several repetitions of low magnitude forces, as is the case with a stress fracture. The clinician who can analyze the mechanics of the injury is better able to evaluate the kind and extent of the injury and therefore provide more appropriate treatment for the patient.

To evaluate an injury accurately, knowledge of the actual mechanism of the injury is essential. For example, stress fractures, bending fractures, compression fractures, sprains, and concussions are all caused by forces, but the mechanism may determine whether the injury is a fracture or a sprain. The type of fracture, in turn, depends on the characteristics of the force involved. Different applications of force may cause either a bending, stress, or compression fracture. The tissues involved are more easily located and the extent of the injury can be better evaluated when one understands how the injury was caused. The importance of knowing the mechanical aspects of injury has been emphasized by many authors (Viano et al., 1989; Krag et al., 1986; Gozna, 1982; Soeur, 1982; Jacobs and Ghista, 1981; Kaufer, 1980; Alms, 1961.)

ERGONOMICS

Understanding and application of biomechanical principles is also essential in the prevention of injuries in the workplace (Chaffin and Andersson, 1984). Ergonomics is a discipline concerned with the design of facilities, tools, equipment, and tasks that are compatible with the anatomic, physiologic, perceptual, behavioral, and biomechanical characteristics of humans. The mechanical analysis of movement and posture during work allows the ergonomist to recognize unsafe acts and unsafe conditions. Factors that affect the safety of the worker include:

1. The worker's body position.
2. The location of the objects that must be handled.

3. The weight of the objects and the force that must be applied to the tools.
4. The nature of how the force is applied (Andersson et al., 1980).

CLINICAL APPLICATIONS

The principles of biomechanics are used in evaluation and treatment in clinical settings at various levels. An overview of clinical areas in which biomechanical principles are applied follows.

Evaluation

Evaluation of injuries and disabilities involves the use of forces and torques to determine the type and extent of the problem. Noyes and associates (1980) believe that the successful interpretation of clinical laxity tests depend upon biomechanical concepts. Varus and valgus test of the knee use the three-point principle (see Chapter 5). Tension and compression are involved in the Apley and Drawer tests (see Chapter 3). Determination of hip subluxation and dislocation involves use of forces in tests evoking the Ortolani and the Barlow signs. Biomechanical evaluation of balance and gait may provide some answers to the role of sensory systems including the proprioceptive, vestibular, and visual systems. Studies by Nashner (1977 and 1980), Nashner and McCollum (1985), Badke and Duncan (1983), Schenkman and Butler (1989), and Lichtenstein and co-workers (1988, 1989, and 1990) have enhanced the ability of the clinician to evaluate the nervous system. Measurements of posture and movement help to determine possible neurologic dysfunction and may provide suggestions for treatment intervention (Craik, 1984).

Manual muscle testing depends upon the skill of the clinician in applying test forces of varying degrees of magnitude in order to gauge the patient's ability to resist these forces. The significance of lever arm lengths involved in the muscle test as well as the force applied must be considered. (See Chapters 5 and 8).

The location of the center of mass of each body part affects the activity of the muscles that support that part. The clinician can evaluate the patient's posture while standing, sitting, and lifting and moving objects. Treatment procedures based on mechanical principles can be developed to overcome posture problems. (See Chapter 8.)

Treatment

Most procedures used to treat musculoskeletal and neurologic problems are based to a great extent on biomechanical principles.

Surgical procedures such as realignment of the patella, total joint replacements, tendon transfers, ligament repair, fracture stabilization, and spinal fixation are a few examples that must use application of force and torques, and knowledge of strength of materials. (See Chapters 3, 4, and 5.) Tension, compression, shearing, bending, and torsion are of major concern and must be carefully considered in order to have a successful surgical result. (See Chapter 3.) Whether to use, for example, joint fusion, osteotomy, or joint replacement in joint repair depends upon the needed movement and stability for that joint (Walker, 1981).

Exercise programs are provided for prevention and rehabilitation of a variety of problems. Each exercise has its advantages and disadvantages. One exercise may be beneficial for a specific situation but may be harmful in other instances. The use of various abdominal strengthening exercises are examples (LeVeau, 1973). A great variety of exercise devices have been developed to determine their value; each should be evaluated biomechanically. Body position, resistance and effort, lever arm length, point of force application, the weight of certain device parts, and pulley arrangement all must be considered in analyzing the effectiveness of any exercise device. (See Chapter 8.)

Various traction procedures utilize force to overcome gravity, friction, and soft tissue resistance. Crutches and canes help relieve forces of gravity on an injured or weak body part. The coefficient of friction between the walking surface and the crutch tips determines the angle at which the crutches can safely contact the ground. (See Chapter 6.) Evaluation and treatment of gait relies upon the mechanical characteristics of displacement, velocity, and acceleration. (See Chapter 7.)

Manual therapy uses such movements as oscillations, glides, distractions, leverage on limbs, and direct force on an area. Soft tissue mobilization uses forces with appropriate direction and rhythm to achieve the desired results. Properly applied forces can influence the formation of new scar tissue. Unwanted cross-links can be stretched or ruptured. Range of motion of various joints can be increased with appropriate uses of forces and torques. Examples of specific forces and direction of forces in manipulation are provided by Donatelli and Wooden (1989), Maitland (1986), Grieve (1984), Bourdillon and Day (1987), and Basmajian (1985).

Work-hardening therapy utilizes physiologic functioning by evaluating one's working ability and then gradually increasing performance by increasing strength, endurance, and tolerance for a specific work action (Hopkins and Smith, 1988). Knowledge and use of biomechanical principles are essential for an effective program.

The proper functioning of orthoses and prostheses require that the laws of biomechanics are obeyed (Cool, 1989). A knowledge of forces and torques along with an understanding of stresses, strains, and bending of beams is important (American Academy of Orthopedic Surgeons, 1985). The strength of a variety of materials must be known. (See Chapter 3.)

For good splint fabrication, knowledge of force magnitude, point of application, and line of application are essential. The individual fabricating the splint must know these force characteristics and how to adjust them to obtain appropriate splinting effectiveness. Static splints may be used to protect weak muscles from being stretched by providing a force to counteract the stronger muscle group. They also may provide support and corrective alignment for various body parts. Dynamic splints apply nearly constant force on a body part as the part moves. The splint provides forces that substitute for absent or decreased muscle force to allow rest, maintain joint function, or prevent anky-losis. The splint must be designed and con-structed to provide specific loading of the part with appropriate direction. Outriggers, for ex-ample, must be placed accurately and secured firmly to the body of the splint. The individual designing and constructing the splint should be aware of the magnitude of force, the line of pull, the pressure of the splint, and the pressure areas. The static base must provide a solid foun-dation to allow proper alignment and to attach prosthetic components (Hopkins and Smith, 1988). (See Chapters 4 and 5.)

Splints and prostheses use elastic force from rubber bands and springs to produce needed loads on the body part or terminal device. The elastic force of a rubber band depends upon its cross-sectioned area and its material properties. Forces of springs depend upon their property characteristics. Knowlege of materials helps the clinician make an intelligent decision in choos-ing the appropriate material for the splint or prosthesis.

A prosthesis must be designed and con-structed so that its kinematics are similar to the normal situation. Size, angle, and properties of materials must be assessed for proper function-ing of joint replacements. Straps, uprights, springs, bars, plates, and stirrups are only a few components that can apply a specific magnitude of force and appropriate direction to correct soft tissue and bony problems. External prostheses must be constructed with overall weight and weight distribution considered. The pressure between the socket and residual limb must be evaluated. The forces involved with slings, straps, cables, cable loops, and other compo-nents must be analyzed to allow proper func-tioning and longevity of the device. (See Chap-ters 4, 5, 7, and 8.)

PROTECTIVE EQUIPMENT

Most sports utilize some sort of protective equipment. The equipment may be worn by the participant or located within the playing area. Protective padding, bandages, and footwear are designed to provide protection to the indivi-dual's body. Playing surfaces, such as grass, ar-tificial turf, and floors for aerobic classes and gymnasiums, are constructed with friction and resilience considered. (See Chapters 3, 6, and 7.)

BODY MOVEMENT

Gait laboratories have been established to ob-jectively analyze gait characteristics. Some of these facilities have been expanded as labora-tories for the analysis of human motion of many varieties. Force platforms, cameras, digitizers, and electromyographic equipment are some ex-amples of devices used to determine the kine-matic and kinetics of various movement. Some examples of activities include walking, falling, lifting, kicking, throwing, jumping, and manual skills. A variety of athletic and work skills have been analyzed to improve performance and provide safety. (See Chapter 7.)

SUMMARY

Examples of biomechanics are abundant in many disciplines. Only a few examples of the immense scope of biomechanics are presented in this text. As you observe procedures and ac-tivities in your specific discipline, you should recognize the biomechanical principles involved and be able to appropriately apply these prin-ciples and to correct situations in which these principles are used incorrectly.

Formula and Units

When studying mechanics, you will become in-volved with mathematical formulas. Don't be afraid of formulas. They are a shorthand method for writing definitions or for solving problems and show relationships among vari-ables, such as proportions.

You should remember the units for each vari-able. You can then use unit analysis to show re-lationships. For example:

$V = s/t$

s units in meters (m) or feet (ft)
t units in seconds (sec)
therefore, v would have units
in m/sec or ft/sec

Various disciplines do not use the same system of units. Although the International System of Units (SI) has become widely accepted, its use by practitioners in the United States is still not widespread. Although the first two editions of this text used the Engineering or English Gravitational System, this edition uses the SI system. Conversions are presented in Table 1–1.

By using the conversions and unit analysis, for example, you may convert miles per hour (mph) to meters per second.

55 miles/hr $\times$ 1 hr/60 min $\times$ 1 min/60 sec
$\times$ 5280 ft/l mile $\times$ 0.3048 m/l ft
= 24.587 m/sec.

The units of miles, hours, minutes, and feet all cancel out; leaving the units of meters per second.

The problems presented in this text should not be considered exact. Several assumptions occur when we attempt to determine force acting on the body:

1. Only two-dimensional figures are used.
2. Calculations of muscle force often refer to a muscle group and not necessarily the force of a single muscle.
3. The mass and weight of body segments are estimates based upon reported research. (See Appendix A.)
4. The lengths of lever arms are estimates based upon reported research. (See Appendix A.)
5. The minimal amount of friction in the joints is disregarded.
6. Effects of ligaments, synergist and antagonist muscles, and other soft tissues are disregarded.

QUESTIONS

1. Define mechanics, biomechanics, statics, dynamics, kinematics, kinetics.
2. Discuss the application of biomechanics to exercise programs.
3. Cite examples of biomechanical principles related to orthopedic appliances and surgical applications.

TABLE 1–1. CONVERSION BETWEEN THE INTERNATIONAL SYSTEM OF UNITS (SI) AND THE ENGINEERING ENGLISH GRAVITATIONAL SYSTEM

Item	SI to English	English to SI
Length	1 meter (m) = 3.281 feet (ft)	1 ft = 0.3048 m
	1 m = 39.37 inches (in)	1 ft = 30.48 cm
	1 centimeter (cm) = 0.3937 in	1 in = 2.54 cm
	1 kilometer (Km) = 0.6214 mile (mi)	1 mi = 1.609 Km
Area	1 m^2 = 10.763 ft^2	1 ft^2 = 0.0929 m^2
	1 cm^2 = 0.155 in^2	1 in^2 = 6.452 cm^2
Velocity	1 m/sec = 3.281 ft/sec	1 ft/sec = 0.3048 m/sec
	1 m/sec = 2.237 mi/hr	1 mile/hr = 0.447 m/sec
Acceleration	1 m/sec^2 = 3.281 ft/sec^2	1 ft/sec^2 = 0.3048 m/sec^2
Mass	1 Kilogram (Kg) = 0.683 slug	1 slug = 14.59 Kg
Force	1 Newton (N) = 0.2248 pound (lb)	1 lb = 4.448 N
	1 Kg(f) = 9.8 N	
Torque	1 Nm = 0.7376 ft-lb	1 ft-lb = 1.3558 Nm
Mass Moment of Inertia	1 Kgm^2 = 0.7373 slug ft^2	1 slug ft^2 = 1.356 Kgm^2
Angle	1 radian (rad) = 57.296 degrees	1 degree = 0.0175 rad
Pressure	1 Pascal (Pa) = 1 N/m^2 = 0.000145 lb/in^2 (psi)	1 lb/in^2 = 6894.8 (N/m^2)
Power	1 watt (Joules/sec) = 0.737 ft-lb/sec	1 ft-lb/sec = 1.356 watt
Work	1 Joule = 0.737 ft-lb	1 ft-lb = 1.356 Joule

4. Discuss in general the biomechanical factors involved in locomotion.

5. What is the value of understanding the biomechanical principles involved in growth and development?

6. Cite examples of biomechanical principles involved in rehabilitation.

7. Give specific examples related to athletic performance and prevention of injury in sports.

8. List disciplines in which biomechanical principles are applied, and cite several specific examples for each.

9. Make the following conversions;
   (a) 12 inches to centimeters
   (b) 10 lb to N
   (c) 5 mph to m/sec
   (d) 50 ft-lb to Nm
   (e) 90° to rad
   (f) 20 cm to inches
   (g) 80 N to pounds
   (h) 15 m/sec to mph
   (i) 200 N to ft-lb
   (j) 6 rad to degrees
   (k) 15,000 psi to GPa

REFERENCES

Alms M: Fracture mechanics. J Bone Joint Surg (Br) 43:162–166, 1961.

American Academy of Orthopedic Surgeons: Atlas of Orthotics: Biomechanical Principles and Application, 2nd ed. St. Louis, C V Mosby, 1985.

Andersson BG, Ortengren R, Schultz A: Analysis and measurement of loads on the lumbar spine during work at a table. J Biomech 13:513–520, 1980.

Badke MB, Duncan PW: Patterns of rapid motor responses during postural adjustments when standing in healthy subjects and hemiplegic patients. Phys Ther 63:13–20, 1983.

Basmajian JV: Manipulation, Traction and Massage. Baltimore, Williams & Wilkins, 1985.

Bourdillon JF, Day EA: Spinal Manipulation, 4th ed. E. Norwalk, CN, Appleton & Lange, 1987.

Brand P: Clinical Mechanics of the Hand. St. Louis, C V Mosby, 1985.

Dunn JW: Scientific Principles of Coaching. Englewood Cliffs, NJ, Prentice-Hall, 1955.

Carter DR, Orr TE, Fyhrie DF: Relationship between loading history and femoral cancellous bone architecture. J Biomech 22:231–244, 1989.

Chaffin D, Andersson GBJ: Occupational Biomechanics. New York, John Wiley & Sons, 1984.

Cool JC: Biomechanics of orthoses for the subluxed shoulder. Prosthet Orthot Int 13:90–96, 1989.

Contini R, Drillis R: Biomechanics. Appl Mechanics Rev 7:49–52, 1954.

Contini R, Drillis R: Biomechanics in Applied Mechanics Surveys. New York, Spartan Books, 1966.

Craik R: Biomechanics: A neural perspective. Phys Ther 64:1810–1811, 1984.

Dillman CJ: A kinetic analysis of the recovery leg during spring running. In Cooper JM (Ed): Selected Topics on Biomechanics. Chicago, The Athletic Institute, 1971.

Donatelli R, Wooden MJ: Orthopaedic Physical Therapy. New York, Churchill Livingstone, 1989.

Eberhart HD, Inman VT, Bresler B: The principal elements in human locomotion. In Klopsteg PE, Wilson PD (Eds): Human Limbs and Their Substitutes. New York, McGraw-Hill, 1954.

Fess EE, Philips CA: Hand Splinting: Principles and Methods. St. Louis, C V Mosby, 1987.

Fung YC, Perrone N, Anliker M (Eds): Biomechanics. Philadelphia, Lea & Febiger, 1972.

Ghista DN: Applied Physiological Mechanics. New York, Harwood Academic Publishers, 1979.

Ghista DN, Roaf R: Orthopaedic Mechanics: Procedures and Devices, vol. 2 New York, Academic Press, 1981a.

Ghista DN, Roaf R: Orthopedic Mechanics: Procedures and Devices, vol. 3. New York, Academic Press, 1981b.

Gozna ER: Biomechanics of Musculoskeletal Injury. Baltimore, Williams & Wilkins, 1982.

Graham JM, Jr: Smith's Recognizable Patterns of Human Deformation, 2nd ed. Philadelphia, W B Saunders, 1988.

Grieve GP: Mobilization of the Spine, 4th ed. New York, Churchill Livingstone, 1984.

Guthrie-Smith OF: Rehabilitation, Reeducation and Remedial Exercise. Baltimore, Williams & Wilkins, 1943.

Hopkins HL, Smith HD: Occupational Therapy, Philadelphia, J B Lippincott Co., 1988.

Isacson J, Grahsberg L, Knutsson E: Three-dimensional electrogoniometric gait recording. J. Biomech 19:627–634, 1986.

Jacobs RR, Ghista DN: A biomechanical basis for treatment of injuries of the dorsolumber spine. In Ghista DN (Ed): Osteoarthro Mechanics. New York, McGraw-Hill, 1981.

Kaufer H: Mechanics of the treatment of hip injuries. Clin Orthop 146:53–61, 1980.

Krag MH, Pope MH, Wilder DG: Mechanisms of spine trauma features of spinal fixation methods. Part I, "Mechanisms" of injury. In Ghista DN (Ed): Spinal Cord Injury Medical Engineering. Springfield, IL, Charles C Thomas, 1986.

LeVeau BF: Movements of the lumbar spine during selected abdominal strengthening exercise. Doctoral Thesis, The Pennsylvania State University, 1973.

LeVeau BF, Bernhardt DB: Developmental biomechanics. Phys Ther 64:1874–1882, 1984.

Lichtenstein MR, Burger MC, Shiavi RG, et al.: Comparison of biomechanics platform measures of balance and videotaped measures of gait with a clinical mobility scale in elderly women. J Geront 45:M49–54, 1990.

Lichtenstein MF, Shields SL, Shiavi RG, et al.: Clinical determinants of biomechanics platform measures of balance in aged women. J Am Geriat Soc 36:996–1002, 1988.

Lichtenstein MF, Shields SL, Shiavi RG, et al.: Exercise and balance in aged women: A pilot controlled clinical trial. Arch Phys Med Rehabil 70:138–143, 1989.

Lord M, Reynolds DP, Hughes JR: Foot pressure measurement. A review of clinical findings. J Biomed Eng 8:283–294, 1986.

Maitland GD: Vertebral Manipulation, 5th ed. Boston, Butterworths, 1986.

Miller DI, Nelson RD: Biomechanics of Sports. Philadelphia, Lea & Febiger, 1973.

Nashner LM: Fixed patterns of rapid responses among leg muscles during stance. Exp Brain Res 30:13–24, 1977.

Nashner LM: Balance adjustments of humans perturbed while walking. J Neurophysiol 44:650–664, 1980.

Nashner L, McCollum G: Organization of postural human movements: A formal basis and experiments synthesis. Behav Brain Sciences 8:135–173, 1985.

Noyes FR, Grood ES, Butler DL, et al.: Clinical laxity tests and functional stability of the knee: Biomechanical concepts. Clin Orthop 146:84–89, 1980.

Plagenhoef SC: Computer programs for obtaining kinetic data on human movement. J. Biomech 1:332–334, 1968.

Radin EL: Relevant biomechanics in the treatment of musculoskeletal injuries and disorders. Clin Orthop 146:2–3, 1980.

Radin EL, Simon SR, Rose RM, et al.: Practical Biomechanics for the Orthopedic Surgeon. New York, John Wiley & Sons. 1979.

Rasch PF: Notes towards a history of kinesiology, parts 1 to 3. J Am Osteopath Assoc 58:572–574, 641–644, 713–714, 1958.

Schenkman M, Butler RB: A model for multisystem evaluation, interpretation, and treatment of individuals with neurologic dysfunction. Phys Ther 69:538–547, 1989.

Schmid-Schönbein GW, Woo SL-Y, Zaaifach BW: Frontiers in Biomechanics. New York, Springer-Verlag, 1984.

Soeur R: Fractures of the Limbs: The Relationships Between Mechanism and Treatment. Springfield, IL, Charles C Thomas, 1982.

Viano DC, King AI, Melvin JW, et al.: Injury biomechanics research: An essential element in the prevention of trauma. J Biomech 5:403–417, 1989.

Walker PS: Biomechanical aspects of artificial joints. In DN Ghista (Ed): Oestoarthro Mechanics. New York, McGraw-Hill, 1981.

Winter DA: The Biomechanics and Motor Control of Human Gait. Waterloo, ON, University of Waterloo Press, 1987.

2

Useful Terms and Concepts

INTRODUCTION

The study of biomechanics is based upon many terms and concepts that must be defined and discussed before delving into the substance of the science. The bases of biomechanics are the concepts of force and motion. In this chapter, force is defined and several types of forces are described. Terms that relate to the concept of force are presented. The concept of motion is briefly discussed with regard to Newton's laws of motion and illustrated with common examples.

FORCE

The study of forces and their effects is fundamental to the understanding of body form and motion. No matter what you do, whatever activity in which you are involved, force is there. You might consider that force is always with you and must be considered in all of your endeavors.

Definition

Force has often been defined as mass times acceleration ($F = ma$), or as the entity that tends to produce motion or to halt or change direction of motion. More simply put, force can be defined as a push or pull.

Characteristics

More than a definition is needed to describe a force. Force should be described by four characteristics: magnitude, line of application, sense, and point of application. Figure 2–1 illustrates these characteristics for a muscle force.

All four of these characteristics must be supplied to completely describe a force acting on an object.

Magnitude (M) represents the amount of force being applied. The International System (SI) unit for force is the newton (N), but force

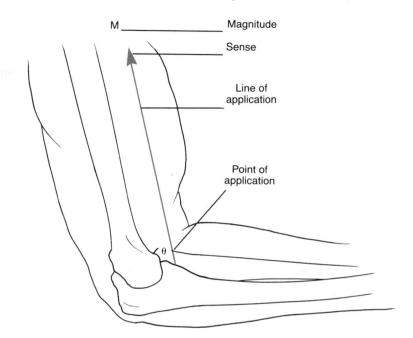

FIGURE 2–1

A force vector and the four characteristics of force.

has commonly been presented in units of pounds, Kilopond, or kilogram force.

The line of application represents an imaginary straight line of indefinite length along which a force is acting. A force can be considered to achieve the same results as it acts anywhere along this line of application. This principle is known as the principle of transmissibility. The orientation of this line is stated as an angular position in regard to a given system, such as the X–Y coordinate system, or in regard to an object, such as bone or supporting surface. The angle of force is represented by θ in Figure 2–1.

The sense along the line of application is also of fundamental importance. The effect will be different if you pull in one direction instead of pushing in the opposite direction. The sense in Figure 2–1 is represented by an arrowhead on the line of application.

The point at which the force is applied is of significance in respect to its effect upon that specific point. A force is often represented by one line and point of application at a specific point, although the force may be represented over a larger surface area.

When a force is present, at least two objects must be involved. One object must always act on another. We most often think of force when two objects are in contact with each other such as when a boxing glove hits an opponent's jaw, when a baseball bat hits a ball, or when two automobiles come together in a collision. Forces, however, may also act between two objects that are not in contact with each other. Examples of such situations include the attractive force of gravity, the attraction and repulsion of electrically charged particles, magnetic force, and the attractive forces of a nucleus that hold an atom together.

Force Diagram

Magnitude alone is a *scalar* quantity, that is, it has no direction. Examples of scalar quantities are speed, length, temperature, and time. A *vector* is a quantity that gives direction as well as magnitude. Force is considered as a vector quantity because it has magnitude and direction and thus can be represented by a vector, which is a directed straight line. When a vector is used to represent a force, its length should be made proportional to the magnitude of the force. If we let 1 cm represent 20 N, a line 2 cm long would represent a force of 40 N. Since the vector drawn to scale indicates magnitude (by the length), action line (by the location of its shaft), and the direction of the force (by its arrowhead), and it is placed on the object at the point of application of the force, the vector can be used to define the force completely. For example, in Figure 2–1, a vector is used to represent the force of the biceps brachii muscle. In mechanics we use vectors consistently since this is the easiest way to deal with forces. The student should become proficient in visualizing *force systems* (any group of two or more forces) as a series of vectors acting in relation to an object or to one another. Any time a vector is used to represent a force, it should be labeled with a letter or number designating its magnitude, as shown in Figure 2–1. If its magnitude in newtons is known, we of course label the vector with the actual force in newtons. If, however, the magnitude of the force is not known, we use a letter such as F or P to designate the magnitude of the force. Capital letters are generally used for this purpose. In order to evaluate the effect of forces, a line drawing of the forces and the body on which the forces are acting is made. Since the object or body may be very complicated, we can represent it by a simplified drawing called a *space diagram.* Only enough details are required on the space diagram to locate the position of the forces properly. Drawing the space diagram in some cases may be quite simple, whereas in other cases it becomes more difficult. A space diagram must contain the necessary dimensions to locate accurately the position of all forces acting on the body. Distances may be designated in actual values, if known, or may be represented by small letters. A more accurate diagram is called the *free body diagram,* which requires that all forces be drawn in the correct proportion. Such a figure of a body shows all the forces that are acting on it, whether their values are known or unknown. The greatest difficulty with the diagram is locating all the forces acting on the body.

TYPES OF FORCES

The forces with which we are most concerned in biomechanics include gravity, muscle contraction, elasticity, contact, inertia, and buoyancy.

Gravity

The force of gravity is always present. It is the mutual attraction between any two objects anywhere in the universe. The magnitude of gravitational force is directly proportional to the product of the two masses and inversely proportional to the square of the distance between them. A gravitational constant (G) is needed to provide numerical and dimensional validity. Hence, gravitational force is given by the equation:

$$F_g = G \frac{m_1 m_2}{r^2}$$

Since the mass of the earth is so much greater than the other objects on earth, the attraction between these other objects is negligible. The line of application of gravitational force is given as the line between the center of mass (center of gravity) of the object and the earth. Since the object is more easily moved than the earth, the sense is given as being toward the center of the earth. The point of application can be considered as the center of mass of the object.

Gravity is the most common force acting on the human body. Our body parts and the object with which we work are under a constant gravitational force we must resist in some way (Fig. 2–2).

Weight is the term used to represent the force of gravity between the earth and an object. The weight (W) of an object depends upon two things: (1) the amount of material of the object or its mass (m) and (2) the strength of the gravitational field that is evident by the acceleration (g) of the object in response to the constant application of the gravitational force. Thus,

$$W = mg$$

Since weight is a force, the units for weight should be presented as units of force, or Newtons. Often in the literature you may see the units for weight in kilograms, which may be representing force or mass. Be sure you know which entity is being presented. One kilogram of force of 1 kg of mass equals 9.8 N, which equals 2.2 lb. The acceleration caused by the force of gravity is approximately 9.8 m/sec.^{2} or 32.2 ft/sec.^{2}

Muscle

Without muscle force we would not be able to maintain an upright posture or move from place to place (Fig. 2–3). Muscle is composed of a large number of myofibrils, which are contractile elements of the muscle. These contractile elements can actively produce force that is transmitted to the bony attachments by way of connective tissue. The magnitude of the muscle force depends upon the amount of neural stimulation and number of motor units activated. The line of action can be placed through the muscle tendons. The points of application are at the bony attachments at each end of the muscle. The sense at each end of the muscle attachments tends to be toward the muscle belly.

In the strict sense, contraction refers to active shortening of a muscle with the distance between the two muscle attachments decreasing. Muscle, however, produces force in three different muscle-lengthening situations. In concentric muscle action, the muscle shortens as the muscle force is greater than the effects of the external forces. With isometric muscle action, the overall length of the muscle does not change. However, the contractile units of the muscle shorten as the series elastic elements of the muscle lengthen a similar amount. The muscle force in this case equals the effects of the external forces. With eccentric muscle action, the effects of the external forces are greater than the force produced by the contractile units of the muscle. The results cause the muscle to lengthen. Such lengthening can be controlled by the contractile muscle units and the series and parallel elastic units within the muscle.

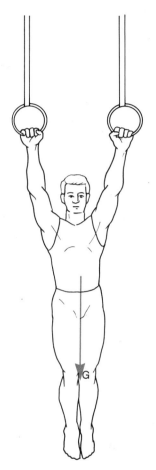

FIGURE 2–2

Gravity acting on a gymnast's body.

Elasticity

Elastic elements within the muscles and other tissues and elastic properties within nonbiological materials provide a restoring force or resistance that tends to bring a material back to its resting size and shape (Fig. 2–4). The formula for elastic force is $F = -Kl$, where K is a constant related to the type of material, and l is the amount of deformation of the object beyond its original size. Muscles in a lengthened position, eccentric contractions, springs, and elastic exer-

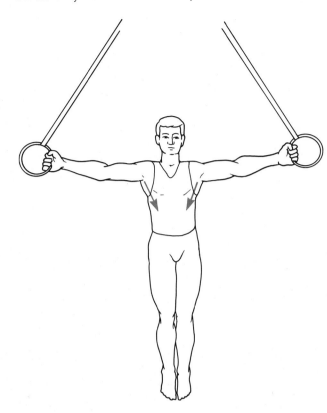

FIGURE 2-3

The use of muscle force to overcome gravity and move the body.

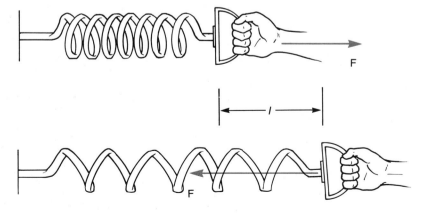

FIGURE 2-4

A stretched spring provides a restoring force to revert to its original length.

$$F = -Kl$$

cise bands are only a few examples of elastic force.

Contact

A force exists between two objects whenever they are in contact (Fig. 2–5). A contact force is not an active force but reacts to outside forces. Contact forces may be readily obvious, such as a book on a desk, buttock contact with a chair, a cane blocking a wheelchair, a torn cartilage in the knee, a bottle containing a liquid, or restraints such as seat belts. Friction, which is a less obvious contact force, resists the sliding of one object past another. The force of static friction (F_s) is related to the coefficient of static friction (μ_s) between the two surfaces and the magnitude of the normal force (N) pressing the two surfaces together:

$$F_s = \mu_s N$$

Inertia

As a person moves body parts, the resistance of inertia must be overcome by a force to begin movement, while force of some kind must be used to stop movement, to reduce the speed of movement, or to change direction of the movement (Fig. 2–6). Inertia is the property of any object to resist the change of state of rest or motion of that object. Its magnitude is related to the mass or amount of material of the object. The greater the mass of the material, the more difficult it is to accelerate (a), start, stop, or change the speed or direction of the object's motion (F = Ma).

Buoyancy

Buoyancy refers to the upward force of any fluid upon an object immersed in it (Fig. 2–7). The magnitude of the buoyant force (B) is equal to the weight of the fluid displaced by the object. The line of action of the buoyant forces passes through the object's center of gravity. The object's center of buoyancy is located at the center of gravity of the volume of fluid before the fluid is displaced. The force, or partial body weight (F), that the feet of a patient must bear as he or she stands in a pool equals the patient's total body weight (W) minus the weight of the water displaced (B), or F = W − B (Fig. 2–8).

FIGURE 2–5

Contact forces exist whenever one object is in contact with another: *A,* Book on a shelf. *B,* Person sitting on a bench.

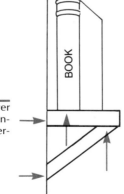

A

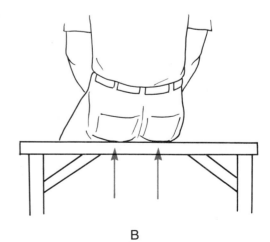

B

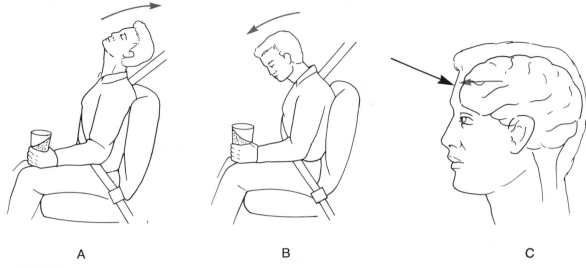

FIGURE 2–6

Effects of inertia: *A,* If an automobile starts rapidly or is hit from behind, the head tends to remain at rest as the body is moved forward. *B,* If an automobile stops rapidly, the head tends to continue moving as the body stops (note the fluid level in the cup). *C,* The inertia of the brain can cause brain and vessel damage if the head is hit or stopped suddenly.

FIGURE 2–7

Buoyancy of a fluid: *A,* Floating object weighing (W) 2 newtons (N) buoyed up by 2 N of force. *B,* Effect of buoyancy on an object that does not float. A 15 N weight is buoyed up (B) by 5 N, giving a scale reading.

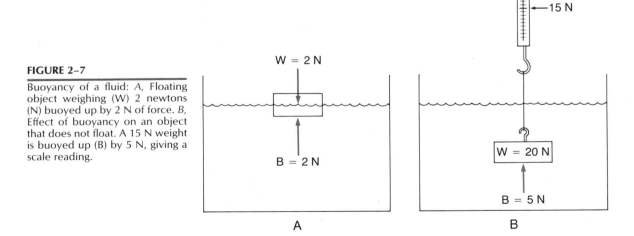

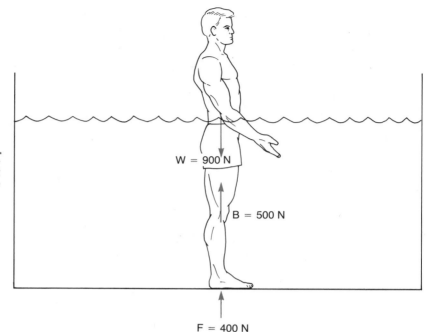

FIGURE 2–8

Buoyancy force (B) acts on an individual standing in a pool so that lower limbs bear less (F) than the total body weight (W).

W = 900 N

B = 500 N

F = 400 N

OTHER TERMS

Load

An outside force or combination of forces acting externally on an object is called a load (Fig. 2–9). The pull of a muscle on a bone provides a load on the bone. Holding a weight in the hand provides a load on many structures of the arm. Standing provides a load on each foot. Lying places loads on the heels, ischial tuberosities, and other bony areas.

Strength

The term *strength* is used in biomechanics in two different ways. In disciplines dealing with muscle physiology, strength is often used to refer to the muscle's ability to produce or resist force. Engineers, on the other hand, relate strength to the ability of an object to resist deformation. Strength in either case cannot be

measured directly. Strength of materials will be considered in more detail later in this chapter.

Pressure

In some instances we must deal with the many separate forces as they are in contact with other objects. *Pressure,* which is an important aspect of force, indicates how the force is distributed over an area. Pressure is defined as the total force per area of force application, as shown in the equation $P = F/A$. This formula yields the average pressure given in units of force per unit area, for example, newtons per square meter, or pascals. If a pressure pad on a back brace exerts an 18 N force over an area 15 cm by 20 cm, the average pressure in the region beneath the pad would be 18 N divided by 300 cm^2, or about 600 N per square meter. What would be the magnitude of the force per unit area if the pad were 7 cm by 10 cm in size?

This principle of force per unit area is utilized

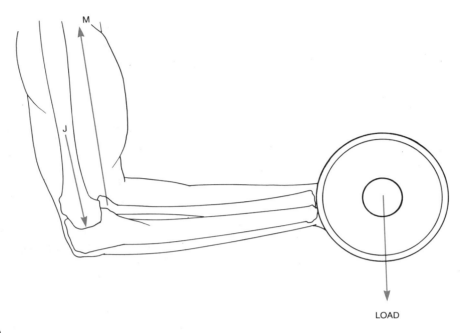

FIGURE 2–9

A hand weight provides a load to the structures of the upper limb. The muscle (M) puts load on the bone. The combined weight and muscle force produce load at joint (J).

in skiing and snowshoeing, making it possible to stand and walk on soft snow (Fig. 2–10). Without the use of skis or snowshoes a person would not be able to support his or her weight on the snow. Because of the small area of the foot, he or she would fall through. With the increased size or surface area of the skis or snowshoes, the body weight is distributed over a larger area and the total force per unit area is decreased, making it possible for the body weight to be supported. If you push with your fist in the palm of the opposite hand, you can withstand considerable force without discomfort. The same amount of force exerted by your thumb into the palm becomes painful because the pressure per unit area is now much greater. An equal force exerted by the point of a needle would be disastrous. In general, to avoid pain and possible injury to the skin, forces should be sustained over as large an area of body surface as possible. Skin breakdown, pressure sores, and ulcerated areas are serious clinical complications that could be

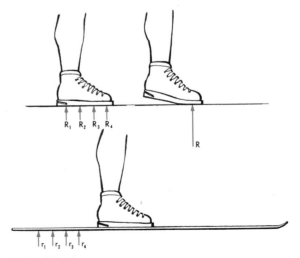

FIGURE 2–10

Distribution of body weight on the supporting surface varies according to the surface contact area. R = reacting force of the floor. (The pressure shown under one area actually acts over the entire length of the ski surface [r].)

easily avoided with the application of the above principle.

Pressure sores occur as a direct result of prolonged pressure that is sufficient to collapse local blood vessels. The position of patients in bed should be changed frequently in order to alternate the skin areas under pressure. This is particularly true in the presence of circulatory or sensory impairment (Nuseibek, 1986). Pressure is a critical factor in the fitting of prosthetic devices for lower extremity amputees, especially those with ischial weight-bearing devices or end-bearing stumps. The socket must be designed so that the contact force is distributed over a large skin area. Padding of bony prominences is important as well in the application of braces and casts.

The "give" or yield of the material contacting and supporting the body surfaces is a primary factor in avoiding dangerous effects of continuous pressure. When force is exerted against the body surface by rigid materials such as wood or metal, pressure is concentrated in the areas of bony prominences. Softer materials such as felt, padding, or sponge rubber allow better equalization of the pressure over the entire contact area and protect the skin over bony prominences. Equalization of pressure has been attempted by inserting an air-filled chamber or water bag of some sort between the two contacting surfaces. Bremner (1959) applied this principle in scoliosis bracing by inserting a water-inflated football (rugby) bladder between a plaster jacket and the thorax at the site of corrective pressure. The advantage of this hydrostatic bag was said to be "automatic pressure distribution and perfect congruity and adaptability of shape," particularly in adjusting to breathing and other trunk movements. Air splints and newer methods for protecting against formation of pressure sores are also based on this equalization of pressure by fluids. Head slings used in neck traction devices should fit snugly so that force will be applied as evenly as possible over a large surface.

Pressure may also be used in treatment as well. Consistent pressure to the surface of an immature hypertrophic scar to reduce scarring is essential to soften, smooth, and maintain elastic skin. Pressure garments are often used in such situations. Certain manual therapy and massage procedures also make use of pressure.

The pressure in a fluid varies with the depth of the fluid. As a diver descends deeper under the surface of the water, the hydrostatic pressure increases. However, the pressure is the same at all points at a specific depth (Fig. 2–11). The pressure at a given depth (y) depends upon

FIGURE 2–11

Pressure on the diver is the same at all points at depth y. As y increases, the pressure also increases.

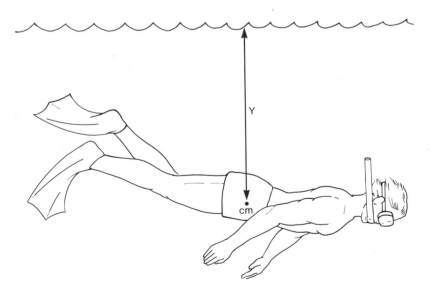

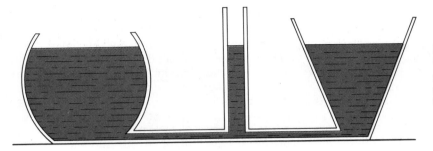

FIGURE 2–12

The pressure of a fluid in a container depends only upon the depth of the fluid and not upon the shape of the container.

the density of the fluid (ρ) and the gravitational acceleration of the object (g). If an object is in a liquid open to the air, the hydrostatic pressure also depends upon the atmospheric pressure (Pa). Thus, the pressure in a liquid open to the air, such as in a whirlpool bath, would be

$$P = Pa + \rho gy$$

The pressure of a fluid in a container depends only upon the depth and not upon the shape of the container (Fig. 2–12).

Gases such as air may be compressed within an enclosed container. In such cases the pressure in the container increases. An example is air in an automobile tire.

For all practical purposes liquids are incompressible. When pressure is applied to an enclosed liquid, that pressure is transmitted equally to every portion of the liquid and to the walls of the vessel containing the liquid. This fact is referred to as Pascal's law. Examples of this situation are the results of compression on intervertebral discs (Fig. 2–13), exercise devices using hydraulics, and a hydraulic joint system in an above-knee prosthesis.

Space

Space is another basic consideration in the study of mechanics. The forces that we deal with may act along a single line in a single plane or in any direction in space. Since we must have some means of locating our forces along a line, in a plane, or in space, it is necessary to provide some reference system. In the two-dimensional system, we do this by dividing the plane into four quadrants by means of two perpendicular

lines or axes. These axes are generally labeled X in the horizontal direction and Y in the vertical direction. The X axis is termed the abscissa, the Y axis the ordinate. The point of intersection of the two axes is known as the *origin* of the system. Measurements along the X axis to the right of the Y axis are positive. Those to the left of the Y axis are negative. Measurements along the Y axis above the X axis are positive, below are negative (Fig. 2–14). Any point on the plane can now be defined by being assigned X and Y values. These numbers, which determine the point location, are called the coordinates of the point. The point A, defined by X = 3, Y = 5, will be found three units to the right of the origin and five units above the origin. The point B, defined

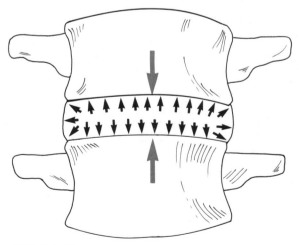

FIGURE 2–13

Pressure within an intervertebral disc resulting from load on the disc.

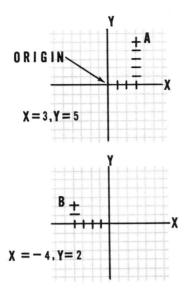

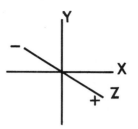

FIGURE 2–15

Addition of the Z axis to the X and Y coordinates permits the location of points in space.

FIGURE 2–14

The location of points in a plane in relation to the X and Y axes. A is 3 units to the right and 5 units upward. B is 4 units to the left and 2 units upward.

by X = −4, Y = 2, is found by moving 4 units to the left of the origin and up two units.

In order to locate points in three dimensions, a third axis must be introduced. This passes through the origin and is perpendicular to the X–Y plane in which the two original axes are found. The third axis is usually labeled Z. All points in front of the original X–Y plane are positive, while those behind the X–Y plane are negative. Now we have the means of locating any point in space. After the position in the X–Y plane is defined, you can locate the points either in front of the plane or behind the plane by means of a positive or negative coordinate (Fig. 2–15).

In setting up such a system of coordinates for the purpose of describing human motion, it is convenient to place the origin at the center of mass of the body, which is approximately anterior to the second sacral vertebrae. Three cardinal planes may then be visualized in relation to the X, Y, and Z coordinates (Fig. 2–16): frontal (or coronal), dividing the body into front and back portions (X–Y plane); sagittal, dividing the body into right and left halves (Y–Z plane); and

transverse (or horizontal), dividing the body into upper and lower portions (X–Z plane). This system of reference coordinates and planes facilitates description of movement of the body segments and allows for an exact definition of

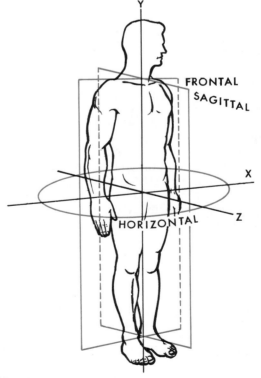

FIGURE 2–16

The three cardinal planes of the body related to the X, Y, and Z axes.

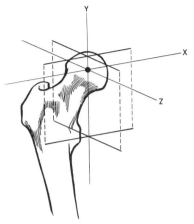

FIGURE 2–17

System of coordinates related to the mechanical axis of the hip joint.

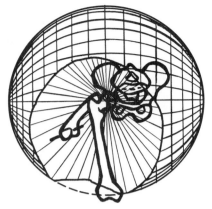

FIGURE 2–18

Example of "globographic" recording of range of motion. (From Strasser H, Gassmann A: Hilfsmittel und Normen zur Bestimmung und Veranschaulichung von Stellungen, Bewegungen und Kraftwiskungen am Kniegelenke. Meckle: Bonnet: Anat Heft 2:6–7, 1893.

any point in space. Fick (1850), who first computed the action of the thigh muscles on the hip joint over a hundred years ago, used such a system. Since he was interested in muscle action relative to the hip joint, he placed the origin of his coordinate system at the axis of the joint, as shown in Figure 2–17. By projecting the action lines of the individual muscles, he could determine their effect in moving the femur in each of the three cardinal planes. For example, a muscle such as the iliacus or pectineus, pulling in a direction anterior to the X–Y plane, flexes the part. The gluteus maximus, pulling posterior to this plane, extends it. The adductor and abductor muscles apply their force from points medial and lateral (respectively) to the Y–Z plane. Rotation is calculated in relation to the Y axis. (This means of computing the values of muscle forces such as these will be considered in Chapter 4.) The method employed by Fick to determine the action of muscles about the center of rotation of a joint has been in general use for many years. Elaborate globe-shaped devices have been designed to measure the position of the body segments in space and to record ranges of motion in joints that move in two or more planes (Fig. 2–18). A number of such examples are cited by Steindler (1955), Morehouse and Miller (1971), and Engin and Chen (1988). For the purpose of kinematic analysis of movements of the upper

extremity, Taylor and Blaschke (1951) have worked out a complex system of angles, axes, and centers. These authors stress that even this elaborate method is somewhat idealized and only approximates the true joint function, which is rather complicated.

Matter

Matter is that which occupies space. In our discussion of biomechanics we will often be dealing with the quantity of matter, or *mass*, to which the force of gravity is applied.

Mass

Mass is the quantity of matter of an object. It depends upon the volume and density of that object. The mass of an object is the same whether it is on earth, on the moon, or on a spaceship. Mass has the important characteristics of offering resistance to change in linear motion. Mass is measured in kilograms or slugs. Mass may be an object, such as an exercise weight, or it may be the entire body or a segment of the body. In order to apply the principles of mechanics to human movement, the concept of *center of mass* of an object must be used constantly. The center of mass, by definition, is that point at the exact center of an object's mass. This is often called the center of gravity. In the case of a square block or a cylinder in which the mass is symmetrically distributed, this point is at the geometric center of the object (Fig. 2–19). However, if the distribution of mass is asymmetrical, as is true of the limbs of the human body, the center of mass will be nearer to the larger and heavier end. The center of mass of the entire human body when the limbs are straight as in ordinary standing lies within the pelvis (Fig. 2–20). This point may vary in position from person to person according to body build, age, and sex. It will also vary within any given person when the arrangement of the segments shifts, as in walking, running, or sitting. Since this point represents the center of the total mass, it will shift when weight is added to or subtracted from some part of the body, as with the addition of a cast or brace or following amputation of an extremity. Weights, centers of mass of the body segments, and joint centers have been determined by Braune and Fischer (1963), Dempster (1955), Clauser and associates (1969), and Webb Associates (1978). Additional characteristics have been reported by Chaffin and Andersson (1984). A summary of these studies is given in Appendix A and will

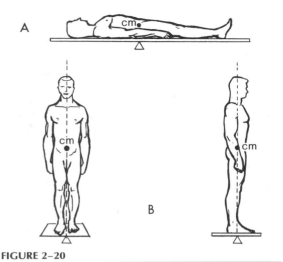

FIGURE 2–20

Center of mass of the entire human body.

be useful in estimating the magnitude and location of gravitational forces as accurately as possible in setting up and solving problems.

The force acting on the entire mass of a rigid object may be considered to be acting as a single vector through its center of mass. This single vector represents the sum of many parallel forces distributed throughout the object. The use of this principle results in simplicity without the loss of accuracy.

Mass Moment of Inertia

Mass moment of inertia ($I = mr^2$) is equivalent to mass in angular motion as it offers resistance to change in rotatory motion. Its value depends upon both the mass of the object and the manner in which the mass is distributed. The value of the moment of inertia depends upon the location of the axis around which the mass is rotated. The units for moment of inertia are kilogram-meters squared or slug-inch squared.

The radius of gyration is similar to center of mass. It is the location in which the sum of the distribution of mass appears to be concentrated without changing its moment of inertia. More discussion concerning moment of inertia will be presented later in this book.

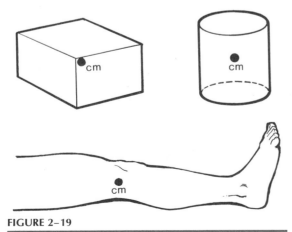

FIGURE 2–19

Center of mass of symmetrical and asymmetrical objects.

NEWTON'S LAWS OF MOTION

The basic laws involved in the areas of statics, kinematics, and kinetics were formulated at the beginning of the eighteenth century by Sir Isaac Newton, an English mathematician. In our discussion we will make use of his three laws of mechanics.

Law of Inertia

The first law, called the *law of inertia*, states that a body remains at rest or in uniform motion until acted upon by an unbalanced or outside set of forces. This body is said to be in equilibrium when these conditions exist. This means that if a body is at rest, the forces acting on it must be completely balanced, and if a body is moving, it will continue to move at a uniform speed until some force causes it to stop moving or to change its rate or direction of motion.

Law of Acceleration

The *law of acceleration,* Newton's second law, is a special case of the first and states that the acceleration of a particle is proportional to the unbalanced force acting upon it and inversely proportional to the mass of the particle. In other words, a large push on a small object will accelerate it rapidly and a small push on a large object will accelerate it slowly.

Law of Reaction

Newton's third law, the *law of reaction,* states that for every action there is an equal and opposite reaction. In any case in which two objects are in contact, the force exerted on the second body by the first must be exactly equal and opposite to the force exerted on the first body by the second (Fig. 2–21). If you push against an object, it pushes back against you with equal force in a direction exactly opposite to that of your push.

Examples

These laws will be considered throughout the text. The reader can think of many instances in which these laws apply. The first two laws are well illustrated in normal walking. The lower limb must be swung forward forcibly by action of the hip flexor muscles so that the foot may be placed ahead of the body as the center of mass travels forward. The leg swing is a ballistic or thrust movement that once begun continues without further muscle effort. The swinging limb must then be stopped or decelerated in a controlled fashion by the hip extensors so that the heel can be brought to the ground at the proper time and place (Fig. 2–22). Gravity is also a force in the acceleration of the limb at the beginning of the swing and in deceleration at the end of the swing. This swinging action of the limb in walking is like that of a damped pen-

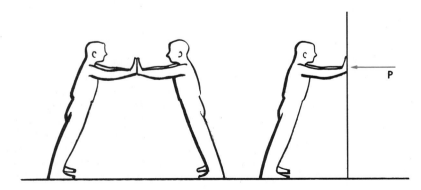

FIGURE 2–21

A push must be opposed by an equal and opposite push. The equal and opposite push of the wall (P) cannot be seen but it is just as real.

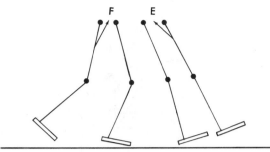

FIGURE 2–22

In the ballistic movement of hip flexion during the swing phase of walking, the thigh is first accelerated by the hip flexor muscles (F) at the beginning of swing and then decelerated by the hip extensors (E) before heel strike.

dulum that is forcibly accelerated and when once started must be forcibly stopped. Without the muscle forces the limb would continue at rest or continue in motion beyond the proper point, making smooth walking impossible. The control of the arm swing by muscles in fast walking or running is another example of muscle activity used to overcome inertia of a body segment.

A body that is stationary or moving at a constant speed is moving in a state of *equilibrium.* A force must be applied to change this state. In the case of a moving object, forces that help to slow down and stop this motion include (1) friction between the object and the supporting surface and (2) air resistance. A patient being moved in a wheelchair may be thrown forward if the wheels suddenly catch on a door sill or the patient's trunk is forced against the back of the chair when someone gives the chair an unexpected shove from behind. We have all had this experience while riding in an automobile when the driver suddenly applies the brake or the accelerator. The property of matter known as inertia causes an object either to resist being set in motion or, if moving, to resist being slowed down or stopped. The inertia of a body is proportional to its weight. If an aide attempts to push a very heavy patient on a gurney, he has difficulty not only getting started but also stopping the movement at the end of the trip. Transporting a child would entail less resistance to

starting and stopping. Likewise, an amputee need overcome less inertia in the control of the remaining portion of a limb than in control of the normal side. On the other hand, a limb in a cast or brace requires more than normal energy to control. The amount of decrease or increase of inertia is directly proportional to the change in mass. This is an important factor in energy expenditure and fatigue. Compare your own arm swing in walking when your hands are free with your swing when you are carrying a briefcase or handbag in one hand.

An example of the effect of inertia frequently seen in the clinic is the trauma sustained by the cervical spine in so-called whiplash injuries, or cervical syndrome (see Fig. 2–6). Because the car in such accidents is usually bumped from the rear, the rider's head is first snapped into extension. This is because it attempts to remain at rest while the trunk is moved violently forward. The head is then thrown into a flexed position as the trunk comes to rest. In this way, the delicate structures on both the anterior and posterior aspects of the neck may be damaged. Brain damage in football injuries is also a similar type of injury caused by the inertia of the brain.

Newton's third law regarding equal and opposite forces is illustrated by the usual floor or ground reaction in standing or walking. The supporting surface pushes upward against the sole of the foot with the same amount of force and along the same line of action as the downward force of the foot (Fig. 2–23). In locomotion the character of the surface may be such that it fails to provide counterforce to the foot and makes progress difficult and tiring, as when one walks on soft sand or gravel. Thin ice may supply the necessary equal and opposite reaction for a small boy, while his older brother will break through the surface. If a crutch or cane is placed on the floor in a vertical position, it is very stable since the floor pushes vertically upward in return. However, if a crutch is placed far out to the side at an angle to the body, the action line of the reaction force is at a corresponding angle with the vertical and the crutch is more likely to slip (Fig. 2–24). A person taking long strides is more apt to slide forward when his heel strikes a slippery floor than one who

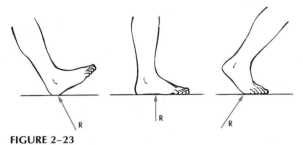

FIGURE 2–23

The ground reaction force R is equal in action line and magnitude to the downward thrust of the foot during walking, but opposite in direction. The force is greater at heel strike than at mid-stance because of the body's momentum, and greater at push-off due to the plantar flexion thrust of the calf muscles driving the body forward.

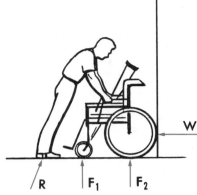

FIGURE 2–25

Counter forces, represented by R, F_1, F_2, and W, are provided by the floor and wall to stabilize the wheelchair as the patient prepares to sit down.

takes shorter steps with his foot coming down in a more nearly vertical direction. Horizontal force, such as that which accompanies the push-off in walking, must be opposed by an equal and opposite force so that the foot is stable and progression can take place. Friction between the sole of the foot and the ground normally supplies the necessary counterforce. Lack of friction, as in walking on a slippery surface, will make normal walking difficult or impossible. In our daily life all posture and movement is constantly influenced by the surface that supports

us. We may not be conscious of this because through experience our adjustments have become largely automatic. Contrast your movement in stepping off a curb into the street with stepping into a small canoe on a lake. Unfamiliar or unstable supporting surfaces require control of movement on a conscious level. A paraplegic patient may face frustration and possible injury if he or she attempts to get on a bed that has freely rolling casters or forgets to lock the wheelchair or back it up against a wall before sitting down in it (Fig. 2–25). He or she cannot plan or execute the movement successfully unless an adequate counterforce from a stable bed or chair is provided.

QUESTIONS

1. If a quantity has only magnitude but not direction is it a vector or a scalar quantity? Give an example of a vector quantity; a scalar quantity.
2. What are the four characteristics of a force that are necessary to define the force completely?

    (a) Describe (by a diagram) the pull of the brachialis muscle on the forearm in terms of these four characteristics.

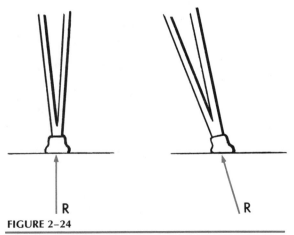

FIGURE 2–24

The direction of floor reaction force R opposing the force exerted by the crutch.

(b) Describe (by a diagram) the pull of gravity on the forearm in these terms: (1) with the forearm hanging at the side; (2) with the forearm horizontal.

3. Make a line drawing of the following:
(a) forces on the foot as the heel strikes the ground in walking, including:
(1) the upward force of the ground against the heel
(2) the downward thrust of the tibia on the talus
(3) the upward pull of the anterior tibial muscle undergoing eccentric contraction (doing negative work).
(b) forces acting on the foot as it pushes off in late stance, including:
(1) the upward pull of the Achilles tendon
(2) the downward thrust of the tibia on the talus
(3) the upward force of the ground against the metatarsal heads.
(c) forces acting on the arm when the patient has flexed it to 90 degrees, including:
(1) the pull of the deltoid acting at the deltoid tubercle
(2) the pull of gravity on the arm (locate the vector at the estimated center of gravity)
(3) the counterforce exerted by the glenoid fossa against the articular surface of the humerus (Newton's third law).

4. What are Newton's three laws of motion?

5. Explain how one or more of Newton's laws is involved in each of the following:
(a) A patient who is seated stands up.
(b) A patient is practicing a "swing through" crutch gait in which he or she leans forward on both crutches, swings both legs forward, and places his or her feet on the floor ahead of the crutch tips.
(c) As an exercise weight is hung on a wall peg, the peg supporting the weight breaks off.
(1) The falling weight smashes a hole through the floor.
(d) A patient who is practicing posture exercises is unable to keep the proper trunk alignment because the table mat is too soft.

6. Suggest some examples of applications of Newton's laws from the clinical area and from sports (e.g., kicking a football or high jumping).

7. Compare walking with running in terms of Newton's laws.

8. How does the force per unit area concept apply to the use of skis and snowshoes? To the size and number of sails on a boat?

9. Compare skin pressure on the sole of the foot in ordinary standing and in tiptoe standing. How does this apply to a patient with an equinus (fixed plantar flexion) deformity of the foot?

10. Why might posture-control chairs, which fix the body position rigidly, be harmful to patients if used for long periods of time?

11. How can the force per unit area concept be applied to the analysis of massage techniques such as pétrissage and friction? Give examples.

REFERENCES

Braune W, and Fischer O: Über den Schwerpunkt des menschlichen Korpers mit Rucksicht auf die Austrustung des deutschen Infanteriste. *In* Krogman WM, Johnston FE (Eds): Human Mechanics—Four Monographs Abridged. Wright-Patterson Air Force Base, Ohio, 1963 (AMRL-TDR 63-123).

Bremner RA: Observations on the ambulant correction of thoracic scoliosis and kyphosis with particular reference to the experimental use of hydrostatic pressure. J Bone Joint Surg (Br) *41B*:96–104, 1959.

Chaffin D, Andersson GBJ: Occupational Biomechanics. New York, John Wiley & Sons, 1984.

Clauser CE, McConville JT, Young JW: Weight, volume and center of mass of segments of the human body. Wright-Patterson Air Force Base, Ohio, 1969 (AMRL-TR-69-70).

Dempster WT: Space requirements of the seated operator. WADC Technical Report *55*:159, 1955.

Engin AE, Chen S-M: On the biomechanics of the hip complex in vivo—I, Kinematics for determination of the maximal voluntary complex sinus. J. Biomech *10*:785–795, 1988.

Fick A: Statistische Berachfung der Muskulature des Oberschenkels. Zeitslirift für Rationelle Medicin *9*:94–106, 1850.

Morehouse LE, Miller AT: Physiology of Exercise, 6th ed. St. Louis, CV Mosby, 1971.

Nuseibek IM: Mechanism and management of pressure sores. *In* Ghista DN (Ed): Spinal Cord Injury. Medical Engineering. Springfield, IL, Charles C Thomas, 1986, pp 269–282.

Steindler A: Kinesiology. Springfield, IL, Charles C Thomas, 1955.

Strausser H, Gassmann A: Hilfsmittel und Normen zur Bestimmung und Veranschaulichung von Stellungen, Bewegungen und Kraftwiskungen am Kniegelenke. Meckle: Bonnet: Anat Heft 2:6–7, 1893.

Taylor CL, Blaschke AC: A method for kinematic analysis of the shoulder, arm and hand complex. Ann NY Acad Sci 51:1123, 1951.

Webb Associates: Anthropometric Source Book, vol. 1. Washington, DC, National Aeronautics and Space Administration (NASA 1024), 1978, pp IV-1–IV-76.

3

Strength of Materials

INTRODUCTION

Materials are often subjected to external forces or loads. The material in turn tends to resist these loads. The ways in which a material responds to a load will be presented in this chapter. You should note how different types of materials are affected by loads. Biological materials behave differently than nonbiological materials. These differences, for example, have major importance in fracture care and joint replacement.

COMMON TERMS

Strain

Whenever a load or force is applied to a material, the material changes size or shape. For some materials, a load of only small magnitude will produce great changes, whereas for others a load of great magnitude may cause only slight changes. In general the changes that occur are called deformations. When the external changes in size or shape are expressed in terms of the original form of the material, these deformations are called strains.

A longitudinal strain (S) (Fig. 3–1) is the change in the dimensions of the material (Δl) divided by its original size (l), or

$$S = \frac{\Delta l}{l}$$

A traverse strain in which layers of the material slide past each other is the change in shape of the body and is often determined by the angle of deformation (Fig. 3–2). Strain has no standard unit of measure, it may be recorded in cm/cm, inches/inch, percent, and so on.

There are three principle strains. The two longitudinal strains are tension (Fig. 3–1A) and compression (Fig. 3–1B). The loads on each are colinear and opposite in direction. In tension, however, the loads are acting away from each other, while in compression the loads are acting toward each other. Biological tissues often undergoing tension strain are tendons, ligaments, muscle, blood vessels, and nerves. Examples of tissues often under compression strain are intervertebral discs, joint cartilage, and vertebrae.

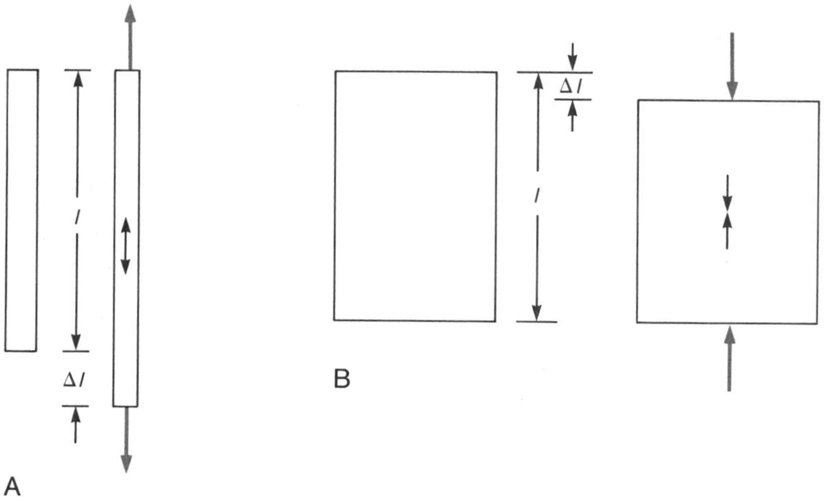

FIGURE 3–1

Longitudinal strains: *A,* Tension. *B,* Compression. Strain S = Δ l/l.

The third strain is shearing. In this case parallel but noncolinear forces acting in opposite directions cause adjacent planes of a material to slide past one another (Fig. 3–2A). Perpendicular lines of the material tend to change their orientation. Examples of shearing strain occur between the fifth lumbar vertebra and the sacrum, at epiphyseal plates of bones, and at joint surfaces.

Other loading situations incorporating the three primary strains are bending, measured by the radius of the curvature of the beam, and torsion, measured by the radius of the rotation of an end face of the object.

Stress

Along with the strains caused by external loads are reaction forces set up within the material. These internal reaction forces are called stresses. Stress is defined as the internal force per unit area upon a cross section that a part of a body on one side of a plane exerts on a part of the body on the other side of the plane. Stress is not visible but can be computed in terms of force per unit area. Longitudinal stress, or normal stress, is perpendicular to the cross section, while transverse stress is parallel or tangent to the surface of the plane.

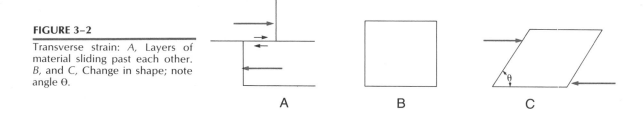

FIGURE 3–2

Transverse strain: *A,* Layers of material sliding past each other. *B,* and *C,* Change in shape; note angle θ.

Bending

Bending occurs when a load is placed upon a supported beam. The beam may be an end-supported beam or a cantilever-loaded beam.

The end-supported beam has a point of support at each end, with the load or loads placed between the two supports (Fig. 3–3A). The beam may often be loaded at three or four points. The amount of bending that occurs depends upon the magnitude of the loads and the distance between the load and supports. As the beam bends, it develops a curvature. The amount of curvature determines the magnitude of bending. The concave side of the beam is away from the two end supports. Within this concave portion, compression stress is developed. On the convex side of the beam, tension stress occurs. On a plane between these portions neither compression nor tension occurs. This plane is called the neutral plane of the beam (Fig. 3–3B). Bearing weight on the foot is an example of loading of a beam in the body (Fig. 3–3C).

The cantilever-loaded beam has one firmly supported end and a load placed at the other end (Fig. 3–4A). In this form of loading the beam tends to bend, with its upper surface being convex and its lower surface being concave. Compression stress is developed in the concave portion, while tension is developed in the convex portion. Shearing will occur parallel to the load and perpendicular to the load (Fig. 3–4B). Weight on the proximal end of the femur is a good example of cantilever loading (Fig. 3–4C).

A column may be loaded with the load directed along the axis of the column (Fig. 3–5A). Compression stress is developed within the column, and shear develops at 45° to the load. If the load is applied away from the center of the column, the loading scheme is termed eccentric column loading (Fig. 3–5B). In this situation bending of the column may occur. The side of

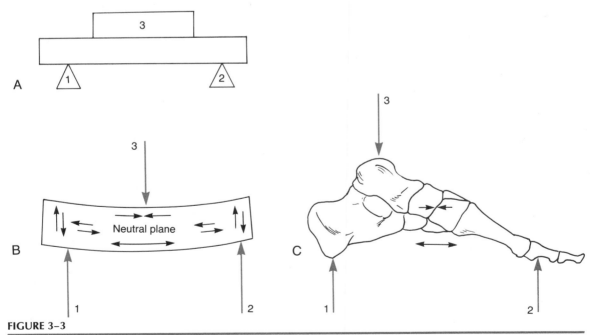

FIGURE 3–3

Loading of end-supported beam with location of stresses: 1 and 2 represent the end supports; 3 represents the load. *A,* Diagrammatic representation. *B,* Representation of stresses. *C,* Anatomical example (foot).

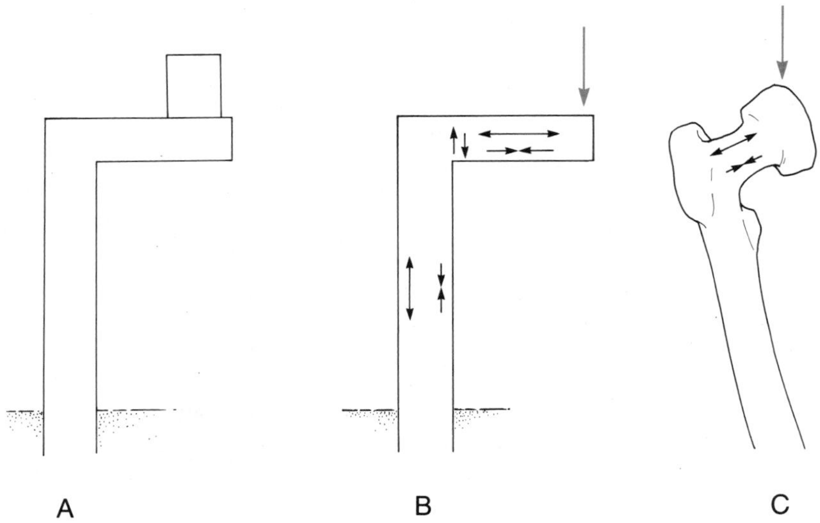

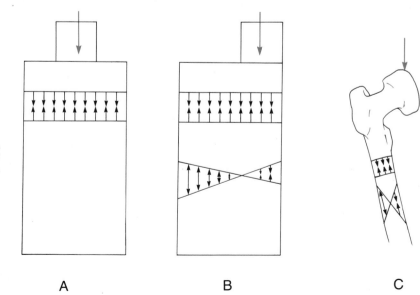

FIGURE 3–4

A, Loading of cantilever beam. *B,* Location of stresses. *C,* Anatomical example (proximal end of femur).

A   B   C

the load becomes concave with additional compression being developed, while the side away from the load becomes convex with tension being developed. The further the load is away from the center of the column, the greater is the bending effect. Loading of the femur and tibia through the proximal end of the femur illustrates eccentric column loading (Fig. 3–5C).

Torsion

Torsion develops when a rod or shaft is loaded so that it tends to twist around its long axis (Fig. 3–6A). The loads are usually applied perpendicular to the long axis of the object. Compression, tension, and shearing stresses are set up within the object (Fig. 3–6B). The magnitude of torsion

FIGURE 3–5

Loading of column: *A,* Center loading. *B,* Eccentric loading. *C,* Loading of femur.

A   B   C

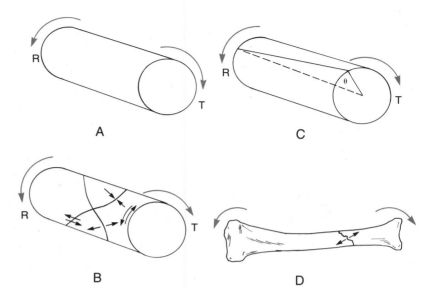

FIGURE 3–6

Torsion: *A,* Forces R and T acting in opposite directions causing twisting. *B,* Stresses during torsion. *C,* Magnitude of torsion determined by angle θ. *D,* Spiral fracture resulting from torsion.

is determined by the amount of rotation that occurs at the end face of the object (Fig. 3–6C). A spiral fracture of the tibia of a skier is an example of the result of a torsion load (Fig. 3–6D).

RHEOLOGICAL PROPERTIES

Elasticity

In a material that exhibits elastic behavior, the material will return immediately to its original dimension. The relationship between load and deformation will be a straight line for loading and unloading. The material will return all the energy applied to it. This type of material may be called a Hookean body (Fig. 3–7A). A spring and rubber band are good examples of elastic-behaving materials.

VISCOSITY

A viscous material does not deform instantaneously from an applied load. The stress will develop, but the strain will be delayed. The stress behavior of a viscous material depends upon the rate of loading. The greater the rate of loading, the greater will be the stress developed.

A constant rate of strain produces a constant stress. In a pure viscous material the deformation is not recoverable. In other words, the material does not return to its original size or slope. The energy is absorbed within the material. Most biological tissues exhibit some viscous behavior. A syringe and a hydraulic door closer are good examples of viscous materials. A viscous-type material may be referred to as a Newtonian body (Fig. 3–7B).

VISCOELASTICITY

Viscoelastic materials demonstrate a variety of combinations of elastic and viscous behaviors. A viscoelastic material will tend to deform slowly in a nonlinear fashion. When the load is removed, the material will tend to slowly and nonlinearly return to its original size and shape. The viscoelastic material demonstrates elasticity as it tends to return to its original size and shape and demonstrates viscous behavior as it responds to the rate of loading. Viscoelastic materials may behave as elastic and viscous elements in a series (a Maxwell body, Fig. 3–7C), in parallel (a Kelvin or Voigt body, Fig. 3–7D), or in a variety of other combinations.

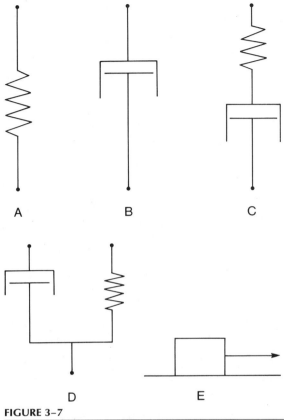

FIGURE 3–7

Rheological models: *A,* Elastic element (Hookean body). *B,* Viscous element (Newtonian body). *C,* Maxwell body. *D,* Kelvin or Voight body. *E,* Plastic element (St. Venant body).

Plasticity

A material that exhibits the property of plasticity retains its change in size and shape when the load causing the change is removed. Unlike an elastic material, no size, shape, or energy recovery occurs. Like the property of elasticity, however, when a load is applied, deformation occurs instantly and continues to occur as long as the load is applied or until the material fails. As opposed to a viscous material, no time delay or loading rate dependency exists. The plastic element is often represented by a block on a surface with friction between the block and surface (a St. Venant body, Fig. 3–7E).

STRESS-STRAIN CURVE

Within limits, the relationship between load and deformation or stress and strain is described by Hooke's law, which states that the deformation increases proportionally to the applied load, or strain increases proportionally to the stress resisting the applied load.

The stress-strain curve (Fig. 3–8) can be used to describe the total relationship between load-deformation or stress-strain.

As a load is applied to a material it begins to deform. The amount of deformation depends upon the magnitude of the load and the ability of the material to resist the load. The stiffness of the material is the property indicating the amount of deformation that occurs in proportion to the load applied. A very stiff material can tolerate a high load or high stress with only a small amount of strain. Steel and dry bone are examples. A less stiff material will have a greater magnitude of strain with less magnitude of load or stress. A rubber band is an example. A stiff material will have a steep slope on the stress-strain curve while a less stiff material will be represented by a less steep slope (Fig. 3–9). The ratio, $E = \sigma/\epsilon$, of stress to strain (ϵ) is termed the *modulus of elasticity* (E). Other terms used for this ratio are Young's modulus for tension, bulk modulus for compression, and shear modulus for shearing. The higher the value of the modulus of elasticity, the stiffer is the material. The area on the stress-strain curve in which this ratio remains proportional may be called the proportional range of the curve. The proportional limit is the point (P) on the curve at which the ratio between the stress and strain no longer remains proportional.

Within certain limits a material may possess the property of elasticity. That is, the material will have the ability to return to its original size and shape after the load has been removed. The elastic limit is the point on the curve beyond which the deformed material will not return to its original size or shape. A permanent deformation will exist. The range of the curve in which the material will return to its original size or shape is the elastic range (A). The range on the curve beyond the elastic limit is called the plastic range (B).

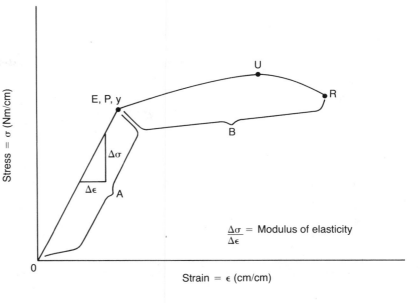

FIGURE 3–8

FIGURE 3–8

Stress-strain curve: Elastic limit = E; proportional limit = P; yield point = y; ultimate strength = U; rupture point = R; elastic range = A; plastic range = B.

Other points on the stress-strain curve are as follows. The yield point is the point at which strain will continue to occur without a similar increase in load or stress (y). The ultimate strength of the material is represented by the highest point on the curve (U). The breaking or rupture strength is the point at which the material breaks (R).

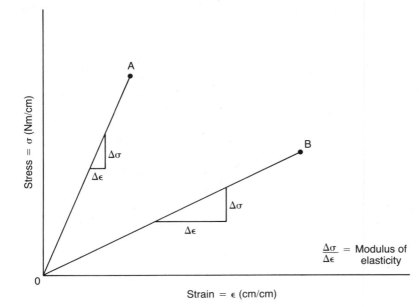

FIGURE 3–9

Representation of stiffness. Line A is stiffer than B.

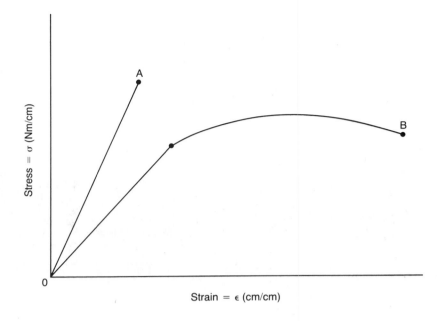

FIGURE 3–10

Representation of brittle (*A*) and ductile (*B*) materials. A brittle material has no or limited plastic deformation.

OTHER MECHANICAL PROPERTIES

Often differentiation between brittle and ductile materials is added (Fig. 3–10). A brittle material is one that has little or no plastic deformation (Fig. 3–10A). The breaking joint of the material is near its elastic limit. A brittle material may have no yield point. Glass and dry bone are good examples of brittle materials. A ductile material is one that has a large plastic deformation before it breaks (Fig. 3–10B). As a material is deformed under tension in the plastic range, the cross-sectional area of the material decreases as the material lengthens. This phenomenon is called *necking*. The ratio of the change in the cross-sectional and axial dimension is referred to as Poisson's ratio. Copper and steel are good examples of ductile materials.

The work done on a material as it is loaded is represented as the area under its stress-strain curve (Fig. 3–11). The area under the elastic range curve represents the stored strain energy (A). As the material is unloaded, all or some of this energy may be recovered.

A material that is loaded demonstrates a certain amount of resilience when the load is removed. Resilience is the ability of a material to rebound to its original size and shape with vigor (Fig. 3–12A). A highly resilient material will return to its original size and shape with the same vigor as it was deformed. Little energy is lost during loading and unloading of a highly resilient material.

Damping is the characteristic of a material to return to its original size and shape with less vigor that it was deformed (Fig. 3–12B). It can be considered to be the opposite of resilience.

A material that exhibits the characteristic of damping has a loss of energy during loading and unloading. When a material undergoes cyclic loading, the phenomenon of the loss of energy related to the difference between loading and unloading behavior is called *hysteresis.* The energy lost in this situation is determined by the area between the loading and unloading curves. If the loading causes the curve to go into the plastic range, a considerable amount of energy may be lost (Fig. 3–12C).

The area of the stress-strain curve under the plastic range, between the elastic limit and the

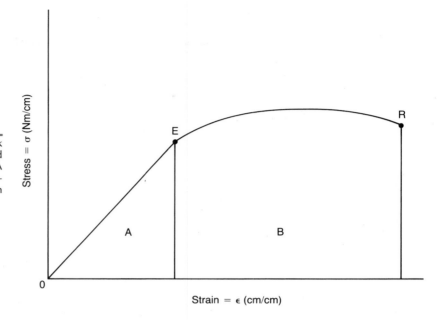

FIGURE 3–11

Work and stored energy. Work done is area under curve. Stored energy is represented in area A under elastic range curve; absorbed energy is represented in area B.

breaking point, represents absorbed strain energy (B). This amount of energy cannot be recovered and is dissipated as the material is permanently deformed.

Any object may fail or break because of mechanical fatigue. Mechanical fatigue is defined as failure of a material caused by repeated cyclic loading of a material. The greater the magnitude of the load, the fewer the cycles that will be needed to break the material. The lower the load, the greater the number of repetitions that will be needed before the material will break. The endurance limit of a material is the load at which an infinite number of cycles may occur without failure (Fig. 3–13). A stress fracture is an example of a bone failing from mechanical fatigue.

A material may also fail because of creep. The phenomenon of creep occurs as a material deforms when it is loaded for a prolonged time (Fig. 3–14). The greater the load, the faster the material will deform toward failure. A low magnitude load may be too small to cause creep followed by breaking of the material.

Stress relaxation is similar to creep. Stress relaxation occurs when a material is strained (deformed) to a given dimension and maintained at that strain. In this situation the stress within the material gradually decreases with time (Fig. 3–15). The difference between creep and stress relaxation is that creep occurs with a constant load applied and strain increases, whereas stress relaxation has a constant strain and stress decreases. Creep and stress relaxation occur during treatment with traction, splints, and serial casts.

MATERIAL PROPERTIES

Now that you have some understanding of the general behavior of materials, we may look more closely at how specific materials respond.

The mechanical properties of material are dependent upon the makeup and arrangement of its constituents. A material may be homogeneous with an even distribution of its components throughout the material. The mechanical properties of this type of material are the same at all points. Most metals are good examples of homogeneous materials. A heterogeneous material, on the other hand, is composed of dissim-

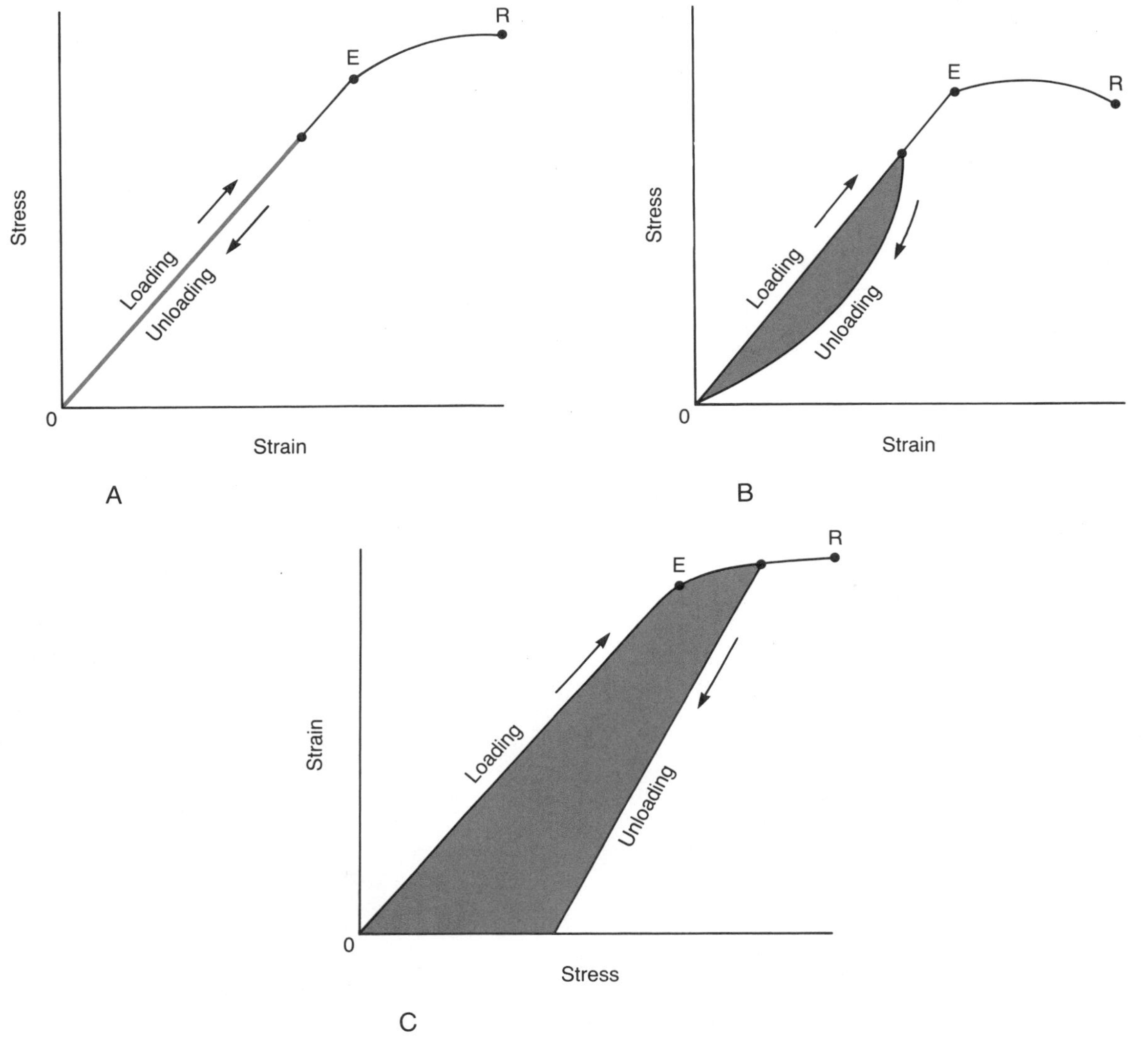

FIGURE 3–12

Resilience and damping during loading and unloading; shaded area represents energy lost. *A,* Resilient material. *B,* Energy lost in less resilient material. *C,* Energy lost when loading takes material into plastic range.

ilar or nonuniform constituents. Its mechanical properties will not be the same for all points. The mechanical properties are unpredictable at various points of a heterogeneous material. Cement, aggregate, and bone are examples of heterogeneous materials.

An isotropic material is one that has no directional alignment of its components and in which the mechanical properties are the same in all directions at any point of the material. The mechanical properties of an anisotropic material that has a directional structure material are different in different directions. Copper, silver, rubber, and certain plastics are examples of isotropic materials. Wood, bone, and ligaments are examples of anisotropic materials.

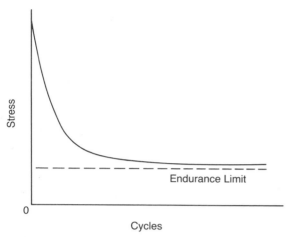

FIGURE 3–13

Mechanical fatigue: Relationship between stress at failure to number of cycles of loading. Endurance limit is level of stress below which an infinite number of cycles will not cause failure.

Biological Materials

Biological tissues exhibit a wide variety of behaviors in response to mechanical loading. Such behaviors are related to the makeup and configuration of the constituents of each individual tissue.

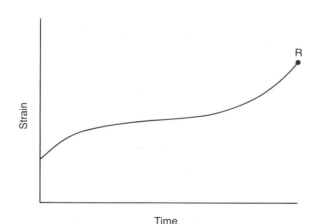

FIGURE 3–14

Creep phenomenon: Increasing strain occurring because of prolonged loading.

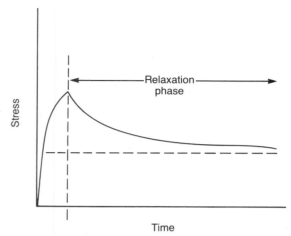

FIGURE 3–15

Stress relaxation: The stress on an object loaded under a constant strain is reduced with length of item loaded.

An understanding of the mechanical properties of biological tissues is important for the evaluation and treatment of trauma and disease. The causes and treatment of fracture, arthritis, and soft tissue injury and the use of prosthetic replacements all depend upon this knowledge.

CONNECTIVE TISSUE

Connective tissues are complex biological tissues made up of varying amounts of collagen, elastin, ground substance, water, and minerals. The relative amounts depend upon the type and age of tissue. The function of connective tissue is predominantly mechanical. Connective tissue has a good ability to withstand tensile stress and recover in size and shape when the load is removed.

Collagen is a fibrous protein that is helical in molecular arrangement. The collagen fibrils made up of the molecules are generally parallel but may differ in organization in different structures. This component is found in most connective tissues including bone, cartilage, tendons, ligaments, skin, blood vessels, the cornea, vitreous humor, the basement membrane, and the framework of all tissues and organs except blood, lymph, and keratinous tissue (Parry and Craig, 1988).

The role of collagen is to provide structural integrity. Its fibrils have a high tensile strength. Tissues with high tensile strength have high collagen content (e.g., tendons and skin), and collagen fibers of 1 mm^2 cross section can withstand a load of 980 N (Buckwalter and Cooper, 1987). Collagen that is highly cross-linked is stiff, while collagen with fewer cross links is less stiff.

Collagen has a tensile strain of approximately 8 to 10 percent and an elastic modulus of 8 $\times$ 10^7 N/m^2 (Parry and Craig, 1988). Although collagen is strong in tension, it is weak in torsion and bending. Therefore, collagen gives connective tissue its ability to withstand high tensile loads.

Elastin is not as widespread as collagen. It is mostly found in arteries, lung tissue, skin, and selected ligaments. An important mechanical property of elastin is its great extensibility and its ability to recover its original size and shape. Elastin can be extended by 1.6 times (Fung, 1981) to double (Parry and Craig, 1988) its original size and recover completely. The elastic modulus of elastin is 6 $\times$ 10^5 N/m^2 (Parry and Craig, 1988), which is much less than collagen. Elastin does not appear to have the ability to creep when loaded for a prolonged time. Extensibility, elasticity, and lack of creep are important properties provided to some connective tissues by elastin.

Glycosaminoglycans (GAG) make up the basic unit of proteoglycans, which are the major macromolecules of connective tissue ground substance (Buckwalter and Cooper, 1987; Montes and Junqueira, 1988). These molecules are composed mainly of carbohydrates and create long polysaccharide chains. The mechanical properties include their ability to fill empty space and to be hydrophilic. Because of the negative electrical charge of the polysaccharide chains, they repel each other, disperse, and fill available space. Their hydrophilic ability allows them to absorb and retain a great amount of water. The contained water provides resistance to compression, resiliency, and joint lubrication. Glycoproteins, which are composed largely of all protein, organize, support, and bind the macromolecules. Dense connective tissue contains very little ground substance, while loose connective tissue is made up of large amounts of ground substance (Fung, 1981).

BONE. The major factors that determine the mechanical responses of bone to loading are the material properties of the bone; the size, geometry, and form of the bone; and the direction, magnitude, and rate of force application. Bone is a nonhomogeneous anisotropic composite structure that behaves viscoelastically. It is composed of organic material, which makes up about 35 percent of its weight (Fung, 1981; Carter and Spengler, 1978). This organized substance is composed of collagen (90 to 95 percent), GAGs (1 percent), and other proteins (4 to 9 percent). The collagen fibers run parallel to each other along the length of a mature bone. Collagen provides the tensile strength of bone. Water makes up about 20 percent of the weight of mature bone, while minerals account for the remaining 45 percent (Carter and Spengler, 1978). The major minerals in bone are calcium phosphate and calcium carbonate. Hydroxyapatite crystals and amorphous calcium phosphate are the main mineral components. Sodium, magnesium, and fluoride are also found in bone in lesser amounts.

The hydroxyapatite crystals provide strength and stiffness to bone. The elastic modulus (E) of these crystals is about 165 GN/m^2 as compared with steel (E = 200 GN/m^2) and aluminum alloy (E = 70 GN/m^2) (Fung, 1981). The stiffness prevents buckling of the bone and gives it the ability to resist shear and compression. With increased stiffness, the bone also has increased brittleness and decreased toughness.

A bone with a larger cross section can distribute the force over a larger area. In this way the stress (force/area) is reduced within the structure. The shape of the bone also influences the distribution of the stresses. A tubular bone, for example, can more evenly distribute the stresses resulting from bending or torsional loads than can a solid cylinder of equal mass (Carter, 1985). Torsion and bending are also resisted more easily if the structural material is distributed at a distance from the central axis. A hollow cylinder distributes the material in such a way.

The form of bone may also affect its mechanical properties. Carter and Spengler (1978) reported that the classification between cancellous and cortical bone is based upon the porosity of the structure. They defined porosity as the proportion of the volume occupied by nonmineralized tissue. Cancellous bone was defined as having a porosity of 30 percent or more, while cortical bone had a porosity of between 5 and 30 percent. Cortical bone is found in the diaphysis of bones. The diaphyses and epiphyses are composed of cancellous bone.

Cancellous (trabecular) bone and cortical (compact) bone are similar in material composition (Carter and Spengler, 1978). A major difference in the structure of these types of bones is their density or porosity. The density of cortical bone is about 1.6 to 2.0 g/cm^3, while the density of trabecular bone ranges from 0.07 to 0.97 g/cm^3 (Albright, 1987). The mechanical properties of cancellous and cortical bone differ to a great extent because of their density and porosity. Carter and Spengler (1978) determined that the compressive strength of a bone specimen was approximately proportional to the square of its apparent density, while its compressive modulus was proportional to the cube of its apparent density. Based upon this information, a person can predict that the strength and compressive modulus of bone will decrease as the density of bone decreases from disuse and with age after 30 to 40 years. One should also be aware that as bone density increases from exercise, these mechanical properties increase (Hayes, 1986). Advani and associates (1979) have stated that the ultimate stress and elastic modulus depend primarily on porosity and that bone porosity should be considered as crucial to its mechanical integrity as mineralization.

Bones are modeled and remodeled in a geometrical pattern to resist loads in a particular direction. Carter (1985) reported that longitudinal loading was approximately 50 percent greater than transverse loading. Bone has also been shown to resist greater loads of compression than tension loads. In turn, bone resists tension loads better than shearing or torsion.

The rate of loading affects the ultimate strength of the bone and its ability to absorb energy. A bone resists rapidly applied loads much better than slowly applied loads (Carter, 1985; Albright, 1987). At fractures following rapidly applied loads, however, the greater absorbed energy causes greater damage to the bone and surrounding tissue. Table 3–1 provides values for various mechanical properties of bone. Note the differences in direction of loading, rate of loading, form of bone, and location of bone. These values differ based upon how the material was tested and which part of the bone was tested.

CARTILAGE. Cartilage is a specialized connective tissue that consists mainly of a solid matrix (20 to 40 percent) of collagen and a proteoglycan gel, water (60 to 80 percent), and some sparsely dispersed cartilage cells (chondrocytes). The proportions of each depend upon the type, location, and health of the cartilage as well as the specific function of the tissue. The collagen fibers that make up about 65 percent of the solid matrix provide high-tensile loading resistance. They are stiff and strong when stretched. The proteoglycan macromolecules (about 25 percent of the solid matrix) being hydrophilic can offer stiffness in compression as they control water content. The water can freely exchange externally to the tissue.

Articular cartilage functions (1) to distribute the force evenly under load, which in turn decreases the compression on the joint; (2) to provide a time-dependent shock absorber; and (3) to reduce friction in the joint.

Since the modulus of elasticity of articular cartilage is about 20 times less than that of trabecular bone, cartilage will deform more than bone (Weightman and Kempson, 1979). This deformation increases the load contact area in the joint and reduces the compressive stress relayed to the subchondral bone. Even distribution of this pressure is a result of the high water content of the cartilage. Remember that according to Pascal's law a load applied to a fluid is transmitted equally in all directions.

During many normal activities loads are applied to joints at fairly high rates. These dynamic loads are resisted by the articular cartilage. The hydrophilic and permeability properties of the proteoglycans, the incompressibility of water, and the high tensile strength of colla-

TABLE 3–1. SELECTED MECHANICAL PROPERTIES OF BIOLOGICAL TISSUES

Tissue	Ultimate Stress *Megapascal (MPa)*	Modulus *Gigapascal (GPa)*	Strain to Fracture *Percent*
Muscle*	0.147–3.50	–	58–65
Fascia*	15	–	–
Tendon*			
Various	50–150	–	9.4–9.9
Various	19.1–88.5	–	–
Achilles	34–55	–	–
Ligament*			
Nonelastic	60–100	0.111	5–14
ACL	37.8	–	23–35.8
Collagen	50	1.2	–
Cartilage (hyaline)			
Tension	4.41	–	10–100
superficial	10–40	0.15–0.5	–
deep	0–30	0–0.2	–
costal	44	–	25.9
Compression	7–23	0.012–0.047	3–17
patella	–	0.00228	–
femoral head	–	0.0084–0.0153	–
costal	–	–	15.0
Shear			
normal	–	0.00557–0.01022	–
degenerated	–	0.00137–0.00933	–
Torsion			
femoral	–	0.01163	
Disc			
Tension	2.7	–	–
Compression	11.0	–	–
Torsion	4.5–5.1	–	–

Data from Carter, 1985; Mears, 1979; Sokoloff, 1966; Kempson, 1979; Woo, 1986; Gelberman, 1987; Frank and Woo, 1985; Reilly and Burstein, 1974; Currey, 1970; Lindahl and Lindgren, 1967b; Kennedy et al., 1976; Advani et al., 1979; Fung, 1981; Albright, 1987.
*Tension.

gen function to control the rate of cartilage response to the load. The proteoglycan gel swells as it attracts the water into the molecule. This swelling stretches the collagen fibers until their tensile stress balances the swelling force. Thus, the collagen fibers are being stressed in unloaded cartilage. This situation provides the compressive rigidity of cartilage.

When a load is applied perpendicularly to the articular cartilage surface, the cartilage offers resistance instantly as the cartilage deforms, causing increased pressure within the cartilage and tension upon the collagen fibers. The first phase following loading is an elastic response, followed by the second phase, which is a creep response. The solid matrix of the proteoglycan gel is porous and permeable. If the load is maintained, water will be allowed to leave the molecule to areas of less pressure. This process, however, is not instantaneous but governed by a frictional drag related to the fluid viscosity as the fluid passes through the pore walls. The process is reversible following removal of the load. The reaction of cartilage to loading is a good example of a viscoelastic response. The water that has been squeezed out of the cartilage may aid in joint lubrication.

FIBROUS TISSUE. Fibrous tissues are tough, flexible, pliant sheets or cords that possess great tensile strength. Their primary solid component is densely packed collagen fibers. These fibers

TABLE 3–1. SELECTED MECHANICAL PROPERTIES OF BIOLOGICAL TISSUES *Continued*

Tissue	Ultimate Stress Megapascal (MPa)	Modulus Gigapascal (GPa)	Strain to Fracture Percent
Annulus			
Tension	15.68	–	–
Skin	8.3–133.9	–	190
Aorta	74.46	–	106
Collagen	–	0.00012	–
Elastin	–	0.0004	–
Bone (cortical)			
Tension			
collagen	50	1.2	–
osteons	38.8–116.6	–	–
axial			
femur (slow)	78.8–144	6.0–17.6	1.4–4.0
(fast)	172	–	–
tibia (slow)	140–174	18.4	1.5
fibula (slow)	146–165.6	–	–
transverse			
femur (fast)	52	11.5	–
Compression			
osteon	48–93	–	–
axial			
mixed	100–280	–	1–2.4
femur	170–209	8.7–18.6	1.85
tibia	213	15.2–35.3	–
fibula	–	16.6	–
transverse			
mixed	106–133	4.2	–
Shear	50–100	3.58	–
Bending	132–181	10.6–15.8	–
Torsion	54.1	3.2–4.5	0.4–1.2

are usually parallel and directed along the axis of tensile loading. Water makes up about 65 to 70 percent of their weight. They contain small amounts of elastin and proteoglycans. The specific amount of each material depends upon the function of the tissue.

Fibrous tissue may be divided into three groups: (1) dense and regular, (2) dense and irregular, and (3) loose and fibrous. The dense and regular tissues are ligaments, joint capsules, and tendons. Fascial layers, blood vessels, reticular layers of dermis, and capsules of organs are composed of dense and irregular tissues. Tissues between muscles and subcutaneous areolar tissue are loose fibrous tissues (Buckwalter et al., 1987).

Ligaments and joint capsules have similar structure and mechanical function. They prevent abnormal joint motion and stabilize the joint. They are predominantly highly organized, densely packed collagen fibers in cords or layers of sheets. The collagen provides tensile strength and stiffness, but these fibers will buckle under axial compression.

Woo (1986) has reported that cruciate ligaments and collateral ligaments have similar water content (65 to 70 percent) and similar collagen (75 to 80 percent of dry weight) and elastin (<5 percent dry weight) content. Cruciate ligaments seem to have over twice the proteoglycan content that the collateral ligaments have.

Tendon appears to be the most specialized of the dense fibrous tissue. This tissue may also vary from broad sheets to thin cords. Tendons must support large muscle forces with minimal deformation. The water and collagen content of tendons is similar to that of ligaments. The elastin content, however, is less, making up less than 3 percent of the dry weight of the tissue. The collagen fibers are arranged parallel and run longitudinally. These fibers, however, are not perfectly straight when relaxed but have a wavy form. This waveform may be the result of the pull of elastin fibers (Proske and Morgan, 1987). When a load is first applied to the tendon, strain occurs with little stress as the fibers are straightened. Following the removal of the wave, the tendon generally has a linear elastic region. A tendon may yield and become plastically deformed if its yield point is exceeded. Proske and Morgan (1987) studied the stiffness of tendons. Note that if a tendon has a low stiffness, the muscle force applied and the load on the body part will cause the tendon to elongate. The efficiency of the motor system would be low.

Proske and Morgan (1987) found that a tendon does stretch and recoil. They determined that at low loads a tendon is much less stiff than at higher loads. A less stiff tendon allows the muscle to shorten at a slightly slower speed, making it more efficient when shortening. A stiffer tendon, however, provides for more brisk and accurate movements. The conclusions by Proske and Morgan (1987) state that if a tendon is allowed to have some stretch, less disturbance of the contracting muscle fibers occurs and elastic energy in the musculotendinous unit may be stored. Such a system can help maintain a lower total energy level.

OTHER FIBROUS TISSUE. The mechanical properties of blood vessels depend upon the balance of content between collagen and elastin fibers. This balance is much different than in the previously discussed fibrous tissues. In general, collagen makes up 25 to 35 percent of the dry weight of the blood vessels, and elastin makes up 40 to 50 percent. In the aorta, elastin is about twice as abundant as collagen, whereas in the vessels farther from the heart the ratio reverses to about 2 to 1. Proteoglycans make up about 2 to 2.5 percent of the vessels's dry weight, with

more in the arterioles than in the veins. Blood vessels are about 60 to 70 percent water.

The collagen is loosely arranged and wavy in appearance. This structure has an important effect on the function of the vessels. When the vessels are loaded at low levels of blood pressure, the elastin responds by stretching and the collagen offers little resistance as they straighten. As the blood pressure increases, however, the collagen fibers are stretched, offering greater stiffness. Therefore, increased blood pressure is met with a nonlinear increase in vessel stiffness.

Skin has a random and loose collagen structure, and collagen makes up about 65 to 70 percent of its dry weight. Elastin fibers make up about 5 to 10 percent and proteoglycans compose about 1.5 to 2 percent of the dry weight. Skin is about 60 to 65 percent water. As skin is elongated the fibers tend to realign along the line of the load. Skin has a greater strain to failure percentage than tendons or ligaments.

MUSCLE

Multinucleated muscle fibers are the basic components of muscles. Within the fibers is an elastic protein known as connectin. Each fiber is surrounded by a lipid bilayer called the sarcolemma, which in turn is enclosed by a protein-polysaccharide coating. Endomysium, a connective tissue composed mainly of collagen with a few elastin fibers, lies between one fiber and the next. The muscle fibers and adjoining tissue are grouped into bundles, or fascicles. A thicker amount of the endomysium connective tissue, the perimysium, encases each fascicle. The entire muscle made up of fascicles is surrounded by an even thicker layer of connective tissue called epimysium. Note that the connective tissue is continuous throughout the muscle and is interspersed between the muscle fibers. Tendon connections to the bone are continuous with the connective tissue of the muscle. The tendon is joined to the muscle as its collagen fibers extend into the sarcolemma (Squire, 1986). Because of this arrangement, tendons lying in series with muscle fibers must carry the same load as the muscle (Proske and Morgan, 1987).

Each muscle fiber consists of a series of contractile units called sarcomeres. Each sarcomere within a muscle fiber is the same length and contracts with the same force. The sarcomere is composed of myosin myofilaments and actin myofilaments that overlap and form cross-bridges when activated. These bridges tend to forcefully shorten the muscle. The myosin and actin filaments maintain their length but slide past each other to shorten the sarcomere. Combined shortening of sarcomeres shorten muscle fibers, which in turn results in total muscle shortening.

The number of bridges capable of forming depends upon the degree of filament overlap (Fig. 3–16A). The potential force that can be generated by a muscle depends upon the number of cross-bridges formed. The greater the number of bridges formed, the greater the potential force produced by the muscle (Gordon et al., 1966; Gans, 1982; Gans and DeVree, 1987; Squire, 1986). Note the force produced in Figure 3–16B as compared with the amount of filament overlap in Figure 3–16A. In position 1 no overlap exists. Therefore, no force is present. Positions 2 and 3 appear to provide the potential for the greatest number of bridges, resulting in the greatest amount of force. As the filaments are positioned so that the sarcomere is shortened (see Fig. 3–16), fewer bridges are formed and the force is less. The force of a muscle is zero when it is about twice its resting length and approaches zero at about 60 percent of its resting length (Jokl, 1987).

Hence, the length of a muscle when it is stimulated or activated has a direct bearing on the force the muscle can produce. Jokl (1987) reported that when body joints are in their neutral position a muscle is considered to be at its resting length. However, in this position muscles tend to be under slight tension and if ruptured will retract about 20 percent.

If the sarcomeres shorten as they are activated, the force produced decreases. The faster the shortening, the greater the drop in force produced.

The combination of the connective tissue and the contractile elements affects the mechanical properties of the muscle. The Hill model establishes the muscle as a viscoelastic material that is responsive to the rate of load application (Gordon et al., 1966). Squire (1986) likens the response of the muscle model to the Voigt element consisting of a spring and dashpot in parallel together in series with a spring (Fig. 3–7D). The model illustrates the effect of both the contractile elements and the series and parallel elastic components. Zajac (1989), however, indicates that the series elastic component may be neglected. A length-tension diagram (Fig. 3–17) shows how total tension may be developed from combined voluntary muscle contraction and passive tension.

Angulation of the muscle fibers with the tendon (pinnation) also affects the amount of force a muscle may effectively transmit and the total excursion of the muscle. If the muscle fibers are parallel with the tendon, the total force produced by the fibers should be applied to the tendon. In this situation the excursion of the muscle is greater than in pinnated muscles. If these muscles change length drastically, the cross-bridges formed may vary considerably, and the consistency of force may be greatly affected. Fibers that insert at an angle to the tendon transmit less than 100 percent of their force to the tendon. As the angle of the fiber insertion into the tendon increases, the less effective the muscle fiber force will be ($F_{tendon} = F_{muscle} \cos \Theta$). This concept will be addressed further in Chapter 4. As a pinnated muscle shortens, the fiber angle increases, which in turn decreases the effective force to the tendon (Gans, 1982; Gans and DeVree, 1987; Otten, 1988). Few muscles are truly parallel with their accompanying tendon.

Nonbiological Materials

Nonbiological materials have been used to take the place of biological tissues for ages. They are used for internal prostheses as well as for external orthotic and prosthetic appliances. A material is selected for its specific use depending on its mechanical, physical, and chemical properties. Often an attempt is made to choose the specific material that most closely resembles the properties of the replaced tissue. The material, however, must also be biocompatible. Several

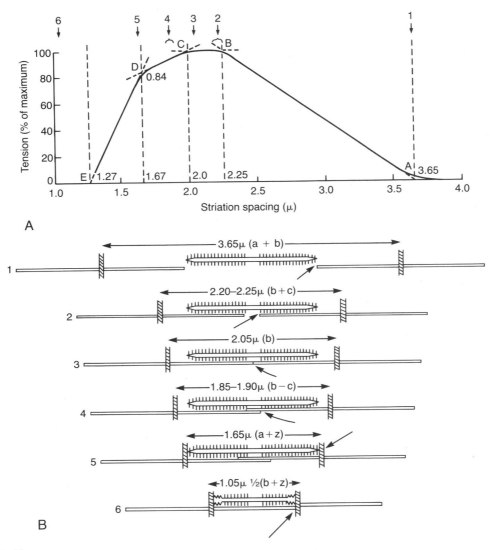

FIGURE 3–16

A, Schematic summary of results of sarcomere shortening. The arrows along the top are placed opposite the striation spacings at which the critical stages of overlap of filaments occur, as in *B*. *B*, Critical stages in the increase of overlap between thick and thin filaments as a sarcomere shortens. (From Gordon AM, Huxley AF, Julian FJ: The variation in isometric tension with sarcomere length in vertebrate muscle fibers. J Physiol *184*:170–192, 1966.)

journals are totally directed toward tissue engineering, biorheology, and biocompatibility. This section will only briefly touch upon the broad subject of materials used as implants, prostheses, and orthoses.

IMPLANT MATERIALS

Materials are implanted into the body for several reasons including fracture stabilization, correcting deformities, and replacement of joints.

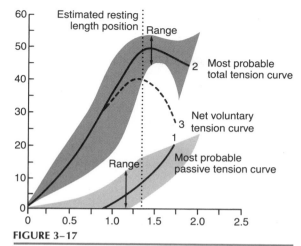

FIGURE 3–17

Isometric length-tension diagram for striated muscle. If passive tension curve (line 1) is subtracted from total tension curve (line 2), maximum muscle tension is developed at the normal resting length of muscle (line 3). The resting length of muscle is about 20 percent longer than the length of an excised, completely relaxed muscle. The horizontal axis represents muscle length; the vertical axis represents force. (From Astrand PO, Rodahl K: Textbook of Work Physiology. New York, McGraw-Hill, 1970.)

The success often depends upon the mechanical properties and design. The materials seem to fail most often from mechanical fatigue (Williams, 1981).

Few types of metals are used as implants. Some cobalt-chromium alloys, titanium and dilute titanium alloys, and stainless steel are the major types most suitable at this time.

A large number of cobalt and chromium alloys exist for surgical implants. Three major groups are cobalt-chromium-molybdenum (Co-Cr-Mo), cobalt-chromium-nickel (Co-Cr-Ni), and cobalt-nickel-chromium-molybdenum (Co-Ni-Cr-Mo). Some of their mechanical properties are shown in Table 3–2. You should compare the properties of the various materials listed in this table.

A pure titanium or dilute titanium alloy can serve as an implant. A common alloy is composed of 6 percent aluminum and 4 percent vanadium. The amount of oxygen dissolved in the material affects its strength. The greater the amount of oxygen, the greater the strength.

Note that according to Table 3–2 the elastic modulus of titanium is about half that of cobalt-chromium and stainless steel, but its strength is similar.

Stainless steel is an iron-carbon alloy that always contains chromium and usually contains nickel. Its mechanical properties are given in Table 3–2. The popularity of stainless steel for implants appears to be being replaced by cobalt-chromium and titanium.

Plastics consist of organic polymer molecules with specific additives. Pure polymers have poor mechanical properties that can be improved by the additives. Many of the additives, however, may be harmful to human tissues.

Polymethylmethacrylate is a polymer with several diverse surgical applications. Its major use, however, is as a bone cement. The material may be molded during polymerization (a mixing process). This mixing creates an exothermic reaction producing a high temperature that may damage tissues. It is the best self-curing bone cement available (Williams, 1981).

An ultra-high molecular weight, high density polyethylene is a common plastic used in metal-plastic joint replacements. High density polyethylene has a high wear resistance and produces few particles from wearing (Williams, 1981).

Polypropylene has mechanical properties similar to polyethylene except that its wear-resistance capability is less. A high fatigue resistance is a major advantage of this material. It can be used in components that undergo repeated flexing (Mears and Rothwell, 1979; Redford, 1986).

Most ceramic materials are crystalline metallic compounds with closely packed anions and smaller metalic ions. The strength of ceramics comes from the strong directional bonding. These materials are usually extremely brittle with a high elastic modulus and high compressive strength but relatively low tensile strength. Aluminum oxide is a ceramic material. An advantage of this material is its compressive strength and resistance to wear. A disadvantage is the marked difference of the elastic modulus between it and bone (Mears and Rothwell, 1979; Redford, 1986).

TABLE 3–2. MECHANICAL PROPERTIES OF NONBIOLOGICAL TISSUES

Material*	Ultimate Stress Megapascal (MPa)	Modulus Gigapascal (GPa)	Strain to Fracture Percent
Polyethylene			
Low-density	4.116–20.58	0.1–0.27	50–800
High-density	20.58–37.73	0.4–1.24	15–130
Polypropylene	27.44–41.16	1.1–1.5	10–700
Tension	19.9–30.9	–	–
Compression	25.4–55.0	–	–
Polystyrene	21.95–54.88	2.6–3.1	1–60
Polymethyl	41.16–82.32	2.4–3.1	2–5
Methacrylate tension	55.0–75.5	–	–
Polymethyl methacrylate (PMMA) tension compression	75.5–130.3	–	–
Polytetra	13.72–48.02	0.41–0.55	100–600
Fluroethylene (Teflon)			
Nylon 66	85	2.1–2.8	50–90
Polyvinal chloride (PVC)			
Tension	34.3–61.7	–	–
Compression	54.9–89.2	–	–
Acrylonitrile-butadiene-styrene (ABS)	20.6–54.9	–	–
Polyester			
Tension (thermosetting)	6.9–377.3	0.00069–13.7	0.3–300
Compression	6.9–411.6	–	–
Urethane tension	0.137–8.9	–	–
Compression	0.137–13.72	–	–
316 Stainless steel	550–700	120–395	35–55
Cobalt-Chromium			
Alloy ASTM F35	651–720	223–240	8
Alloy ASTM F90	892	188–652	50
MP 35 N	1670	240	13
Titanium			
Pure	400–710	110–274	15–30
Alloy 6Al4V	1000–1200	110	12–16
Aluminum			
Pure	70	70	60
Alloy	100–550	70–79	1–45
Wood	30–70	10–14	
Rubber	7–20	0.0007–0.004	100–800
Vitallium FHS	1502–1681	–	18–29

Data from Askeland, 1984; Mears, 1979; Williams, 1981; Gere and Timoshenko, 1984; Scheller et al., 1982; Redford, 1986; Lynch, 1975.
*MP 35 = special alloy code; 6Al4V = 6% aluminum and 4% vanadium.

ORTHOTICS AND PROSTHETICS

Metals are commonly used in the construction of orthoses and prostheses. The most common metals at this time are steel and aluminum. Stainless steel contains at least 12 percent chromium. The advantages of steel are its strength and the variety of alloys available. Its disadvantage is its weight. Aluminum has an advantage of a high strength-to-weight ratio, but it cannot endure repeated bending. It fails quickly from mechanical fatigue.

Polymeric materials are composed of giant organic molecules. Various types exist, but they are commonly grouped into three categories: thermoplastic, thermosetting, and elastomers.

Thermoplastics are polymeric materials that have their form changed following heating, without having their structural properties changed. Their mechanical characteristics generally include viscoelastic properties, creep, increased ductility, low elastic modulus, and less strength than the thermosetting polymers. Thermoplastic materials are often tough and resilient. Common examples of thermoplastic polymers are acrylics, polyethylene, polypropylene, acrylonitrile-butadiene-styrene, and polyvinyls (Askeland, 1984; Redford, 1986).

Thermosetting polymers cannot be reformed by heating. They generally have greater strength and modulus of elasticity than thermoplastic polymers, but they are less ductile. They tend to be hard and rigid. Common thermosetting polymers are some polyesters, polyamides, urethanes, amino resins, and phenolic resins. Some forms of these materials may also be thermoplastic (Mears and Rothwell, 1979; Redford, 1986).

Elastomers are either natural or synthetic rubber. They have an excellent ability to deform and to recover completely. They are tough and resilient (Askeland, 1984).

Polymers commonly found in fiber form are some polyamides (nylon), polyethylene terephthlate (Dacron or terylene), and polytetrafluorethylene (PTFE). These materials have tensile strength in the direction of their fibers and are often used as surgical sutures.

Other materials commonly used are plaster of Paris and fiberglass tape. Plaster of Paris can be very brittle, but this property is decreased if it is rubbed smooth. Fiberglass tape is stronger and lighter than plaster. It is also water-tolerant. Fiberglass tape, however, is more expensive, has a longer application time, may have sharp edges, and is more difficult to remove (Mears and Rothwell, 1979).

EXAMPLES FROM THE LITERATURE

Biological Tissues

Many factors influence the biomechanical properties of biological tissues (see Table 3–1). Some of these factors are age (Table 3–3), sex, and the amount and type of loading.

AGE AND SEX

The skeleton undergoes continuous changes over the lifespan. We see the changes in form, percent of constituents, and mechanical properties as the bone matures. The changing of bone, however, does not stop at maturity. Constant remodeling occurs.

In the 1960s, Weaver and Chalmers (1966) studied cancellous bone, while Lindahl and Lindgren (1967a and 1967b) evaluated cortical bone in relation to changes with age. Weaver and Chalmers (1966), while studying the vertebra and calcaneus, found that the mineral content and compression strength of the trabeculae increase rapidly before the age of 30 and slowly decrease after the age of 40. Below the age of 50 these cancellous bone characteristics for men and women were similar. After 50, however, the strength and mineral content of women's trabeculae decreased more rapidly than for the calcaneus. Lindahl and Lindgren (1967a and 1967b) studied the cortical bone of the femur and humerus. They found that the humerus had an ultimate stress value 10 percent greater than the femur, but the density of the femur was greater than that of the humerus. Structurally, the outer diameter of the cortical bone increased with age, with men having about 13 percent greater diameter than women. The density of the cortical tissue increased for men but remained relatively the same for women. Men had a greater density in the femur than did women; however, the density of the humerus was similar between the sexes. The cross-sectional area of cortical bone was greater in men than in women, but it decreased with age in men. The mechanical properties generally showed no differences between men and women. In both, the ultimate strength decreased about 10 percent over the span of 15 to 89 years. The strain to failure decreased about 35 percent. The modulus of elasticity, however, showed no changes with age. Currey and Butler (1975) looked at a younger group of subjects (2 to 48 years old) and studied the mechanical properties of bending a bone. They found that

TABLE 3–3. CHANGES IN SELECTED MECHANICAL PROPERTIES WITH AGE

Tissue	Age							
	0–9	*10–19*	*20–29*	*30–39*	*40–49*	*50–59*	*60–69*	*70–79*
Bone								
Ultimate tension (MPa)	–	116.0	125.0	122.0	114.0	95.0	88.0	88.0
Ultimate compression (MPa)	–	–	170.0	170.0	164.0	158.0	148.0	–
Ultimate percent elongation	–	1.5	1.4	1.4	1.3	1.3	1.3	1.3
Ultimate percent compression	–	–	1.9	1.8	1.8	1.8	1.8	1.8
Bending (femur) (MPa)	174.6	193.3	202.1	198.5	221.9	–	–	–
Bending (femur) (MPa)	–	–	212.0	212.0	199.0	190.0	181.0	165.0
Cartilage								
Ultimate tension (MPa)	4.6	4.6	4.5	4.2	3.6	2.5	1.5	1.3
Ultimate compression (Mpa)	–	11.6	9.9	9.6	8.2	7.2	7.2	–
Ligament								
Tensile strength (MPa)	–	–	37.8	–	–	13.3	–	–
Elastic modulus (MPa)	–	–	111.0	–	–	65.3	–	–
Ultimate percent elongation	–	–	44.3	–	–	30.0	–	–
Tendon								
Tensile strength (MPa)	53.0	56.0	56.0	56.0	56.0	56.0	53.0	44.0
Muscle (rectus abdominis)								
Tensile strength (MPa)	–	0.19	0.15	0.13	0.11	0.10	0.09	0.09

Data from Yamada, 1970; Currey and Butler, 1975; Noyes and Grood, 1976; Burstein et al., 1976.

while bending strength and modulus of elasticity for bending increased with age, the ability for the bone to absorb energy decreased. This characteristic is related to the child having a greater plastic deformation than the adult.

Burstein and associates (1976) evaluated the mechanical properties of the femur and tibia. They also found no differences in mechanical properties of bone between men and women. They noted that the tibia had greater ultimate strength, stiffness, and strain than the femur. They also found that the femur responded differently during aging. The femur decreased with age in the properties of yield stress, ultimate tensile and compression stress, elastic modulus, ultimate strain, and energy absorption. The tibia decreased in only ultimate strain and energy absorption. The authors stated that the most important change in the mechanical properties during aging was the decrease in strain that leads to decreased energy absorption. Currey (1979) studied the changes in energy absorption and related it to the increase in the mineralization of the bone tissue.

Two recent reviews of the mechanical properties of bone tend to provide a more complete picture of what is occurring in bone during aging (Sanders and Albright 1987; Martin and Burr, 1989). Certain structural changes affect these mechanical properties. A simplified pattern can give a general idea of what happens. The outer diameter of the cortex increases continuously from osteoblastic activity, while the internal diameter increases from osteoclastic activity. Before the age of 30 years, the osteoblastic activity may be more active than the osteoclastic, which provides an increase in the cortex thickness. After about 40 years of age, the osteoblastic activity slows down, while the osteoclastic activity may continue at the same rate. This activity results in a slow decrease in the cortical thickness. The decrease appears to be faster in women than in men. The cross-sectional area of bone tissue tends to decrease. In the vertebrae the trabeculae decrease in total mineral content as the number of trabeculae decrease. The remaining trabeculae may hypertrophy to resist compressive loads. In a span of 50 to 60 years, women may lose 50 percent of their trabeculae, while men may lose only 25 percent (Sanders and Albright, 1987). Martin and Burr (1989) summarized the material property changes. They noted that after 30 years of age cortical bone decreases its tensile strength about 4 to 5 percent per decade. Torsion and compression strength decrease at about half that rate. Ultimate strain decreases only a small amount. The energy to failure was reported to decrease about 6.8 percent per decade in the femur and 8.4 percent per decade in the tibia.

The results of these bone studies indicate that changes are occurring in the mechanical properties of bones even in healthy individuals. We must be aware that these changes occur at different times and to different degrees in different bones. The bone tissue in men and women seems to have similar mechanical properties before the age of 50 years, but men have a greater amount of this tissue. Therefore, their bones can tolerate greater loads.

As you may remember from the earlier description, cartilage responds elastically and viscoelastically. A major contributor in its ability to resist loading is its ability to control the flow of its water content. This control is related to its permeability. Armstrong and Mow (1982) studied the changes of cartilage permeability and the compressive modulus of cartilage with age. Both properties were found to be highly correlated with the water content of the cartilage but not significantly with age. The authors suggest that more study related to the mechanical properties of cartilage, its detailed biochemical composition, and natural aging is needed.

The mechanical properties of ligaments related to age were studied by Noyes and Grood (1976). They obtained anterior cruciate from trauma victims, above-knee amputees, and cadavers. A younger group was 16 to 26 years old. The older group was 48 to 86 years old. One of their purposes was to define the mechanical properties needed for a cruciate ligament prosthesis. They found major declines in mechanical properties of the anterior cruciate ligament with age. The ultimate strength of younger ligaments (1730 N, or 390 lb) was more than double the strength from the older group (734 N or 165 lb). The elastic modulus for the younger ligaments

(111 MPa) was almost twice as much as the older ligaments (65.3 MPa). Energy to failure and strain energy failure were approximately three times greater in the younger group than in the older group. Stiffness was also greater in the younger ligaments. The mode of failure between the two groups was different. The younger ligaments failed with ligamentous disruption. Failure of the older specimens occurred as avulsion fraction of the bone beneath the ligament insertion site. Previous studies using cadavers and specimens from older humans may have provided major underestimations of replacement tissue properties for the anterior cruciate ligament.

LOADING

The mechanical properties of tissues depend upon the loads applied to them. Deprivation and enhancement of stress within a tissue influence its structure and mechanical characteristics. You probably know that a muscle that is not used becomes smaller and weaker. A muscle that is exercised becomes larger and stronger. Connective tissue is also dependent upon stress and will atrophy or hypertrophy depending upon its loading history.

Carter and co-workers (1987) used loading and mechanical property values determined by other researchers to develop a computer model to predict the major features of skeletal morphogenesis. Their model described how loading from the first contractile elements of the muscular system in the embryo and muscular activity of the mother can affect skeletal development. It further related mechanical loading to development of the diaphysis and narrow cavity, the metaphyseal and epiphyseal bone, the location and geometry of the epiphyseal plate, the development of secondary ossification centers, and the growth of articular cartilage. The results of this study emphasize the importance of mechanical stresses in early skeletal development. The model supports the findings of others that immobilization can delay the appearance of the secondary ossific nucleus. It describes how the growth plate is aligned to avoid shear stress. It shows that if intermittent loads are not applied to the joint, ossification would continue toward the articular cartilage. This would result in progressive cartilage thinning and finally complete degeneration and ossification of the cartilage.

Bone mineral loss has been observed during immobilization in patients with paralysis or fracture. Donaldson and co-workers (1970) investigated the rate of bone loss that could occur from immobilization by restricting three healthy males to complete bed rest for 30 to 36 weeks. At the end of the bed-rest period, mineral loss in the calcaneus ranged between 25 and 45 percent. With resumption of ambulation, bone mineral was restored at the same rate that it was lost. The authors concluded that bone loss occurs in prolonged absence of weight-bearing and that the process is reversible. Lindgren and Mattsson (1977) found different results when studying 80 adult rats. After nine weeks of immobilization, the rats demonstrated osteoporosis in the femur and tibia. After ten weeks of remobilization, the bones remained osteoporetic. These authors concluded that bone loss from immobilization shows no signs of being reversible. Studies of weightlessness during space flight (Smith et al., 1977; Nicogossian, 1985) revealed that mineral loss in the weight-bearing bones is caused by reduced loading. Smith and colleagues (1977) concluded that these mineral losses follow the same pattern as that seen in bed rest. Later data (Nicogossian, 1985) showed that during bed rest most bone mineral is lost in the first five weeks and that the loss gradually decreases after that time. In space flight the loss of bone mineral does not plateau, and this may become a major limiting factor for long space missions. Exercise to load the bones was recommended as a measure to reduce the bone mineral loss.

The recommendation of exercise is consistent with a study done by Rubin and Lanyon (1984) who found that the removal of a load-bearing stimulus resulted in loss of bone mass. However, loading the bone prevented bone mineral loss. Other studies have also provided evidence that bone mineral increases in response to increased exercise.

Jones and co-workers (1977) described the differences in upper limb cortical bone thickness between the playing and nonplaying sides of tennis players. In males the cortical thickness on the playing side was 34.9 percent greater than on the opposite side. In women the cortical thickness on the playing side was 28.4 percent greater than on the other side. Similar results were found in older male tennis players compared with age-matched controls (Huddleston et al., 1980).

Muscle-strengthening exercises seem to affect the bone as well. Colletti and associates (1989) compared a group of men who consistently participated in weight-training exercises for more than one year with a larger group of age-matched controls. The bone mineral density in the lumbar spine, trochanter, and femoral neck was significantly greater in the weight-training group. Although the training program included upper limb exercises, the bone mineral density of the mid-radius was no different between the two groups. Colletti concluded that exercise can increase bone mass and prevent loss of bone and the development of osteoporosis.

Although the previously cited studies support the idea that exercise may increase bone mass, or at least prevent bone loss, not all studies support this. Cavanaugh and Cann (1988) compared the spinal bone loss of a group of early postmenopausal women on a 52-week walking program with a group of similarly aged women who were not on a walking program. Their results showed that both groups lost a similar amount of bone mineral density. Their conclusion was that a brisk walking program for one year does not prevent spinal bone loss in early postmenopausal women.

In contrast, Smith and associates (1989) found that exercise reduces bone loss in both premenopausal and postmenopausal women. They investigated the effect of a four-year aerobic exercise program, including light weights and other loading of the upper limbs, on the bone mineral content of middle-aged women. The exercised subjects lost significantly less bone in the left and right radii and ulnae than the control group. An important question is why exercise seemed to affect the upper limb bone mass of women (Smith et al., 1989) and did not affect the upper limb bone mass of men (Colletti et al., 1989). Several factors in these studies should be considered. The intensity, frequency, and duration of the exercise; the bone part exercised; and the exercise history of the subjects may all affect the bone loss. In following chapters you will see how the loads on body parts may be determined for various activities.

Immobilization of a synovial joint may lead to joint contracture and possible deterioration of the soft tissues of the joint (Frank et al., 1985). Articular cartilage of the joint can severely deteriorate with immobilization. Bed rest or other unloading of the skeletal system or joint immobilization appears to increase the risk of degenerative joint disease (Helminen et al., 1987). The degenerative changes that occur include cartilage thinning, irregularities and fibrillation of the cartilage surfaces, and finally encroachment of the joint space by fibrofatty connective tissue (Akeson et al., 1987a and 1987b; Chvapil, 1988). Palmoski and associates (1979) found that proteoglycan synthesis decreased in the articular cartilage of dogs after six days of immobilization. These proteoglycans are the main components offering resistance to compressive loads and deformation in cartilage (Myers et al., 1988). The magnitude of loss of the proteoglycans varies with the location in the cartilage (Tammi et al., 1987). Thus, the mechanical properties may change at different locations in the cartilage and degeneration may occur more quickly in certain areas. (Tammi et al., 1987).

Maintenance of normal proteoglycan content is vital for the health of the articular cartilage (Tammi et al., 1987). The maintenance of this component of cartilage appears to occur with motion and compression of the joint (Akeson et al., 1987a and 1987b; Tammi et al., 1987; Sokoloff, 1987). Increased compression may enhance the mechanical properties of articular cartilage, unless the load is too great and the load is continuously applied.

Copray and co-workers (1985a and 1985b) demonstrated support for this concept on mandibular cartilage of the rat. They found that a continuous compression of more than 3 g stopped the growth of cartilage. However, growth continued at a slow rate up to a load of 8 g during intermittent compression. Tammi and colleagues (1987) summarized the results of several animal studies related to cartilage load-

ing. In general, elevated weight-bearing and moderate running tended to increase tissue proteoglycan content, thicken the cartilage, increase stiffness, and improve biomechanical properties. On the other hand, strenuous running reversed the beneficial effects found in moderate exercise.

Both decreased and increased loading can alter the biological properties of cartilage (Helminen et al., 1987). The magnitude at which the loading becomes harmful is not yet known. The manner in which the load is applied may also be important (Radin and Rose, 1986). Being able to determine joint forces as presented in Chapter 7 should help provide a better understanding of how to prevent cartilage damage.

Several animal studies have been performed to determine the effects of immobilization and exercise on the mechanical properties of ligaments. A few of these will be presented in the following paragrapshs.

Noyes and co-workers (1974) showed that after eight weeks of immobilization the anterior cruciate ligament–bone complex of monkeys decreased in maximum stress by 39 percent and in energy absorbed to failure by 32 percent and increased in strain to failure. After five months of exercise after the same period of only partial recovery of ligament–bone strength (79 percent) and energy to failure (78 percent) occurred. However, the strain was nearly normal (96 percent). An exercise program used in the study had little effect on the mechanical properties of the ligament during immobilization. In 1977 Noyes reported the results of a study that included a 12-month reconditioned group. His results showed that after 12 months the ligament had still not recovered (maximum stress, 91 percent; energy absorbed, 92 percent).

Woo and associates (1987a and 1987b) studied the effects of immobilization and reconditioning on the medial collateral ligaments of dogs and rabbits. Their results demonstrated a similar trend as the studies by Noyes and co-workers (1974) and Noyes (1977). They found deteriorated mechanical properties following immobilization with an improvement in these properties following reconditioning.

These studies indicate that a ligament–bone complex may take much more time to return to normal mechanical properties than the period of immobilization. Woo and associates (1987a) noted that the ligament substance may heal at a similar rate to that of decline, but the ligament insertion site into bone has a prolonged recovery time. The results of these studies indicate the need to know the loading that a material can safely withstand and the load that is applied to the material during various daily and athletic activities. They also show that the clinician should be aware of the prolonged healing time that may be needed.

Immobilization is not necessary for healing dense fibrous tissue. In some instances immobilization may be harmful. Early motion of injured and repaired tendons seems to prevent the formation of adhesions and reduce the deleterious effects of the mechanical properties that occur with immobilization. Buckwalter and co-workers (1987) report several studies that show early passive motion increases the strength of damaged fibrous tissue. They state that carefully applied loading and motion accelerated tissue healing and improved the quality of the repaired tissue.

Ligaments and tendons appear to respond to increased loading in a similar manner. Tipton and colleagues (1975) found that ligaments in exercised animals were heavier, but the collagen content per weight/length unit was not increased. Total collagen content increases following exercise were reported by Viidik and Gottrup (1984). In exercised animals the mass of the ligament increased giving more total collagen, but the amount per weight was not different.

The type of exercise also influences biomechanical tissues. A single bout of exercise and sprint training showed no change in ligament and ligament–bone junction strength, but endurance exercise increased ligament strength, junction strength, and energy absorbed to failure (Tipton et al., 1975).

The tissue function or location also appears to influence change in response to exercise. Woo and associates investigated the effect of exercise on the digital extensor tendons (1980b) and digital flexor tendons (1981) of swine. They used two different training periods (three months and 12 months). Little or no change in mechanical

properties occurred in either flexor or extensor tendons compared with a nonexercised control group. After 12 months of training, the extensor tendons had a 22 percent increase in tensile strength. The flexor tendons, however, demonstrated no statistical change in mechanical properties or mass. Flexor tendons have a higher collagen concentration and greater tensile strength than extensor tendons. With exercise the collagen content of the flexor tendons did not change, but it increased in the extensor tendons (Woo et al., 1981). The amount of collagen is directly related to the tensile strength of the tendons. In contrast to this study, Blanton and Biggs (1970) found only a slightly higher strength in unembalmed flexor tendons than extensor tendons from adult human lower limbs.

Hubbard and Chun (1988) studied the responses of tendons to three repeated 30-minute elongation cycles interspersed with two 30-minute rest periods. The results indicate that from the beginning to the end of the testing session the peak load to obtain the desired elongation decreased, the energy lost for each loading cycle decreased, and the tendon became more slack. The major changes occurred with the first cycle of elongation. During the rest periods the tendon recovered only a small amount of its ability to resist extension. The importance of this study can be related to prevention and treatment of injuries that require reduction of resistance to extension and increased mobility. Much more study in this area is needed.

Movement is important to maintain healthy tissue, but too little or too much loading is harmful. Loading response appears to be tissue and body area specific. More research is necessary to determine how exercise and treatment programs following injury should be constructed.

For protection against joint injuries and an enhanced healing rate, knowledge of biomechanical properties of joint tissues and the demands that activities place upon them is necessary (Frank et al., 1985).

The following chapters will give you tools to understand better the motion of and the forces being applied to the joints.

Prosthetics and Orthotics

You should remember that bone that is loaded maintains or increases its mineral content, while bone that is not loaded loses its mineral content. Rigid fixation devices for fracture stabilization or total joint prostheses may disrupt the loading on the limb so that loads normally carried by the bone would be carried by the implant. Such a situation would result in loss of bone in the unloaded bony area. The phenomenon is known as stress shielding. Using fixation plates on the femurs of beagles, Uhthoff and Finnegan (1983) showed that the longer the plate remained implanted, the more bone was lost and the slower was bone remodeling. A study by Szivek and co-workers (1981) demonstrated that more bone mineral was lost under a stiffer implant material. Implants should have mechanical properties that provide the needed support for the bony problem but do not cause reduction of bone strength.

Because of the high incidence of ligament injuries, more interest has developed in the use of ligament replacements. The mechanical properties of these materials have been compared with those of human ligaments. In 1976 Grood and Noyes evaluated a polyethylene ligament implant. They found that its strength was about 25 percent of the human anterior cruciate ligament. They also found that the implant progressively elongated under repetitive loading if sufficient rest was not allowed. The researchers concluded that caution is required in the use of this specific type of implant.

More recently, fiber-augmented biological tissues have been studied for use as ligament replacements. Mendes and co-workers (1985) implanted a carbon fiber tow in dogs and patients. The carbon fiber tow consisted of a core of carbon fiber surrounded by layers of fibroblasts and collagen fibers. In the dogs the ultimate tensile strength of the implant was about 88 percent of the natural tissue. Their conclusion was that the material was biocompatible and biomechanically sufficient.

Sabiston and associates (1990a and 1990b) evaluated the mechanical behavior of fresh autographs (the patient's own tissue) and frozen/thawed allografts (donor tissue). The autografts (Sabiston et al., 1990a) showed early deterioration to about 65 percent of the control tissue strength 24 weeks after surgery. The autograft strength recovered to about 10 percent of the control at 48 weeks following the surgery. The allograft (Sabiston et al., 1990b) did not appear to be as successful. The strength at about 12, 24, and 48 weeks had plateaued at about 60 to 75 percent of control ligaments. The long-term fate for any of the grafts, either biological or nonbiological, is still unknown.

Participation in running and other aerobic exercises and certain job requirements may result in lower limb overuse syndromes. Radin (1987) suggested that viscoelastic shoe inserts, thick rubber mats, or seat shock-absorbing material be used to improve symptoms of patients with osteoarthritis. Several researchers have investigated different styles of running shoes to evaluate their shock-absorbing effect (Bates et al., 1983; Komi et al., 1987; Nigg et al., 1987; Nigg et al., 1988; Cinats et al., 1987; and Jorgensen and Ekstrand, 1988). One material called Sorbothane when tested by mechanical devices was estimated to reduce stress on the foot by more than 10 percent (Cinats, 1987). The general trend of most of these studies indicate that the properties of the shoe or shoe insert are not the major factors in limiting the impact on the foot as it hits the ground. Since Sorbothane was not tested in the same manner as the others, it could not be directly compared. Jorgensen and Ekstrand (1988) determined that the use of a heel counter to confine the heel pad resulted in an 8.8 percent increase in shock absorption. They suggested further kinetic study to determine the heel counter effect on muscle activity.

Menard and Murray (1988) reported that energy-storing prosthetic feet designed for running could possibly be used for walking. They observed that very late in the stance the energy-storing prosthetic foot that they were studying delivered an accelerating force. A medical heel whip appeared to compensate for this action. Their gait analysis was limited. Kinematic and kinetic analysis would help provide more precise information. The mechanical characteristics of materials used in the Carbon Copy II prosthetic foot were described by Arbogast and Arbogast (1988).

The development of new thermoplastic materials for prosthetic components is discussed in articles by Coombes and Greenwood (1988), Coombes and MacCoughlan (1988), and Nakamura and Hatano (1988). The testing procedures and material properties were presented.

The detailed findings by these authors illustrate the importance of research on material properties for those who work with prosthetics and orthotics.

QUESTIONS

1. Differentiate and relate:
   (a) load, stress, strain
   (b) fatigue, creep, stress, relaxation
   (c) tension, compression, shear
   (d) elasticity, viscoelasticity
   (e) beam loading, torsion loading, column loading
   (f) brittle, ductile
2. Draw and label a stress-strain curve for a:
   (a) stiff brittle material
   (b) less stiff ductile material
3. Compare the following:
   (a) failure of bone at slow and fast loading rates
   (b) failure of a ligament at slow and fast loading rates
   (c) compression strength of bone and titanium
   (d) bending strength of bone and cobalt alloy
   (e) elastic modulus of various biological and nonbiological materials
4. Graph the effect of age on:
   (a) bone compression
   (b) tendon strength
   (c) muscle tensile strength
   (d) cartilage compression strength

REFERENCES

Advani SH, Martin RB, Powell WR: Mechanical properties and constitutive equations of anatomical materials. *In* Ghista DN (Ed): Applied Physiological Mechanics. New York, Harwood Academic Publishers, 1979, pp 31–103.

Akeson WH, Amiel D, Abel MF, et al.: Effects of immobilization on joints. Clin Orthop *219*:28–37, 1987a.

Akeson WH, Amiel D, Woo SL-Y: Physiology and therapeutic value of passive motion. *In* Helminen JH, Kiviranta I, Tammi M, et al. (Eds): Joint Loading: Biology and Health of Articular Structures. Bristol, England, Wright, 1987b, pp 375–394.

Albright JA: Bone: Physical properties. *In* Albright JA, Brand RA (Eds): The Scientific Basis of Orthopedics. Norwalk, CT, Appleton and Lange, 1987, pp 213–240.

Arbogast R, Arbogast CJ: The Carbon Copy II—from concept to application. J Prosthet Orthot *1*:32–36, 1988.

Armstrong CG, Mow VC: Variations in the intrinsic mechanical properties of human articular cartilage with age, degeneration and water content. J Bone Joint Surg *64A*:88–94, 1982.

Askeland DR: The Science and Engineering of Materials. Monterey, CA, Wadsworth, 1984, p 745.

Astrand PO, Rodahl K: Textbook of Work Physiology. New York, McGraw-Hill, 1970.

Bates BT, Osternig LR, Sawhill JA, et al.: As assessment of subject variability, subject shoe interaction and the evaluation of running shoes using ground reaction force data. J Biomech *16*:181–191, 1983.

Blanton PL, Biggs NL: Ultimate tensile strength of fetal and adult human tendons. J Biomech *3*:181–189, 1970.

Buckwalter JA, Maynard JA, Vailas AC: Skeletal fibrous tissues: Tendon, joint capsule, and ligament. *In* Albright JA, Brand RA (Eds): The Scientific Basis of Orthopedics. Norwalk, CT, Appleton and Lange, 1987, pp 387–405.

Buckwalter JA, Cooper RR: The cells and matrices of skeletal connective tissue. *In* Albright JA, Brand RA (Eds): The Scientific Basis of Orthopedics. Norwalk, CT, Appleton and Lange, 1987, pp 1–30.

Burstein AH, Reilly DT, Martens M: Aging of bone tissue: Mechanical properties. J Bone Joint Surg *58A*:82–86, 1976.

Butler DL, Grood ES, Noyes FR, et al.: Biomechanics of ligaments and tendons. *In* Hutton RS (Ed): Exercise and Sports Sciences Reviews. Washington, DC, Franklin Institute Press, 1978, pp 125–181.

Carter DR: Mechanical loading histories and cortical bone remodeling. Calcif Tissue Int *36*:519–524, 1984.

Carter DR: Biomechanics of bone. *In* Nahum AM, Melvin J (Eds): The Biomechanics of Trauma. Norwalk, CT, Appleton-Century-Crofts, 1985, pp 135–165.

Carter DR, Spengler DM: Mechanical properties and composition of cortical bone. Clin Orthop *135*:192–217, 1978.

Carter DR, Orr TE, Fyhrie DP, et al.: Influences of mechanical stresses on prenatal and postnatal skeletal development. Clin Orthop *219*:237–250, 1987.

Cavanaugh DJ, Cann CE: Brisk walking does not stop bone loss in postmenopausal women. Bone *9*:201–204, 1988.

Chvapil M: Method of treatment of fibrotic lesions by topical administration of lathyrogenic drugs. *In* Nimni ME (Ed): Collagen. Vol II: Biochemistry and Biomechanics. Boca Raton, FL, CRC Press, 1988, pp 161–175.

Cinats J, Reid DC, Haddow JB: A biomechanical evaluation of Sorbothane. Clin Orthop *222*:281–288, 1987.

Colletti LA, Edwards J, Gordon L, et al.: The effects of muscle-building exercise on bone mineral density of the radius, spine, and hip in young men. Calcif Tissue Int 45:12–14, 1989.

Coombes AGA, Greenwood CD: Memory plastics for prosthetic and orthotic applications. Prosthet Orthot Int 12:143–151, 1988.

Coombes AGA, MacCoughlan J: Development and testing of thermoplastic structural components for modular prostheses. Prostet Orthot Int 12:19–40, 1988.

Copray JCVM, Jansen HWB, Duterloo HS: An in vitro system for studying the effect of variable compressive forces on the mandibular condylar cartilage of the rat. Arch Oral Biol 30:305–311, 1985a.

Copray JCVN, Jansen HWB, Duterloo HS: Effects of compressive forces on proliferation and matrix synthesis in mandibular condylar cartilage of the rat in vitro. Arch Oral Biol 30:299–304, 1985b.

Currey JD: The mechanical properties of bone. Clin Orthop 73:210–231, 1970.

Currey JD: Changes in the impact energy absorption of bone with age. J Biomech 12:459–469, 1979.

Currey JD, Butler G: The mechanical properties of bone tissue in children. J Bone Joint Surg 57A:810–814, 1975.

Donaldson CL, Hulley SB, Vogel JM, et al.: Effect of prolonged bed rest on bone mineral. Metabolism 19:1071–1084, 1970.

Frank CB, Amiel D, Woo SY-L, et al.: Joints: Clinical and experimental aspects. In Nahum AM, Melvin J (Eds): The Biomechanics of Trauma. East Norwalk, CT, Appleton-Century-Crofts, 1985, pp 369–397.

Frank CB, Woo SL-Y: Clinical biomechanics of sports injuries. In Nahum AM, Melvin J (Eds): The Biomechanics of Trauma. Norwalk, CT, Appleton-Century-Crofts, 1985, pp 181–204.

Fung YC: Biomechanics: Mechanical Properties of Living Tissues. New York, Springer-Verlag, 1981.

Gans C: Fiber architecture and muscle function. In Terjung RL (ED): Exercise and Sports Sciences Reviews. Washington, DC, Franklin Institute Press; 1982, pp 160–207.

Gans C, DeVree F: Functional basis of fiber length and angulation in muscle. J Morphol 192:63–85, 1987.

Gelberman R, Goldberg V, An K-N, Barnes A: Tendon. In Woo SL-Y, Buckwalter JA (Eds): Injury and Repair of the Musculoskeletal Soft Tissues. Park Ridge, IL, American Academy of Orthopedic Surgeons, 1987, pp 5–40.

Gere JM, Timoshenko SP: Mechanics of Materials, 2nd ed. Boston, PWS Engineering, 1984, p 768.

Gordon AM, Huxley AF, Julian FJ: The variation in isometric tension with sarcomere length in vertebrate muscle fibers. J Physiol 184:170–192, 1966.

Grood ES, Noyes FR: Cruciate ligament prosthesis: Strength, creep and fatigue properties. J Bone Joint Surg 58A:1083–1088, 1976.

Hayes WC: Bone mechanics: From tissue mechanical properties to an assessment of structural behavior. In Schmid-Schonbein GW, et al. (Eds): Frontiers in Biomechanics. New York, Springer-Verlag, 1986, pp 196–209.

Helminen JH, Jurvelin J, Kiviranta I, et al.: Joint loading effects on articular cartilage: A historical review. In Helminen HJ, Kiviranta I, Tammi M, et al. (Eds): Joint Loading: Biology and Health of Articular Structures. Bristol, England, Wright, 1987, pp 1–46.

Hubbard RP, Chun KJ: Mechanical responses of tendons to repeated extensions and wait periods. J Biomech Eng 110:11–19, 1988.

Huddleston AL, Rockwell D, Kulund BN, et al.: Bone mass in lifetime tennis athletes. JAMA 244:1107–1109, 1980.

Hukins DWL, Aspden RM: Composition and properties of connective tissues. Trends. Biochem Sci 10:260–264, 1985.

Jokl P: Muscle. In Albright JA, Brand RA (Eds): The Scientific Basis of Orthopedics. Norwalk, CT, Appleton and Lange, 1987, pp 407–422.

Jones HH, Priest JD, Hayes WC, et al.: Humeral hypertrophy in response to exercise. J Bone Joint Surg 59A:204–208, 1977.

Jorgensen U, Ekstrand J: Significance of heel pad confinement for shock absorption at heel strike. Int J Sports Med 9:468–473, 1988.

Kempson GE: Mechanical properties of articular cartilage. In Freeman MAR (Ed): Adult Articular Cartilage, 2nd ed. London, Pitman Medical, 1979, pp 333–414.

Kennedy JC, Hawkins RJ, Willis RB, et al.: Tension studies of human knee ligaments. Yield point, ultimate failure, and disruption of the cruciate and tibial collateral ligaments. J Bone Joint Surg 58A:350–355, 1976.

Komi PV, Gollhofer A, Schmidtbleicher D, et al.: Interaction between man and shoe in running; considerations for a more comprehensive measurement approach. Int J Sports Med 8:196–202, 1987.

Lai WM, Mow VC, Roth V: Effects of nonlinear strain-dependent permeability and rate of compression on the stress behavior of articular cartilage. J Biomech Eng 103:61–66, 1981.

Lindahl O, Lindgren AGH: Cortical bone in man: I. Variation of the amount and density with age and sex. Acta Orthop Scand 38:133–140, 1967a.

Lindahl O, Lindgren AGH: Cortical bone in man: II. Variation in tensile strength with age and sex. Acta Orthop Scand 38:141–147, 1967b.

Lindgren U, Mattsson S: The reversibility of disuse osteoporosis. Calcif Tissue Res 23:179–184, 1977.

Lynch CT: CRC Handbook of Materials Science, vol. III. Boca Raton, FL, CRC Press, 1975.

MacConaill MA, Basmajian JV: Muscles and Movements. Baltimore, Williams & Wilkins, 1969.

Martin RB, Burr DB: Structure, Function, and Adaptation of Compact Bone. New York, Raven Press, 1989.

Mears DC: Materials and Orthopedic Surgery. Baltimore, Williams & Wilkins, 1979, pp 29–74.

Mears DC, Rothwell GP: The structure and properties of materials. In Mears DC (Ed): Materials and Orthopedic Surgery. Baltimore, Williams & Wilkins, 1979, pp 29–73.

Menard MR, Murray DD: Subjective and objective analysis of an energy-storing prosthetic foot. J Prosthet Orthot 1:220–230, 1988.

Mendes DG, Iusim M, Angel D, et al.: Histologic pattern of biomechanical properties of the carbon-fiber-augmented ligament tendon. Clin Orthop 196:51–60, 1985.

Montes GS, Junqueira LCU: Histochemical localization of collagen and of proteoglycans in tissue. In Nimni ME (Ed): Collagen. Vol. II. Biochemistry and Biomechanics. Boca Raton, FL, CRC Press, 1988, pp 41–72.

Mow VC, Kvei SC, Lai WM, et al.: Biphasic creep and stress relaxation of articular cartilage in compression: Theory and experiments. J Biomech Eng 102:73–84, 1980.

Mow VC, Holmes MH, Lai WM: Fluid transport and mechanical properties of articular cartilage: A review. J Biomech 17:377–394, 1984.

Myers ER, Mow VC: Biomechanics of cartilage and its response to biomechanical stimuli. In Hall BK (Ed): Cartilage, vol 1. New York, Academic Press, 1983, pp 313–341.

Myers ER, Zhu W, Mow VC: Viscoelastic properties of articular cartilage and meniscus. In Nimni ME (Ed): Collagen. Vol. II. Biochemistry and Biomechanics. Boca Raton, FL, CRC Press, 1988, pp 267–288.

Nakamura T, Hatano E: Process of development and application of porous plastic to prosthetic sockets. J Prosthet Orthot 1:202–210, 1988.

Nicogossian AE: Biomedical challenges of spaceflight. In DeHart RL (Ed): Fundamentals of Aerospace Medicine. Philadelphia, Lea & Febiger, 1985, pp 839–861.

Nigg BM, Bahlsen HA, Luethi SM, et al.: The influence of running velocity and midsole hardness on external impact forces in heel-toe running. J Biomech 20:951–959, 1987.

Nigg BM, Herzog W, Reid LJ: Effect of viscoelastic shoe insoles on vertical impact forces in heel-toe running. Am J Sports Med 16:70–76, 1988.

Noyes FR: Functional properties of knee ligaments and alterations induced by immobilization. Clin Orthop 123:210–242, 1977.

Noyes FR, Grood ES: The strength of the anterior cruciate ligament in humans and rhesus monkeys. J Bone Joint Surg 58A:1074–1082, 1976.

Noyes FR, Torvik PJ, Hyde WB, et al.: Biomechanics of ligament failure. J Bone Joint Surg (Am) 56:1406–1418, 1974.

Otten E: Concepts and models of functional architecture in skeletal muscle. Exer Sport Sci Rev 16:89–137, 1988.

Palmoski M, Perricone E, Brandt KD: Development and reversal of a proteoglycan aggregation defect in normal canine knee cartilage after immobilization. Arthritis Rheum 22:508–517, 1979.

Parry DAD, Craig AS: Collagen fibrils during development and maturation and their contribution to the mechanical attributes of connective tissue. In Nimni ME (Ed): Collagen. Vol. II. Biochemistry and Biomechanics. Boca Raton, FL, CRC Press, 1988, pp 1–23.

Proske U, Morgan DL: Tendon stiffness: Methods of measurement and significance for the control of movement. A review. J Biomech 20:75–82, 1987.

Radin EL: Osteoarthrosis: What is known about prevention. Clin Orthop 222:60–65, 1987.

Radin EL, Rose RM: Role of subchondral bone in the initiation and progressions of cartilage damage. Clin Orthop 213:34–40, 1986.

Redford JB: Orthotics Et Cetera, 3rd ed. Baltimore, Williams & Wilkins, 1986.

Reilly DT, Burstein AH: The mechanical properties of cortical bone. J Bone Joint Surg 56A:1001–1022, 1974.

Rubin CT, Lanyon LE: Regulation of bone formation by applied dynamic loads. J Bone Joint Surg 66A:397–402, 1984.

Sabiston P, Frank C, Lam T, et al.: Transplantation of the rabbit medial collateral ligament, I. Biomechanical evaluation of fresh autografts. J Orthop Res 8:35–45, 1990a.

Sabiston P, Frank C, Lam T, et al.: Transplantation of the rabbit medial collateral ligament, II. Evaluation of frozen/thawed allografts. J Orthop Res 8:46–56, 1990b.

Sanders M, Albright JA: Bone: Age-related changes and osteoporosis. In Albright JA, Brand RA (Eds): The Scientific Basis of Orthopaedics, 2nd ed. Norwalk, CT, Appleton and Lange, 1987, pp 267–288.

Scheller AD Jr, Mitchell SB, Barber FC: Femoral component fracture in revision hip arthroplasty. In Turner RG, Scheller AD (Eds): Revision Total Hip Arthroplasty. New York, Grune & Stratton, 1982, pp 147–179.

Skinner HCW: Bone: Mineralizaton. In Albright JA, Brand RA (Eds): The Scientific Basis of Orthopaedics. Norwalk, CT, Appleton and Lange, 1987, pp 199–211.

Smith EL, Gilligan C, McAdam M, et al.: Deterring bone loss by exercise intervention in premenopausal and postmenopausal women. Calcif Tissue Int 44:312–321, 1989.

Smith MC Jr, Rambaut PC, Vogel JM, et al.: Bone mineral measurement—Experiment M078. In Johnston RS, Diellein LF (Eds): Biomedical Results from Skylab. Washington, DC, National Aeronautics and Space Administration, 1977, pp 183–195.

Sokoloff L: Elasticity of aging cartilage. Fed Proc 25:1089–1095, 1966.

Sokoloff L: Loading and motion in relation to aging and degeneration of joints: Implications for prevention and treatment of osteoarthritis. In Helminen HJ, Kiviranta I, Tammi M, et al. (Eds): Joint Loading: Biology and Health of Articular Structures. Bristol, England, Wright, 1987, pp 1–46.

Squire JM: Muscle: Design, diversity and disease. Menlo Park, CA, Benjamin-Cummings Publishing Co., 1986, p 379.

Szivek JA, Weatherly GC, Pilliar RM, et al.: A study of bone remodelling using metal-polymer laminates. J Biomed Mater Res 15:853–865, 1981.

Tammi M, Paukkonen R, Kiviranta I, et al.: Joint loading–induced alterations in articular cartilage. In Helminen HJ, Kiviranta I, Tammi M, et al. (Eds): Joint Loading: Biology and Health of Articular Structure. Bristol, England, Wright, 1987, pp 64–88.

Tipton CB, Matthes RD, Maynard JA, et al.: The influence of physical activity on ligaments and tendons. Med Sci Sports 7:165–175, 1975.

Uhthoff HK, Finnegan M: The effects of metal plates on post-traumatic remodelling and bone mass. J Bone Joint Surg 65B:66–71, 1983.

Viidik AV, Gottrup F: Mechanics of healing soft tissue wounds. In Schmid-Schönbein GW, et al. (Eds): Frontiers in Biomechanics. New York, Springer-Verlag, 1984, pp 263–279.

Von Worvern N: Bone mineral content of mandibles: Normal reference values—rate of age-related bone loss. Calcif Tissue Int 43:193–198, 1988.

Weaver JK, Chalmers J: Cancellous bone: Its strength and

changes with aging and an evaluation of some methods for measuring its mineral content. J Bone Joint Surg *48A*:289–299, 1966.

Weightman B, Kempson GE: Load Carriage in Adult Articular Cartilage, 2nd ed. London, Pitman Medical, 1979, pp 291–329.

Williams DF: The relationship between design and material selection in orthopedic implants. *In* Ghista DN, Roaf R (Eds): Orthopedic Mechanics: Procedures and Devices. vol. 2. New York, Academic Press, 1981, pp 200–302.

Woo SL-Y: Biomechanics of tendons and ligaments. *In* Schmid-Schönbien GW, et al. (Eds): Frontiers in Biomechanics. New York, Springer-Verlag, 1986, pp 180–195.

Woo SL-Y, Sites TJ: Current advances on the study of biomechanical properties of tendons and ligaments. *In* Nimni ME (Ed): Collagen. Vol II. Biochemistry and Biomechanics. Boca Raton, FL, CRC Press, 1988, pp 223–241.

Woo SL-Y, Simon BR, Kvei SC, et al.: Quasi-linear viscoelastic properties of normal articular cartilage. J Biomech Eng *102*:85–90, 1980a.

Woo SL-Y, Ritter MA, Amiel D, et al.: The biomechanical and biochemical properties of swine tendons—long-term effects of exercise on the digital extensors. Connect Tissue Res *7*:177–183, 1980b.

Woo SL-Y, Gomez MA, Amiel D, et al.: The effects of exercise on the biomechanical and biochemical properties of swine digital flexor tendons. J Biomech Eng *103*:51–56, 1981.

Woo SL-Y, Gomez MA, Sites TJ, et al.: The biomechanical and morphological changes in the medial collateral ligament of the rabbit after immobilization and remobilization. J Bone Joint Surg *69A*:1200–1211, 1987a.

Woo SL-Y, Inoue M, McGurk-Burleson E, et al.: Treatment of the medial collateral ligament injury. Am J Sports Med *15*:22–29, 1987b.

Yamada H: Strength of Biological Materials. Baltimore, Williams & Wilkins, 1970.

Zajac FE: Muscle and tendon: Properties, models, scaling, and application to biomechanics and motor control. Crit Rev Biomed Eng *17*:359–411, 1989.

4

Composition and Resolution of Forces

INTRODUCTION

In solving biochemical problems we must take into account all the forces that are acting upon the object. The problem may consist of analyzing a single force system or a combination of force systems. For setting up these problems, the analysis of the forces involved may be approached by two procedures. First, the composition of forces method is used when we have two or more forces acting in the same plane (coplanar) and on the same point (concurrent), and we wish to show their combined effect as a single force, the resultant. Second, occasionally we must replace a single force by two or more equivalent force components. This process is called the resolution of forces. Both approaches may be solved by graphic or algebraic methods.

COMPOSITION OF FORCES

Experimental results have shown that any set of coplanar concurrent forces may be replaced by a single force having the same effect as that of the given forces. This single force obtained by combining the given forces is called their resultant. The following two sections show how the graphic and algebraic methods can be used to determine the resultant from two or more forces.

Graphic Method

The graphic method uses precise measurements of magnitude and direction to obtain the resultant of many vectors or the components of one vector. The graphic method of combining forces utilizes the vector diagram. In the vector diagram, the forces are displayed by arrows, with the length of the arrow representing the magnitude of the force and the arrowhead representing the direction in which the force is acting. Using the graphic method requires that the magnitude be drawn exactly to scale and that the direction be indicated precisely.

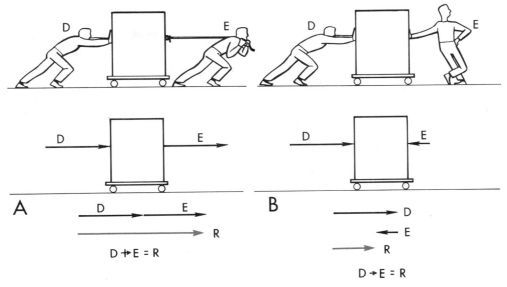

FIGURE 4–1

Addition of vectors to find the total effect of two linear forces. In *A*, forces D and E are added to find the resultant, R. In *B*, E must be subtracted from D since the forces are opposed. (—⊩→ indicates addition of vectors; → represents vector subtraction.)

LINEAR FORCE SYSTEM

The simplest system to analyze is the case in which parallel forces that are coplanar and concurrent are also colinear, or acting along the same line. This system is often called a linear system of forces. Figure 4–1 illustrates the graphic solution of the linear system. In Figure 4–1A, the two boys (D and E) are acting in the same direction. Arrows representing their respective forces are drawn to determine the resulting effects of their combined effort. Vector D is drawn to scale, indicating the magnitude of the force exerted by D. A second vector, representing the force of E, is placed at the tip of the first arrow and points in the direction of the action of E. The distance from the tail of D to the tip of E yields the resultant of the two combined forces. Since these forces are acting along the same line, they may be added together to obtain the resultant.

The two boys are acting along the same line but in opposite directions in Figure 4–1B. The solution, however, is determined by the same procedure. The vector D is drawn with its correct magnitude and direction. The tail of vector E is placed at the tip of D and drawn in the proper direction. Although the two boys are acting along the same line, we cannot draw the vectors end to end because they would lie on top of one another. Therefore, one vector is drawn slightly below the other. As in A, the resultant force is drawn from the tail of the first vector to the tip of the second.

Similar to Figure 4–1A, the two vectors are added. In this case, however, E is acting in the opposite direction. By convention, we can consider all forces acting to the right or upward as positive and those acting to the left or downward as negative. The sign of the resultant indicates its direction. Thus, a − E is added to D to obtain the resultant, which in this case is positive.

CONCURRENT FORCE SYSTEM

The polygon figure may be used to graphically determine the resultant when two or more forces are concurrent (Fig. 4–2). With this procedure, we represent one vector (F_1) quantity by an arrow drawn to the length proportional to its magnitude and in the proper direction, and draw from the tip of this arrow a second arrow of proper length and direction representing a second vector (F_2). A third vector (F_3) is drawn from the tip of the second vector and so on for the remaining force (F_4). Their combined effect, the resultant (R), may be determined by drawing an arrow from the end of the first vector to the tip of the final vector. This last step encloses the polygon. The triangle is a special case used in which only two forces are involved (Fig. 4–3). The force Q is placed with its tail at the arrow tip of force P. The line R drawn from the tail of P to the tip of Q represents the resulting force of the two forces. In this triangle, the angle ϕ is the angle between the two forces.

A parallelogram, which is similar to the triangle, may also be used to determine the resultant from two vectors (Fig. 4–4). By using the

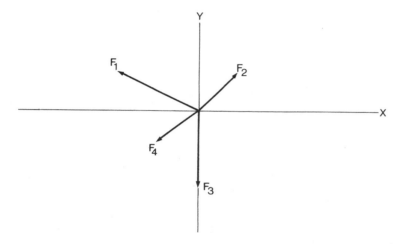

FIGURE 4–2

Solution giving the resultant of forces by the polygon method.

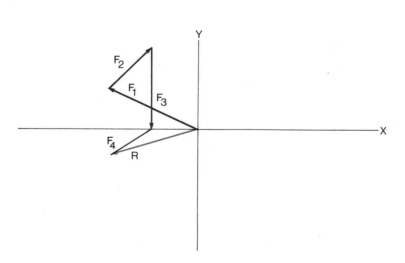

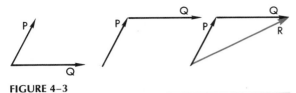

FIGURE 4–3

Use of the Triangle Law in composition of vectors P $\rightarrow$ Q = R.

parallelogram instead of placing the force vectors end to end, the two vectors are drawn to scale in their proper direction from the same point, usually the point of application.

Suppose we wish to find the resultant of two forces whose action lines intersect at an angle theta (θ). The magnitudes of the forces are P and Q. Composition (or addition) of the two forces can be accomplished by constructing a parallelogram with the forces as its sides (Fig. 4–4). From a selected point, we draw vectors representing each of the two forces. The vectors must be drawn in such a fashion that both arrows are directed away from the selected point. The length and direction of the vectors must accurately represent the original forces. Now the other two sides of the parallelogram can be constructed.

A line Q^1, representing Q, equal in magnitude and drawn parallel to force Q, is placed at the tip of force P. A line P^1, representing P, equal in magnitude and drawn parallel to force P, is placed at the tip of force Q. Line Q^1 and P^1 will intersect at a point opposite the originally selected point. Angle ϕ will be formed by line P and line Q^1.

A line drawn from the initially selected point to the opposite corner of the parallelogram gives the magnitude and direction of the resultant force (R), which will have exactly the same effect on the object as the two original forces combined. In Figure 4–5, if P is 6 newtons, Q is 6 newtons, and the angle θ between them is 135°, we can construct the figures so that R equals 11 newtons.

A graphic illustration of composition has been suggested in which nurse N pushes due north on a child's crib while nurse E is pushing it east with slightly more force (Fig. 4–6). They will together move the crib in the same direction as nurse F alone who pushes in a northeasterly direction. The parallelogram in Figure 4–6 demonstrates that in moving the crib a given distance, the combined magnitudes of the forces of the nurses pushing north and east are greater

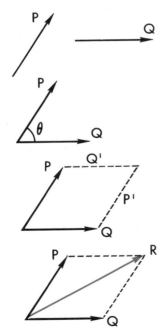

FIGURE 4–4

Construction of a parallelogram to determine resultant vector (R) of two forces, P and Q, whose action lines form angle theta (θ).

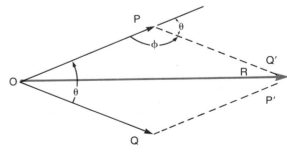

FIGURE 4–5

Graphic solution of two forces, P = 6 newtons and Q = 6 newtons, acting at a 45° angle (θ). Angle ϕ is 180° − 45° or 135°.

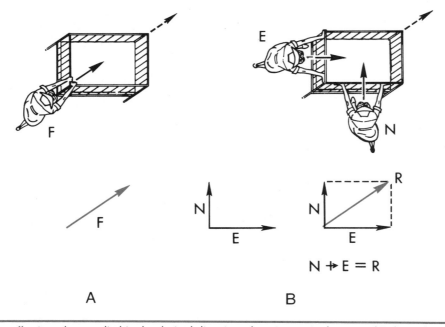

FIGURE 4–6

A force is most effective when applied in the desired direction of motion, as in the case of F shown here. Two or more forces can be combined to obtain the desired direction, N ⤏ E = R. Broken arrow indicates direction of motion of the object. (Adapted from Flitter H: An Introduction to Physics in Nursing. St. Louis, Mosby, 1948.)

than the single equivalent northeasterly force, F. In other words, part of a force is "wasted" when its action line is not in the exact direction of movement of the object.

Algebraic Method

The algebraic method makes use of algebraic equations and utilizes trigonometric concepts. Similarly to the graphic method, it is desirable to have a free body diagram that shows all the forces that are acting. However, some of the forces will be known in magnitude and possibly also unknown in direction. The first step is to draw the figure and place all the known forces on it in their proper locations. Then we determine where an unknown force might be acting on the figure. To aid us here we use Newton's third law, which says that for every action there must be an equal and opposite reaction. If an object is touching our figure at a certain point

and we remove this object, we must place a force at the point of contact to give us the same effect as the object had at that point.

Since we do not know the magnitude of the forces that exist between several bodies in contact and since in some cases we don't know whether they exert a pull or a push on the body under consideration, it becomes necessary to introduce a vector to represent the force. Here, we must assume a direction for the force. This assumed direction may be incorrect, but the correct direction will be revealed when we obtain the sign in the algebraic solution of the problem.

LINEAR FORCE SYSTEM

The linear force system uses the simple algebraic equations of addition. As stated earlier, all forces acting to the right and upward are positive and those acting to the left and down are negative. We may algebraically calculate the resulting force graphically, as determined in Figure 4–1A and B. If the force that D applies is 9 newtons to the right and the force E applies is 6 newtons to the right, then

$$D + E = R$$
$$9\,N + 6\,N = 15\,N$$

As in Figure 4–1B, if the force that D applies is 9 newtons to the right and the force that E applies is 3 newtons to the left, then

$$D + (-E) = R$$
$$9\,N + (-3\,N) = 6\,N$$

For example, let's assign force values to the tug-of-war contestants shown in Figure 4–7A so that F equals 100 N, G equals 200 N, L equals 100 N, M equals 100 N, and N equals 150 N. The direction of the resultant will indicate the winning team. Although it makes no difference in which order the vectors are considered, for convenience we will take the forces acting toward the right (L, M, and N) and then the forces F and G acting toward the left. Figure 4–7B illustrates the graphic solution. Using this method, we must select a convenient scale such as 1 cm equals 50 N. By taking the forces in the order L, M, and N, we draw an arrow representing 2 cm in length with the arrow tip pointing toward the right. The force M, also 2 cm, is drawn toward the right, starting at the tip of the preceding force, L. Likewise, the third force, N, is extended 3 cm toward the right. The total length of the three vectors, 7 cm, represents a single resultant force of 350 N toward the right. The same procedure is used to determine the total forces of F and G pulling toward the left. A 4 cm line representing the 200 N force of G is extended from the tip of the 2-cm long vector representing F. Thus, a combined vector 6 cm long represents a total resultant force of 300 N

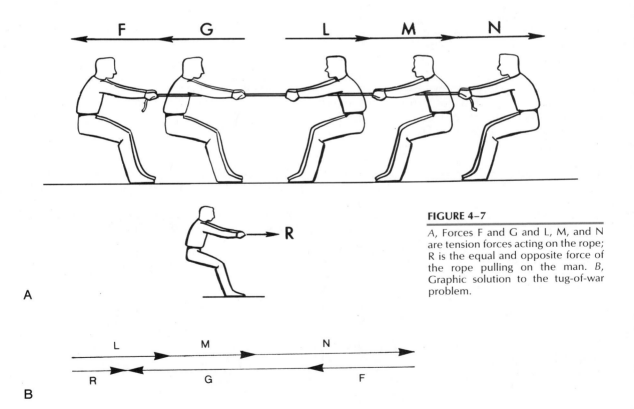

FIGURE 4–7

A, Forces F and G and L, M, and N are tension forces acting on the rope; R is the equal and opposite force of the rope pulling on the man. *B*, Graphic solution to the tug-of-war problem.

toward the left. As in the previous problem, we cannot draw the vectors representing the teams end to end because they would lie on top of one another. So, as shown in Figure 4–7B, one is drawn slightly below the other. A vector drawn from the tail of the first vector, representing team L, M, and N, to the tip of the second vector, F and G, represents a resultant force of the two teams as 1 cm or 50 N. The system would not be in equilibrium, and team L, M, and N would win the contest.

Since all the forces are acting along the same line of action, to solve this problem algebraically, their magnitudes are added together: L + M + N + F + G = R, or 100 N + 100 N + 150 N + (−100 N) + (−200 N) = 50 N. This answer is in agreement with the one determined graphically.

CONCURRENT FORCE SYSTEM

In the preceding section, the vectors were colinear. Often forces are coplanar and concurrent but not colinear. This system is a concurrent force system. The same procedures used to determine the resultant in the linear system, however, may be employed whatever the relative direction of the vectors may be.

Algebraically we may solve for the resultant for noncolinear forces by using the cosine law for triangles (Fig. 4–3). That is,

$$R = \sqrt{P^2 + Q^2 - 2PQ \cos \phi}$$

where P and Q are the original force magnitudes and ϕ is the angle between them. In the special case in which the angle between the two forces is 90°, the Pythagorean theorem, which states that R equals the square root of the quantity $P^2 + Q^2$ (or $R = \sqrt{P^2 + Q^2}$), would be used. To find the resultant of several forces in the polygon method, the same equations are used, taking two forces at a time.

The angle ϕ is determined in the following manner. The angle between lines P and Q is given as 45°. If we used the angle 45° in the law of cosine equations, we would be solving for the side Z in Figure 4–8A. We do not want that value. We want the value of R, which is the side opposite the angle ϕ (Fig. 4–8B). Therefore, line Q^1 is drawn parallel to Q with the tail at the tip

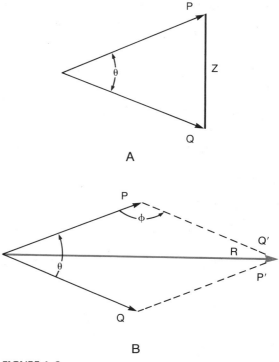

FIGURE 4–8

Use of cosine law for determination of resultant of forces P and Q. *A*, Using θ as the angle between P and Q does not provide the proper resultant value. *B* shows the appropriate resultant vector.

of line P. The angle ϕ is formed between P and Q^1. The value of ϕ is calculated from the theorem stating that the sum of the interior angles formed when two parallel lines intersected by a straight line equals 180°. Therefore,

$$\theta + \phi = 180°$$

The calculations then are

$$45° + \phi = 180°$$

Subtract 45 from both sides of the equations. Then

$$\phi = 180° - 45°$$

or

$$\phi = 135°$$

In the algebraic solution of problems involving rectangular components, we use the trigonometric functions called sine, cosine, and tangent (abbreviated sin, cos, and tan). These are based on the constant relationship of the two sides of a right triangle to the hypotenuse when one angle is specified.

A series of triangles illustrate these relationships and how they vary with a change in the angle concerned (Fig. 4–9). If this principle is clear so that the sine and cosine values can be used with understanding, you will be less likely to make mistakes than if you merely copy the values from a table or from a calculator without visualizing these relationships. The sine of the angle specified is the ratio of length of the "side opposite" the angle to the hypotenuse. In the figure shown,

$$\text{sine } 15° = \frac{\text{side opposite}}{\text{hypotenuse}} = 0.258$$

In other words, the side opposite the angle is 0.258 times the length of the hypotenuse when the given angle is 15°. When the specified angle is 30°, the "side opposite" is 0.500 times the hypotenuse.

In these examples, the "side adjacent" to the angle specified also bears a relationship to the hypotenuse, which is expressed as the cosine of the angle:

$$\cos 15° = \frac{\text{side adjacent}}{\text{hypotenuse}} = 0.965$$

When the angle is 30° the cosine becomes 0.866. The third relationship is the ratio of

$$\frac{\text{side opposite}}{\text{side adjacent}} = \frac{\sin}{\cos}$$

This is known as the tangent of the angle.

No matter what scale is used to represent values of length or force, the ratio of the respective sides of the right triangle remains the same for any specified angle (Fig. 4–10). This relationship is what interests us in dealing with rectangular components of a force.

The sines and cosines of angles in Table 4–1 are useful to know.

If values of one angle and one side or the hypotenuse of a right triangle are known, the rest

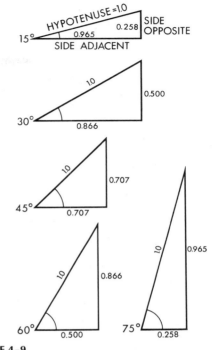

FIGURE 4–9

Ratio of sides of a right triangle corresponding to given angles. The value of the hypotenuse is 1.0.

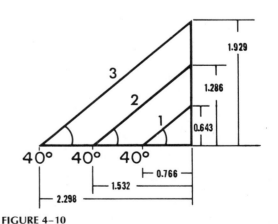

FIGURE 4–10

Ratios of sides are constant for a given angle in right triangles of any size.

TABLE 4–1. SINE AND COSINE VALUES FOR SELECTED ANGLES

Angle	Sine	Cosine
0°	0	1.000
15°	0.258	0.965
30°	0.500	0.866
45°	0.707	0.707
60°	0.866	0.500
75°	0.965	0.258
90°	1.000	0

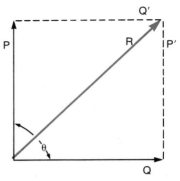

FIGURE 4–11

Forces P and Q acting perpendicular to each other.

of the triangle may be determined. Since tables of the values of sin Θ, cos Θ, and tan Θ are available for Θ equal to any angle, we make use of this in finding rectangular components of a force.

In Figure 4–8B, if $P = 6$ N, $Q = 6$ N, and $\phi = 135°$, we may solve the problem algebraically using the law of cosines:

$$R = \sqrt{(6)^2 + (6)^2 - 2(6)(6)\cos 135}$$
$$R = \sqrt{36 + 36 - (-50.9)}$$
$$R = \sqrt{122.9}$$
$$R = 11.09 \text{ N}$$

If we have P and Q at a 90° angle to each other (Fig. 4–11), then we can use the Pythagorean theorem to solve for the resulting force:

$$P = 6 \text{ N}$$
$$Q = 6 \text{ N}$$
$$\Theta = 90°$$
$$\phi = 90°$$
$$R = \sqrt{P^2 + Q^2}$$
$$R = \sqrt{(6)^2 + (6)^2}$$
$$R = \sqrt{36 + 36}$$
$$R = \sqrt{72}$$
$$R = 8.48 \text{ N}$$

Examples of Composition

When Russell traction is used to immobilize a fractured femur (Calderwood, 1943), the patient's limb is suspended as shown in Figure 4–12. The thigh is maintained at an angle of 20°

with the horizontal plane, or with the bed, so that the relation of the pulley ropes to the alignment of the limb remains constant. In the case of an adult patient, a load of 35 to 50 newtons is applied to the pulley system. The force distal to the foot is nearly doubled by the arrangement of the ropes (Q and S). This force reaches the femur through the leg, while an upward force (P) is applied directly to the knee by means of a sling.

The vector diagram shows that the resultant force is in line with the femur. The counterforce balancing the pulley rope is provided by the patient's weight and the pull of the thigh and leg muscles. How would the resultant force on the femur be affected if the patient were allowed to slide down toward the foot of the bed? Why would it be dangerous to allow this to happen?

We may use the triangle law to find the resultant pull of two parts of a muscle or of two synergistic muscles. For example, consider the pectoralis major muscle (Fig. 4–13). Vector S in Figure 4–14, representing the sternal portion of the muscle, is placed at the tip of vector C, which represents the clavicular part. The resultant of both forces is then a vector from the beginning of C to the tip of S.

In his study of hip abduction muscle force, Inman (1947) determined the action lines of the gluteus minimus, gluteus medius, and tensor fasciae latae by inserting wires in cadaver muscles and making roentgenograms. (The problem involved only forces in the frontal plane.) Mag-

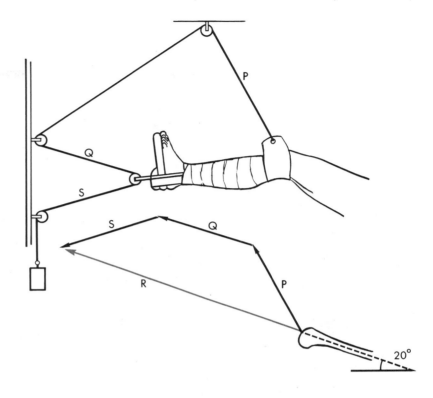

FIGURE 4–12

Russell traction for immobilizing femoral fractures. The resultant traction force applied to the femur is determined by the ropes P, Q, and S. Force R, acting on the limb, is obtained graphically by a vector diagram. (Adapted from Flitter H: An Introduction to Physics in Nursing. St. Louis, Mosby, 1948.)

nitudes of force were then determined by weighing the muscles and computing their average ratios of mass. That is, the mass of each was compared with the total muscle mass of the group. These ratios were found to be:

Tensor fasciae latae, 1:7
Gluteus medius, 4:7
Gluteus minimus, 2:7

The action line and magnitude of the resultant force were then used to compute the torque applied by the hip abductor musculature and il-

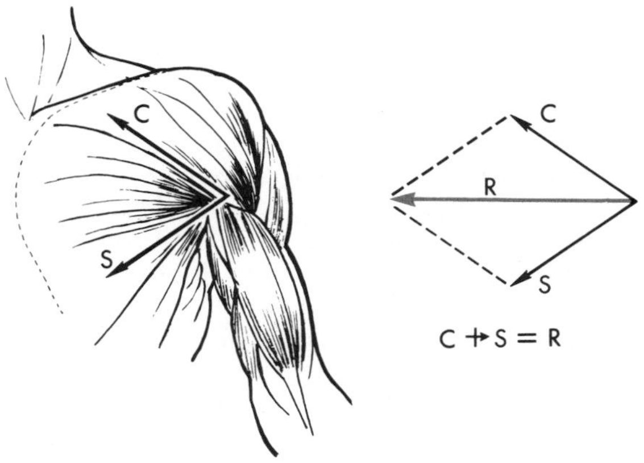

FIGURE 4–13

Clavicular and sternal portions of pectoralis major together produce a single force acting horizontally across the chest (C ⊹→ S = R).

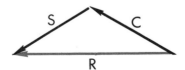

FIGURE 4–14

Use of the triangle law to find a resultant: C ⊹→ S = R. The diagram is based on Figure 4–13.

iotibial band in stabilizing the pelvis in the frontal plane. Figure 4–15 shows the pelvis tilted upward 15°. In this position the moment of gravity is said to be resisted by the muscles alone, with no assistance from the iliotibial band. The figure shows the magnitude and direction of the resultant force being applied to the pelvis by the three muscles.

A complicated example of many forces acting at a point was first presented by Braus (1954) and has been updated by Volz and co-workers (1980). Figure 4–16 shows the direction of force exerted by individual muscles passing over the wrist joint. The figure shows that many combinations of forces can be applied to move the hand. The directions of motion possible are limited only by the joint structures. Volz and associates determined that the summation of all the muscle forces crossing the carpus would tend to place the wrist in a position of flexion and ulnar deviation.

Some examples of composition of forces in the action of muscles are the following:

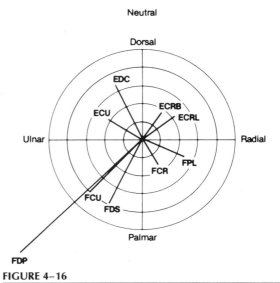

FIGURE 4–16

The magnitude and direction of the mean vector forces for the various muscles crossing the wrist are calculated with reference to the instant center of motion located within the proximal pole of the capitate with the wrist in a neutral position. All forces are expressed in relationship to planes of movement encompassing dorsal and palmar flexion and radial and ulnar deviation. (From Volz RG, Lieb M, Benjamin J: Biomechanics of the wrist. Clin Orthop *149*:112–117, 1980.)

1. Pennate muscles attaching to the tendon at an angle do not utilize their entire force as tension on the tendon (Fig. 4–17). With this arrangement, however, a greater number of fibers are anatomically available.

2. The anterior and posterior parts of the deltoid muscle acting alone will flex and extend the arm in the sagittal plane (Fig. 4–18). By their combined action, pulling on the deltoid tubercule of the humerus, the two portions of the muscle can abduct the arm in the frontal plane.

3. The clavicular and sternal portions of the pectoralis major muscle, acting together, can draw the arm across the trunk in horizontal adduction (Fig. 4–14). Notice the similarity to the structure and action of the trapezius muscle on the posterior chest wall.

4. The two heads of the gastrocnemius muscle, pulling in lateral and medial directions, together exert an upward force on the Achilles

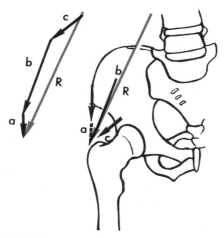

FIGURE 4–15

Single resultant (R) of the three hip abductor muscles stabilizing the pelvis in the frontal plane: vectors *a*, *b*, and *c* represent force of tensor fasciae latae, gluteus medius, and gluteus minimus, respectively. Here the pelvis is tilted upward 15°, a position in which the moment of gravity on the pelvis in unilateral weight-bearing is said to be resisted by muscles alone without help from the iliotibial tract. (From Inman VT: Functional aspects of the abductor muscles of the hip. J Bone Joint Surg *29*:607–619, 1947.)

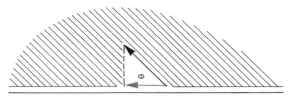

FIGURE 4–17

Muscle fibers attach at an angle to the tendon in a pennate muscle and produce a component of force along the tendon.

tendon (Fig. 4–19). Compare this with a dorsal interosseus muscle (Fig. 4–20).

5. The pull of the quadriceps muscles on the patella guides the patella through the path of motion (Fig. 4–21).

Quadriceps muscle force and patellar tendon force may also direct the patella laterally (Fig. 4–22A). The greater the angle between the longitudinal axis of the femur and longitudinal axis of the tibia, the greater the magnitude of the resultant force directed laterally.

Forces on the patellofemoral joint lead to resultant contact force on the two bones or lateral movement between them (Fig. 4–23). The quadriceps muscle tendon acts as a cord traveling across the pulley of the femoral condyle. The patella lies within the tendon to reduce the compression and friction upon the tendon. As the

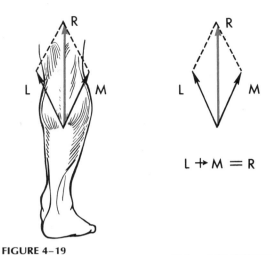

FIGURE 4–19

Medial (M) and lateral (L) heads of gastrocnemius together pull upward on the tendon of Achilles.

knee is placed in a different position, the forces developed in the muscles and patellar tendon produce a resultant force that directs the patella against the femoral condyles. As the angle of the knee increases from 0° flexion, the resultant force increases.

During erect standing with the arm hanging at the side (Fig. 4–24), the supraspinatus is active in order to resist downward dislocation of the humerus (Basmajian, 1967). The weight of the limb (W) and the horizontal pull of the supraspinatus and the tightening of the superior part of the joint capsule (M) produce a resultant force toward the glenoid fossa.

Many additional examples of muscle pairs or separate divisions of the more complex muscle arrangement could be cited here. Muscles that act together to create a resultant force in the manner described have been termed "helping synergists" in the field of kinesiology (from the Greek, *syn*, with, and *ergon*, work, thus "to work with"). Synergistic action is characteristic of fan-shaped muscles and certain opposing groups, such as:

1. Anterior and posterior parts of the gluteus medius in hip abduction.

2. Evertors and invertors of the foot in dorsiflexion or plantar flexion.

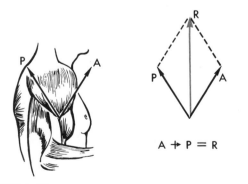

FIGURE 4–18

Example of composition of muscle forces to produce a single resultant force. P and A represent the pull of the posterior and anterior deltoid muscle fibers to produce arm elevation.

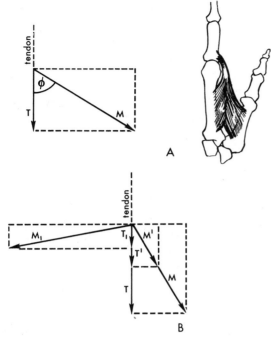

FIGURE 4–20

Relation of tendon shortening to muscle contraction in pennate fiber arrangement. Fiber M contracts with force T in the direction of the central tendon. In *B*, Rose and Wallace (1952) have applied this concept in analyzing typical hand deformity in arthritis, where:

M = normal fiber of first dorsal interosseus muscle

M^1 = force of fiber weakened by disuse

M_1 = force of opposing fiber, after adaptive changes

T = force exerted by normal fiber along tendon

T^1 = force exerted by M^1 in direction of tendon

T_1 = force of M_1 in direction of tendon.

(From Rose DL, Wallace LI: A remedial occupational therapy program for the residuals of rheumatoid arthritis in the hand. Am J Phys Med *31*:5–13, © by Williams & Wilkins, 1952.)

3. Abductors and adductors of the wrist acting in wrist flexion or extension.

4. Upper and lower trapezius muscles in scapular adduction.

Note that in the preceding examples the smaller the angle between the forces, the greater is the resultant (Fig. 4–25). Two or more forces pulling in a similar direction are more effective than if these forces pull in opposite directions.

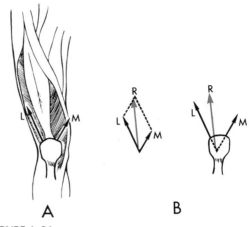

FIGURE 4–21

In locating the single resultant vector (R) of the combined vastus lateralis (L) and medialis (M) muscle forces on the patella, their action lines are extended to the point of intersection.

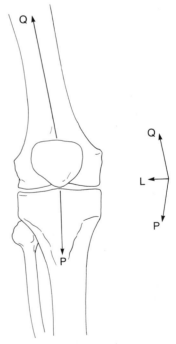

FIGURE 4–22

Force vectors of quadriceps muscles resultant and patellar tendon can give lateral resultant to produce subluxation or dislocation.

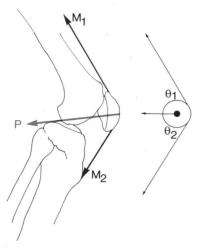

FIGURE 4-23

Tendinous attachments to the patella that produce a resultant force on the patellofemoral joint.

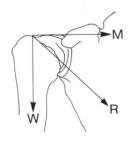

FIGURE 4-24

Static forces on the glenohumeral joint during erect standing.

FIGURE 4-25

Resultant (R) of two forces; note the change in the resultant value as the angle between forces F and P changes: $A < B < C$. Resultant force changes: $A > B > C$.

RESOLUTION OF FORCES

The process of resolving a force into two or more components is just the reverse of composition. Here we replace the original force by two or more equivalent forces. We have seen in the previous section that any pair of concurrent forces has a resultant. Conversely, any single force can be considered to be the resultant of a pair of concurrent forces, but in this case there is endless variety. That is, parallelograms can be constructed about the original force in many ways so that infinite pairs of components are possible. Each component may in turn be resolved into two or more components so that three or more forces may be the equivalent of the original force (Fig. 4–26). The only rule is that components, when added in a vector diagram, must begin where the original force begins and end where the original force ends. The forces from the vector diagram will have to be moved to a parallel position, intersecting at a common point on the action line of the original force in the space diagram. There is absolutely no limitation to the magnitude or direction of the components. One or more may be greater than the original force. The selection and arrangement of components of a force are determined by the problem to be solved.

In Figure 4–27, force F of 10 newtons may be acting at 30° with the horizontal. The two rectangular components may be determined graphically or algebraically.

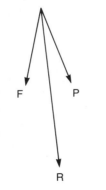

A

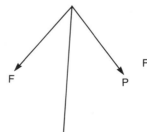

B

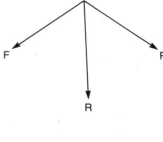

C

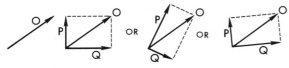

FIGURE 4-26

Rectangular components P and Q of force O.

Algebraically, the calculations are as follows when Q is horizontal and P is vertical. To solve for Q:

$$Q/F = \cos 30° = \sin 60°$$

Multiply both sides by F

$$Q = F \cos 30°$$

Substitute in known values

$$Q = (10)(0.866)$$

Solve

$$Q = 8.66 \text{ newtons}$$

To solve for P

$$P/F = \sin 30° = \cos 60°$$

Multiply both sides by F

$$P = F \sin 30°$$

Substitute in known values

$$P = 10(0.5)$$

Solve

$$P = 5 \text{ newtons}$$

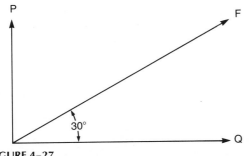

FIGURE 4-27

Determination of the rectangular for components P and Q of force F acting at 30° angle to the horizontal.

These values may be checked graphically, as shown in Figure 4–27.

In our work the most useful resolution of forces involves the determination of rectangular components. Rectangular components lie at right angles to each other. When two lines are drawn forming a right angle, the original force becomes the hypotenuse of a right triangle (Fig. 4–27). Rectangular components must always be smaller in magnitude than the original force. Since we are always dealing here with a right triangle, we may use the laws of trigonometry in arriving at algebraic solutions to problems.

Examples of Resolution

SLIDING A BOX

When we slide a box along the floor, we may observe that the effectiveness of the force acts in a direction other than that of the force itself. In Figure 4–28, the boy is using a rope to pull a box along the floor. His force is acting along the line formed by the rope. However, the effective motion is parallel to the surface of the floor. Thus, some of the force he is applying is being used to slide the box, while another part of his force is being used to lift the front edge of the box.

MUSCLE COMPONENTS

The action line of muscles acting on the bony segments is fixed by their anatomic attachments. Thus, they must often pull in a line other than in the direction of movement, and some of their efficiency is reduced.

When the biceps brachii tendon is applied at right angles to the forearm, the entire force tends to rotate the part about the elbow (Fig. 4–29A). However, when the tendon is applied at a 75° angle to the long axis of the part (Fig. 4–29B), most of the force is acting in the direction to produce rotation of the segment, while some is pulling the forearm upward toward the elbow joint. The component that tends to rotate the part is called the "rotational," or "rotatory," component; the other is the "nonrotatory" com-

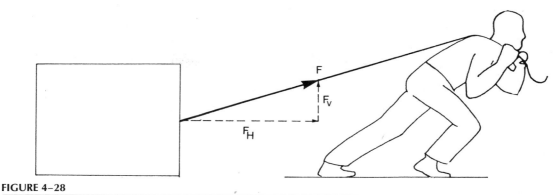

FIGURE 4–28

Forces acting to slide a box along the floor.

ponent, which compresses the joint surfaces or, in some cases, pulls them apart. We will label these components of the original force R and NR, respectively.

In Figure 4–29C, in which the angle of force application is 45°, component vectors R and NR are equal in magnitude. When the angle of application of the force is 30° (Fig. 4–29B), a proportion of the force is available for rotation, but more is applied as compression of the joint.

At 15° a small component tends to effectively rotate the limb, while a large component is directed toward the joint (Fig. 4–29A).

If the limb is above the horizontal, the nonrotatory component of the muscle is directed away from the joint (Fig. 4–29F).

In constructing the parallelogram, the original force is shown as a localized vector drawn to scale on a line diagram, as in Figure 4–29. Rectangular components are then drawn to determine the proportion of the force acting in the direction of movement of the part, and the force is in line with the segment. Component R is drawn at a right angle to the long axis of the part and thus forms one side of a right triangle. Component NR lies parallel to the segment and shows us the compression or tension force in the joint. The scale values of R and NR correspond to that of the original force in the graphic solution of problems. (Can you see that R is equivalent to the "side opposite" the angle we are dealing with in the right triangle formed and that NR is the "side adjacent"?)

Algebraically, the procedure to determine these values is as follows:

Rotatory component

$$R/F = \sin \theta = \cos \phi$$
$$R = F \sin \theta = F \cos \phi$$

Nonrotatory components

$$NR/F = \cos \theta = \sin \phi$$
$$NR = F \cos \theta = F \sin \phi$$

The values you can calculate for the component of each situation are shown in Table 4–2. Note the change in component as the insertion angle of the muscle changes.

The effectiveness of a muscle force rotating a body segment increases as the angle of application to the part approaches 90°. Notice that this is not a linear increase. The rotatory component equals half the original force when the angle at which the force is applied is only 30°.

TABLE 4–2. ROTATORY (R) AND NONROTATORY (NR) COMPONENTS OF MUSCLE FORCE FOR SELECTED FOREARM ANGLES

Muscle Insertion	Muscle Force	R	NR
15°	100 N	25.9 N	96.6 N
30°	100 N	50.0 N	86.6 N
45°	100 N	70.7 N	70.7 N
75°	100 N	96.6 N	25.9 N
90°	100 N	100.0 N	0
120°	100 N	86.6 N	50.0 N

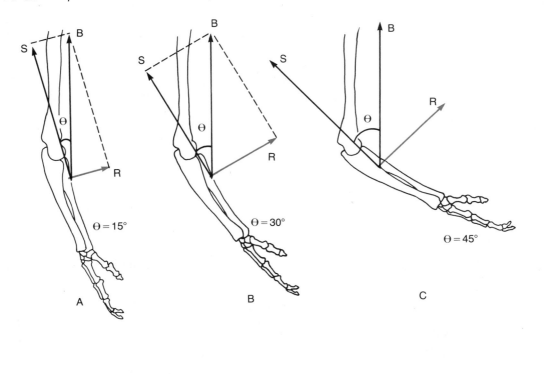

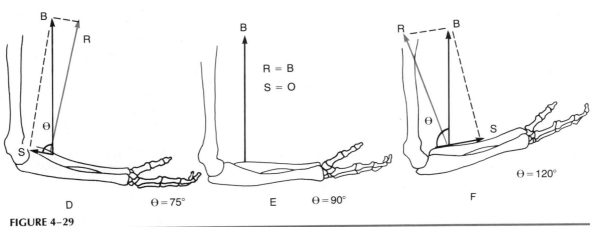

FIGURE 4–29

The rotatory component (R) of force B increases as the body segment moves about its anatomical axis, but its increase is not linear. Forearm flexion: $A = 15°$, $B = 30°$, $C = 45°$, $D = 75°$, $E = 90°$, and $F = 120°$.

When the angle reaches 45° the rotatory component is 70.7 percent of the original force, and the rate of increase per unit of joint movement declines toward 90°. These relationships can be seen by reading down the columns of the sine and cosine tables.

Suppose we wish to find the rotational and compressional forces resulting from the ham-

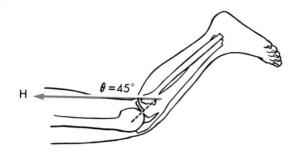

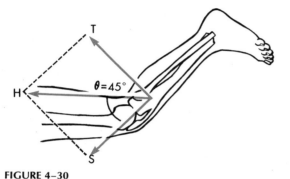

FIGURE 4–30

Rectangular components of the hamstring muscle group, which is pulling on the leg at an angle of 45°. T = rotating and S = stabilizing components of H.

strings acting at a 45° angle with the long axis of the leg. Rectangular components for the hamstrings are constructed in Figure 4–30 to show the characteristics of the two components of H. In this case, they are equal in magnitude.

Consider the deltoid muscle pulling on the abducted arm with a force of 500 N. The action line makes a 20° angle with the humerus (Fig. 4–31). We wish to find the vertical (rotatory) and horizontal (stabilizing) components of this force. If we call the vertical component Fx and the horizontal component Fx, then

$$Fy = D \sin 20° = 500 \times 0.342 = 171.0 \text{ N}$$
$$Fx = D \cos 20° = 500 \times 0.939 = 469.5 \text{ N}$$

It may seem strange that the sum of the magnitudes of the two components of the original force is greater than the force itself. Recall that the square of the hypotenuse of a right triangle

is equal to the sum of the squares of the two sides, or

$$R^2 = Fx^2 + Fy^2$$
$$R = \sqrt{Fx^2 + Fy^2}$$

Let us now review some of the previous examples, which were presented graphically, and supply algebraic solutions. In Figure 4–29, angle ϕ equals 45°, and forces R and NR are each therefore 0.707 × B. If B represents a pull of 50 N, a force of 35 N is acting to rotate the part, and another force of 35 N is compressing the elbow joint surfaces. When angle ϕ equals 30°, R equals 0.500 × 50, or 25 N, and NR equals 0.866 × 50, or 43.3 N. In Figure 4–30, if the hamstrings pull with a force of 150 N on one leg, both the rotational compressional components, T and S, equal 0.707 × 150, or 106 N.

GRAVITATIONAL COMPONENTS

The rotatory effect of a body part or a weight held by that body part depends upon the position of the body part with respect to gravity.

The gravitational force, action line, and direc-

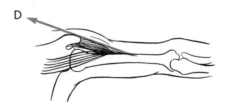

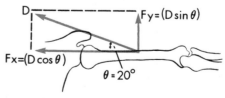

FIGURE 4–31

Resolution of deltoid force (D) into rotatory component (Fy) and stabilizing component (Fx). Angle of force application (θ) is 20°.

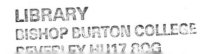

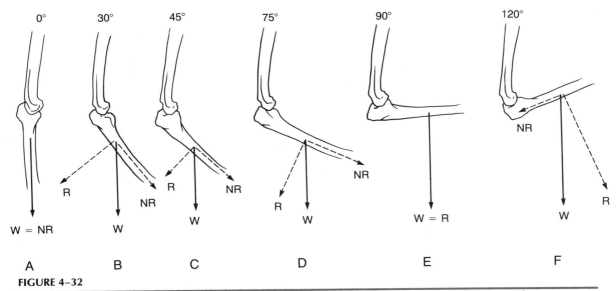

FIGURE 4–32

The change in gravitational components of the forearm as it moves through the range of motion. Forearm flexion: $A = 15°$, $B = 30°$, $C = 45°$, $D = 75°$, $E = 90°$, and $F = 120°$.

tion can never be changed from vertical and downward. As a body segment moves through space, the action line of gravity constantly changes with respect to the long axis of the moving segment. When the part is horizontal, gravity pulls at a right angle; in other positions the angle is less than 90°.

Figure 4–32 illustrates the gravitational effects on the forearm as it is placed in different positions with respect to gravity. As was done for the components of muscle force, the effects may be graphically or algebraically determined.

Table 4–3 shows the changes in the gravitational force components for different limb positions.

GAIT COMPONENTS

The thrust of the heel against the ground at the beginning of the stance phase in walking can be resolved into rectangular components (Fig. 4–33). The horizontal force (X) must be opposed by frictional ground force, and the vertical component (Y) must be opposed by an adequate upward force of the ground or floor. Note the ef-

fect of a longer step (Fig. 4–33B). There is no change in the magnitude of the component vector Y, as shown in the diagram, since this force is determined by body weight. However, the direction and magnitude of O and X are affected by step length.

Since the weight of the man remains constant, Y is constant in direction and magnitude, and O and X must be obtained from Y. The value of Y for an average man might be 1000 N.

TABLE 4–3. ROTATORY (R) AND NONROTATORY (NR) COMPONENTS OF GRAVITATIONAL PULL ON THE FOREARM AT VARIOUS POSITIONS

Limb Position with Respect to Vertical	Gravity	R	NR
0°	15 N	0	15 N
30°	15 N	7.5 N	13 N
45°	15 N	10.6 N	10.6 N
60°	15 N	13 N	7.5 N
90°	15 N	15 N	0
120°	15 N	13 N	7.5 N

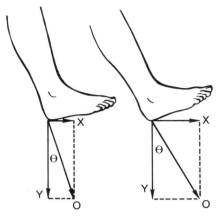

FIGURE 4–33

Vertical (Y) and horizontal (X) components of force O acting against the ground at heel strike in walking. Relative magnitudes of the components depend on the angle of force application, which is related to step length. The angle made by O and Y is θ.

In the first figure, the force O can be obtained from the relation

1000 N = O cos 20°, or

O = 1000 N/cos 20° = 1000 N/0.939
    = 1065 N

The horizontal component will be

X = O sin 20° = 1065 N × 0.342 = 364.2 N

With a longer step, as angle θ becomes 30°, the direction and magnitude of the reacting force O change:

O = 1000 N/cos 30°

        = 1000 N/0.866 = 1155 N

and the horizontal component

X = O sin 30° = 1155 N × 0.5 = 577 N

From this it may be seen that with a longer step length, the relative increase in magnitude of the horizontal component X is larger than the increase in the total ground reaction force O. Frictional force at the heel must be much greater when the step is longer than when it is short.

SPLINT COMPONENTS

The finger cuff of a splint is used to apply force to a bony segment. The force applied may be resolved into a pair of rectangular components. One component perpendicular to the body part provides a force to produce joint rotation. The other component is parallel to the bony part and tends to produce joint distraction or compression. The greater the parallel component, the less the ability of the splint to correct the deformity. The parallel component also causes the cuff to migrate in the direction of the pull. Malalignment of the cuff and tissue breakdown are possible results of such a situation.

Suppose a finger cuff is applied to the middle phalanx of a finger with a force of 2.23 newtons (Fig. 4–34). Let's set the force on the cuff at a 90° angle to the bony part. We may then calculate the rectangular components. The angle between the rotatory component and the applied force would be 0°. The angle between the rotatory component and the axis of the bone would be 90°. The calculations then would be as follows:

R/F = sin 90° = cos 0°
R = F sin 90°
R = (2.23)(1)
R = 2.23 newtons

NR/F = sin 0° = cos 90°
NR = F sin 0°
NR = (2.23)(0)
NR = 0 newtons

If the force of the cuff is set at 75° to the bony part, the rotatory (R) and nonrotatory (NR) components are as follows:

R/F = sin 75° = cos 15°
R = F sin 75°
R = (2.23)(0.966)
R = 2.15 newtons

NR/F = sin 15° = cos 75°
NR = F sin 15°
NR = (2.23)(.259)
NR = 0.58 newton

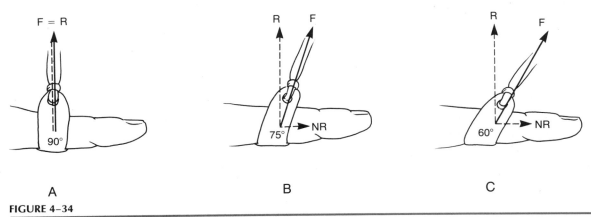

FIGURE 4–34

Force components of finger cuff applied at 90° (*A*), 75° (*B*), and 60° (*C*).

If the force of the cuff is set at 60° to the bony part, the rotatory (R) and nonrotatory (NR) components will be:

$$R/F = \sin 60° = \cos 30°$$
$$R = F \sin 60°$$
$$R = (2.23)(0.866)$$
$$R = 1.93 \text{ newtons}$$
$$NR/F = \sin 30° = \cos 60°$$
$$NR = F \sin 30°$$
$$NR = (2.23)(0.5)$$
$$NR = 1.115 \text{ newtons}$$

Note that as the angle moves farther away from being perpendicular to the bony part, the rotatory component decreases and the nonrotatory component increases. This concept is also true concerning pads from other types of splints and braces.

CERVICAL TRACTION COMPONENTS

Cervical traction provides examples of composition of force. Cervical traction is often provided in either the sitting position (Fig. 4–35A) or the supine position (Fig. 4–35B).

As shown in Figure 4–35A, the upward directed force acts in the opposite direction of the weight of the head and changes the load on the cervical structures.

In Figure 4–35B the vertical component of the traction force opposes the weight of the head while the horizontal component changes the load on the cervical structures.

LUMBAR SPINE COMPONENTS

The lumbar spine is greatly affected by the loads placed on the area. An example of resolution of forces at the lumbosacral (L_5S_1) motion segment is shown in Figure 4–36. As an individual is standing in the superincumbent position, body weight (W) is directed downward. This force can be divided in a force component perpendicular to the upper surface of the sacrum and one parallel to the surface of the sacrum. If the sacral angle is in a normal position of about 45°, the S and C components will be equal. If the lumbar spine is flat and the sacral angle is decreased, the S component will decrease and the C component will increase. If the lumbar spine has increased lordosis, the reverse will occur.

COMPOSITION AND RESOLUTION OF FORCES

In the previous sections we have discussed composition and resolution of forces separately. However, the composition of forces may be used as a step to determine the resultant of two or more forces (Fig. 4–37A).

A rectangular coordinate system may be constructed in any arbitrary direction. For simplifi-

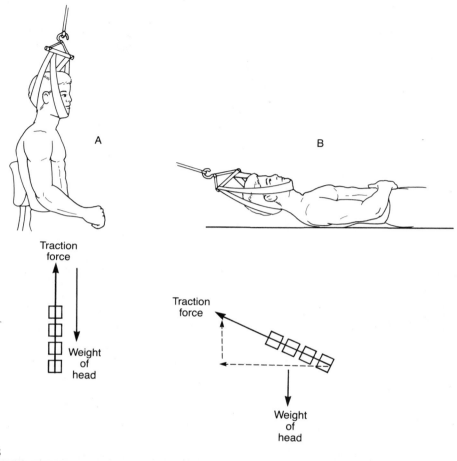

FIGURE 4–35

Forces involved during cervical traction: *A*, Vertical traction. *B*, Horizontal traction.

cation, however, we can make an axis coincide with one of the forces. In Figure 4–37B, the Y axis coincides with force F3. We then resolve each force into its x and y components. Those extending up or to the right are positive, and those directed down or to the left are negative. The force components along the separate axes are added as in the linear system.

As shown in Figure 4–37B, the components for F_1 are $F_{1x} = F_1 \cos \Theta_1$ and $F_{1y} = F_1 \sin \Theta_1$; for F_2 they are $F_{2x} = F_2 \cos \Theta_2$ and $F_{2y} = F_2 \sin \Theta_2$; and for F_3 they are $F_{3x} = F_3 \cos \Theta_3$ and $F_{3y} = F \sin \Theta_{3y}$. Thus, the total X component (F_x) equals $F_{1x} + F_{2x} + F_{3x}$, and the total Y component (F_y) equals $F_{1y} + F_{2y} + F_{3y}$. F_x and F_y are the sides of the triangle, and the hypotenuse (R) is the resultant of the three forces. Using the Pythagorean theorem, we determine the values of R as

$$R = \sqrt{F_x^2 + F_y^2}$$

The direction of R with the X axis is determined by taking any of the trigonometric functions,

$$\tan \Theta = F_y/F_x$$
$$\cos \Theta = F_x/R$$
$$\sin \Theta = F_y/R$$

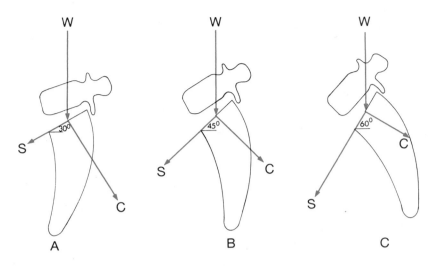

FIGURE 4–36

Change in the compression and shearing force components with the change in the sacral angle.

Let's assign values to the three forces so that $F_1 = 75$ N and $\theta_1 = 30°$, $F_2 = 15$ N and $\theta_2 = 15°$, and $F_3 = 25$ N and $\theta_3 = 90°$. Solve for their resultant:

$$F_{1x} = F_1 \cos 30°$$
$$= 75 \text{ N} \times 0.866 = 65 \text{ N}$$
$$F_{1y} = F_1 \sin 30°$$
$$= 75 \text{ N} \times 0.5 = 37.5 \text{ N}$$
$$F_{2x} = F_2 \cos 15°$$
$$= 15 \text{ N} \times 0.965 = 14.5 \text{ N}$$
$$F_{2y} = F_2 \sin 15°$$
$$= 15 \text{ N} \times 0.258 = 3.87 \text{ N}$$
$$F_{3x} = F_3 \cos 90°$$
$$= 25 \text{ N} \times 0 = 0$$
$$F_{3y} = F_3 \sin 90°$$
$$= 25 \text{ N} \times 1 = 25 \text{ N}$$

Since F_{2x} is to the left and F_{3y} is downward, they will have negative values.

$$F_x = F_{1x} + F_{2x} + F_{3x}$$
$$= 65 \text{ N} + (-14.5 \text{ N}) + 0 = 50.5 \text{ N}$$

$$F_y = F_{1y} + F_{2y} + F_{3y}$$
$$= 37.5 \text{ N} + 3.87 \text{ N} + (-25 \text{ N})$$
$$= 16.37 \text{ N}$$
$$R = \sqrt{F_x^2 + F_y^2}$$
$$= \sqrt{(50.5)^2 + (16.37)^2}$$
$$= \sqrt{2550 + 268}$$
$$= \sqrt{2818}$$
$$= 53.1 \text{ N}$$
$$\tan \phi = 16.37 \text{ N}/50 \text{ N}$$
$$= 0.32432$$
$$\phi = 18°$$

To further illustrate the procedure, suppose we have three forces of 120, 100, and 50 N, as shown in Figure 4-38A. We construct the X and Y axes and proceed to replace each force by rectangular components. Beginning with the horizontal components,

$$R_x = \Sigma F_x = \Sigma F \cos \theta$$
$$= 100 \cos 30° + 50 \cos 45°$$
$$- 120 \cos 60°$$
$$= (100 \times 0.866) + (50 \times 0.707)$$
$$- (120 \times 0.500)$$
$$= 86.6 + 35.3 - 60$$
$$= 61.9 \text{ N}$$

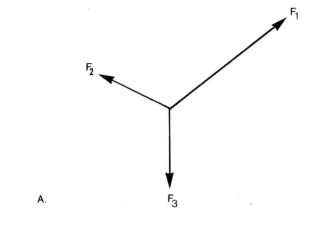

A.

FIGURE 4–37

Method of using the composition of forces to help determine the resultant of two or more forces.

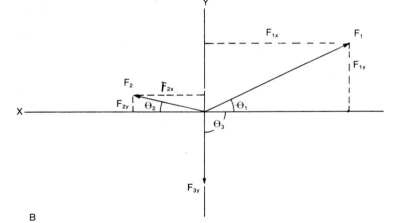

B

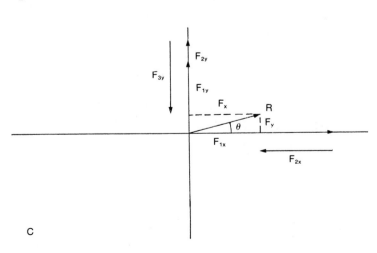

C

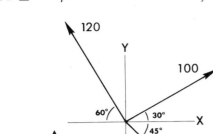

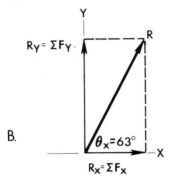

FIGURE 4–38

Vector diagram for algebraic determination of resultant of concurrent force system.

To determine components along the Y axes,

$$R_y = \Sigma F_y = \Sigma F \sin \theta$$
$$= 100 \sin 30° - 50 \sin 45° + 120 \sin 60°$$
$$= (100 \times 0.500) - (50 \times 0.707)$$
$$+ (120 \times 0.866)$$
$$= 50 - 35.3 + 103.9$$
$$= 118.6 \text{ N}$$

The single force that is the resultant of these two rectangular components is the hypotenuse of the triangle of which the values R_x and R_y are the sides.

Then,

$$R = \sqrt{R_x^2 + R_y^2}$$
$$= \sqrt{(61.9)^2 + (118.6)^2}$$
$$= 133.78 \text{ N}$$

and the angle the resultant makes with the horizontal will be obtained from

$$\sin \theta_x = \Sigma F_y/R \text{ or } \cos \theta_x = \Sigma F_x/R$$
$$\sin \theta_x = 118.6/133.78$$
$$\sin \theta_x = 0.886$$
$$\theta_x = 63°$$

We cannot determine from the angle alone whether the force is directed upward or downward from the X axis or to the right or left. We draw a diagram of F_y and F_x in their proper directions according to their signs, and the direction of the force is given by the diagonal, as shown in Figure 4–38B.

In the graphic solution, lines representing the forces are drawn in order, with the tail of one touching the tip of the preceding one (Fig. 4–39). The resultant will be the line drawn from the tail of the first to the tip of the last. The resultant force must pass through the point of concurrence where the original forces of the system meet. In this way the resultant force is completely defined.

EXAMPLES FROM THE LITERATURE

Diagrams of rectangular components of a force appear frequently in the literature. Often these do not include specific values but are used to demonstrate by graphic means relative magnitudes of forces that are resolved into component parts. For example, Steindler's kinesiology text (1955) has a number of such drawings. In Figure 4–40, the force of the knee flexor muscles (e.g.,

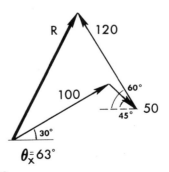

FIGURE 4–39

Graphic solution for resultant of concurrent force system shown in Figure 4–38.

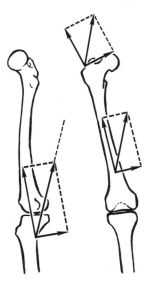

FIGURE 4–40

Example of graphical resolution of forces. Muscles represented are the hamstrings, hip abductors, and adductors, shown with their respective rectangular components. (Adapted from Steindler A: Kinesiology. Springfield, Ill., Charles C Thomas, 1955.)

lution of forces technique. A thigh and pelvis from a cadaver were suspended by Fick in a triangular frame, with the thigh in the anatomic position. The action line of each muscle was estimated from its anatomic location and was extended until it intersected one or more of the three planes that converged at the axis of the hip joint. The force was then divided "according to the parallelopiped of forces" into its components, acting in the respective planes. The action line of an individual muscle was considered to be the resultant of all the small component forces within the muscle, with an equal number of fibers on either side of the line.

As a further example of resolution of a force, Inman and associates (1944) observed that the upper part of the trapezius (F) pulls in a diagonal direction on the shoulder, providing both a supportive component (F_y) and an adductory component (F_x) (Fig. 4–41). From observations of shoulder function these authors concluded that:

Owing to the changes in position of the scapula during elevation, the resultant of the supportive and rotatory components supplied by the upper portion of

semitendinosus or sartorius) in the sagittal plane is shown. The rotatory component flexes the leg; the translatory component compresses the knee joint. In the second figure, a vector represents the force of the hip adductor muscle group. This force both adducts the limb and pushes it upward into the acetabulum. The abductor muscle group pushes the femoral head into the acetabulum as well as swinging the leg out to the side.

Steindler has emphasized the usefulness of the "wasted" or stabilizing components of muscle forces, such as those that serve to protect the joint structures—capsules and ligaments—from wear and tear. They are also an important factor in postural stability and therefore do not deserve the term "wasted." The magnitude of the stabilizing component is far greater than the rotatory component of most muscle forces because the majority of muscles insert at very small angles to the long axis of the segments.

The method used by Fick (1850) to determine force components of the hip muscles in the three cardinal planes is explained by the reso-

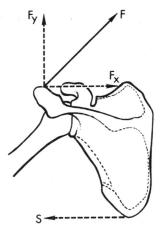

FIGURE 4–41

Resolution of upper trapezius force (F) into supporting component (F_y) and adductory component (F_x). Abductor force (S) of serratus anterior muscle is shown below. (Adapted from Inman VT, Saunders JB, Abbott LC: The function of the shoulder joint. J Bone Joint Surg 26:1–30, 1944.)

the trapezius ... fluctuate[s] in its angle of action. This fluctuation reveals an interesting mechanism in the action of the trapezius. In the resting position, the muscle is entirely supportive. With the first 35 degrees of [arm] elevation, the angle of action of the muscle changes, so that its force is equally divided between the supportive and rotatory roles. From 35 to 140 degrees, the muscle is increasingly more effective as a rotator, with its maximum power at 90 degrees, and beyond 140 degrees its rotatory efficiency decreases and its supportive rises. This complicated mechanism of action of the upper trapezius is achieved by simple elevation of the shoulder girdle as a whole.

An interesting application of resolving a force has been made by Rose and Wallace (1952) in an analysis of typical hand deformity resulting from arthritis. In accounting for the characteristic ulnar deviation of the fingers, these authors review the general scheme of dorsal interosseous muscle action on the fingers. The mechanics of the first dorsal interosseous muscle are then considered, wherein fibers converge to act on a centrally located tendon (see Fig. 4–20).

According to the description given, M represents the force of a muscle fiber, and if the angle ϕ at which the fibers approach the tendon is 60°, cos ϕ is 0.500, and thus R, the component of M acting in the direction of the central tendon, is ½M. If the angle ϕ increases, component T will decrease and vice versa. This analysis can be applied to any bipennate or unipennate arrangement of muscle fibers. The authors go on to point out that in arthritic hand deformities, the intrinsic muscles become weakened from disuse (see Fig. 4–20). The index finger becomes deviated ulnarward, and fiber M, although having a more acute angle of insertion into the central tendon, becomes further weakened from constant stretch. The opposing fiber M_1 shortens adaptively. Thus M_1 has a poor angle of insertion. "Any corrective exercise must balance the bipennate components, yet keep the forces acting in the direction of the tendon as large as possible" (Rose and Wallace, 1952).

The principles involved in the composition and resolution of forces will be used repeatedly in the following chapters. Knowledge of these ideas is essential for understanding the effect of forces acting upon a body.

QUESTIONS

1. Define sine, cosine, and tangent.
2. What is the sine of 0°, 8°, 30°, 45°, 60°, 81°, and 90°?
3. What is the cosine of 0°, 17°, 30°, 45°, 60°, 78°, and 90°?
4. What is the tangent of 0°, 12°, 39°, 45°, 63°, 72°, and 90°?
5. What angle to the nearest 0.5° has a tangent of 2.15, 0.20, 0.38, and 1.45?
6. Mention an example of composition of forces in body movement that has not already been suggested; give an example of resolution of forces too.
7. Which requires stronger ropes to support 150 lb., a swing or a hammock? Explain your answers.
8. Find the vertical and horizontal components of a 10 lb. force pulling at a 30° angle from the horizontal.
9. A girl wishes to canoe across a river having a velocity of 8 miles per hour. If she starts straight across the river at 5 miles per hour, what will be her resultant direction with the river bank? If the river is 400 feet wide, how far downstream will she be before she reaches the opposite bank?
10. What percentage of the muscle force produces effective rotational motion if the muscle inserts at an angle of 25°? 73°? What percentage of the muscle force is directed toward the joint as a stabilizing force in the above problem?
11. How does the resultant change as the angle between two concurrent forces increases? What angle provides the maximum resultant?
12. Four muscles all pull on the patella simultaneously, applying the following forces:

Rectus femoris, 150 N at an angle of 15° to the left of vertical.
Vastus lateralis, 200 N at an angle of 30° to the left of vertical.
Vastus intermedius, 200 N at an angle of 10° to the left of vertical.
Vastus medialis, 230 N at an angle of 40° to the right of vertical.

(a) What is their resultant force?

(b) If the patellar tendon attaches at a 0° angle with the vertical, what is the resultant force on the patella?

(c) What happens to this resultant if the patellar tendon is moved 4° medially?

(d) What would happen to the resultant of the patella if the vastus medialis were strengthened to pull 250 N in the (a) part of the problem?

(e) Relate the above problem to a rehabilitation program.

REFERENCES

Basmajian JV: Muscles Alive, 2nd ed. Baltimore, Williams & Wilkins, 1967.

Benedek GB, Villars FMH: Physics, vol. 1. Reading, MA, Addison-Wesley Publishing Company, 1973.

Bila D, Bottorff R, Merritt P, et al.: Core Mathematics. New York, Worth Publishers, 1975.

Braus H: Anatomie des Menschen. Berlin, Springer-Verlag, 1954, p 360.

Brinkerhoff RF, Cross JB, Lazarus A: Exploring Physics, rev. ed. New York, Harcourt, Brace & World, 1959.

Broer M: Efficiency of Human Movement, 3rd ed. Philadelphia, W. B. Saunders, 1973.

Cailiet R: Low Back Pain Syndrome, 2nd ed. Philadelphia, F. A. Davis, 1968.

Calderwood C: Russell Traction. Am J Nurs 43:1–6, 1943.

Campney HK, Wehr RW: An interpretation of the strength differences associated with varying angles of pull. Res Quart 36:403–412, 1965.

Craig AS: Elements of kinesiology for the clinician. Phys Ther 44:470–473, 1964.

Elliott LP, Wilcox WF: Physics: A Modern Approach. New York, Macmillan, 1957.

Fick A: Statistische Berachtung der Muskulature des Ober-schenkels. Zeitschrift für Rationelle Medizin 9:94–106, 1850.

Flitter HH: An Introduction to Physics in Nursing. St. Louis, C. V. Mosby, 1948, p 22.

Frankel VH, Burstein AH: Orthopedic Biomechanics. Philadelphia, Lea & Febiger, 1970.

Halliday D, Resnick R: Fundamentals of Physics. New York, John Wiley & Sons, 1974.

Hart WL: Preparation of Calculus. New York, Intext Educational Publishers, 1971.

Inman VT: Functional aspects of the abductor muscles of the hip. J Bone Joint Surg 29:607–619, 1947.

Inman VT, Saunders JB, Abbott LC: The function of the shoulder joint. J Bone Joint Surg 26:1–30, 1944.

Kelley DL: Kinesiology. Englewood Cliffs, NJ, Prentice-Hall, 1971.

Larson RF: Forearm positioning on maximal elbow-flexor force. Phys Ther 49:748–756, 1969.

MacConaill MA, Basmajian JV: Muscles and Movements. Baltimore, Williams & Wilkins, 1969.

Miller F, Jr: College Physics, 3rd ed. New York, Harcourt, Brace, Jovanovich, 1974.

Nachemson A: The effect of forward leaning on lumbar intradiscal pressure. Acta Orthop Scand 35:314–328, 1965.

O'Connell AL, Gardner EB: Understanding the Scientific Basis of Human Movement. Baltimore, Williams & Wilkins, 1972.

Rose DL, Wallace LI: A remedial occupational therapy program for the residuals of rheumatoid arthritis of the hand. Am J Phys Med 31:5–13, 1952.

Sears FW, Zemansky MW: University Physics, 2nd ed. Reading, MA, Addison-Wesley Publishing Company, 1955.

Spitbart A, Bardell RH: Plane Trigonometry, 2nd ed. Cambridge, MA, Wesley Publishing Company, 1964.

Steindler A: Kinesiology. Springfield, IL, Charles C Thomas, 1955.

Stewart JDM: Traction and Orthopedic Appliances. New York, Churchill Livingstone, 1975.

Volz RG, Lieb M, Benjamin J: Biomechanics of the wrist. Clin Orthop 149:112–117, 1980.

Wells KR: Kinesiology, 5th ed. Philadelphia, W. B. Saunders, 1971.

5

Static Equilibrium

INTRODUCTION

A body is in equilibrium when, as stated in Newton's first law, it remains at rest or is in motion with constant velocity. If it is at rest, with the velocity equaling zero, it is said to be in *static equilibrium*. With a constant velocity other than zero the equilibrium is called *dynamic equilibrium*. This chapter will deal with the condition of static equilibrium.

FIRST CONDITION OF EQUILIBRIUM

Statics is the study of bodies in static equilibrium as a result of forces acting upon them. We must consider all forces acting on a body when dealing with problems in statics, which include any reaction forces which Newton referred to in his third law. When all the forces that are acting on a body simultaneously have their combined effect cancelled and their resultant is zero, such a body is said to be in *translational equilibrium*. Therefore, the first condition of equilibrium is $\Sigma F = 0$, or the sum of all the forces equals zero. When using the x-y coordinate system, we would then have:

$$\Sigma Fx = 0$$
$$\Sigma Fy = 0$$

Linear Force System

The simplest force system to analyze using the first condition of equilibrium is the linear system in which the forces are coplanar, concurrent, and colinear. This system was discussed briefly in Chapter 4.

▶ PROBLEM 5–1

We can take an example of a 50 N box resting on a table (Fig. 5–1A). Gravity pulls downward on the box with a force of 50 N. Since the box is not moving, a force must be acting to balance the force of gravity. To solve this problem we must first draw a free body diagram showing all the existing forces (Fig. 5–1B). Then, by using the first condition of equilibrium, that

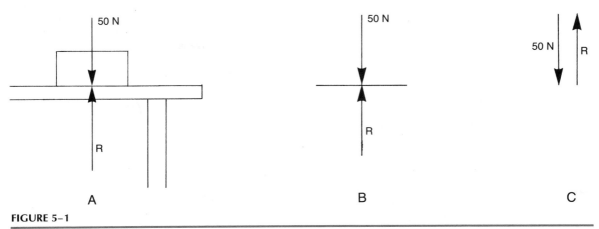

FIGURE 5–1

A linear force system.

the sum of all the forces acting on a body equals zero, we can determine the reaction force necessary to support the box. Since gravity is pulling the box downward, the 50 N will be given a negative sign. We may write algebraically:

$$\Sigma F = 0$$
$$(-50\ N) + R = 0$$
$$R = 50\ N$$

Since the force of gravity and the reaction force of the table have opposite signs, they must be acting in opposite directions. A graphic solution (Fig. 5–1C) confirms the algebraic solution.

In the linear force system, if two forces are acting on a body, to be in equilibrium the forces must be equal in magnitude and opposite in direction. For the tug-of-war teams discussed in Chapter 4 (see Fig. 4–7), equilibrium would result if the resultants of the individual teams were equal in magnitude; their combined resultant would be zero. It is not difficult to think of other examples: for instance, a person standing on one foot, supported by the upward thrust of the floor, a pocketbook or briefcase held in the hand, or a lamp resting on a table.

In a clinic situation, the Sayre sling suspension, some arrangements of skeletal traction, and many pulley weight exercise devices fall into this classification. A series of exercise weights loaded on a weight pan or hanging on a storage peg constitutes a linear force system. Their total force would obviously be determined by adding them together, and the opposing force of the weight pan or peg would have to be equal to the total sum of the weights. A patient preparing for sandbag exercises for the quadriceps muscles may sit with his or her leg over the edge of the plinth while the exercise load is applied. Before the beginning of the exercise, if the foot is dangling, the ligaments of the knee are obliged to support the total weight of the leg, the boot, and the applied weights. When a walking cast or brace is applied to the foot, it exerts an added downward force that must be opposed by the ligaments and muscles passing across each of the lower extremity joints that are proximal to the cast. In this case, the longitudinal tension on the structures of each joint involved equals the weight of the distal part plus the added weight of the cast or brace.

The linear system of forces is an extremely simple one. About the only difficulty one is apt to have in the solution of problems is in giving an incorrect sign to a force to accompany its magnitude. However, it is important that a complete and clear understanding of the principles involved be obtained in dealing with this system, since other, more complicated systems that we shall consider are based on extensions of the principles made use of in the linear system.

Concurrent Force System

Often forces acting on a body do not lie along the same line of action, as they do in the linear system of forces. One such force system, the concurrent force system, occurs when all the forces meet at a point. Whenever three forces act upon an object, they must be concurrent or parallel.

If two coplanar, nonparallel forces are acting on a rigid body (Fig. 5–2A), a third force must act to maintain equilibrium. To determine the magnitude and direction of the third force, the resultant of the two original forces must be found. The third force is its equilibrant (Fig. 5–2B). The third force must pass through the point of intersection of the original forces. Hence, to be in equilibrium, the three coplanar, nonparallel forces must be concurrent. Otherwise rotation will occur, and although the system is in translation equilibrium, it would not be in rotational equilibrium. Note that the action lines of the forces may be extended and the point of application may be located anywhere along the line of action of the force.

Often the magnitude and direction of two of the three concurrent forces are not known. To illustrate the concurrent system, which commonly occurs in the body, let's examine Figure 5–3A. Suppose a 10.2 Kg or 100 N weight (W) is supported by a cord and is resting on a plane inclined 30°. We may wish to determine the

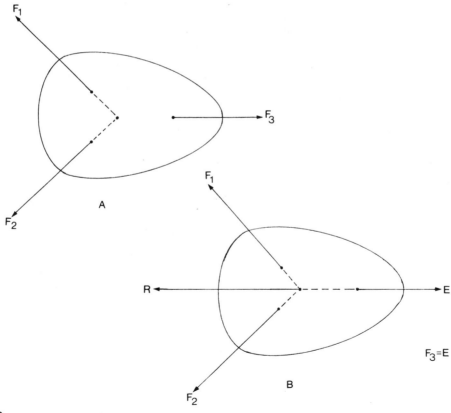

FIGURE 5–2

Concurrent forces: *A*, F_1 and F_2 act on the object. F_3 balances these two forces. *B*, R is resultant of F_1 and F_2. E is equilibrant of R.

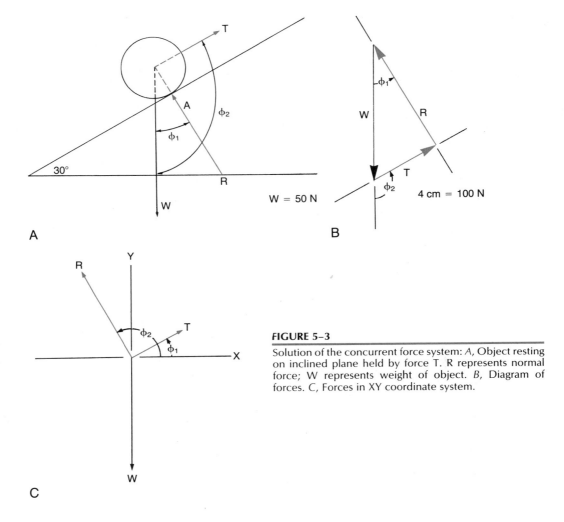

FIGURE 5–3

Solution of the concurrent force system: *A*, Object resting on inclined plane held by force T. R represents normal force; W represents weight of object. *B*, Diagram of forces. *C*, Forces in XY coordinate system.

tension (T) in the cord and the reaction force (R) at the point of support (A) on the inclined plane. In this situation the magnitude of only one force is known. However, the direction of all three forces may easily be determined. The force of the weight is produced by the pull of gravity and acts vertically downward. The direction of the line of force (T) produced by the cord may be observed directly. Remember that if three forces acting on a body are in equilibrium, they must be concurrent. Thus, the direction of the reaction force (R) is determined by constructing a line between the point of contact between the weight and plane (A) and the point of intersec-

tion of the lines of force of the weight (W) and the cord (T). Suppose $\phi_1 = 30°$, and $\phi_2 = 120°$. We may now draw a vector diagram and solve for the magnitudes of the tension in the cord and the reaction force of the plane (Fig. 5–3B). We first draw the weight vector (W) to scale. For example, 4 cm equals 100 N. To the head of this vector we may draw the line of action representing the tension in the cord. This line may be extended in both directions. Next, the line of action representing the reaction force is drawn at the tail of the weight vector. This line may also be extended in both directions. As this line intersects the line of action of the cord, a triangle is formed by the three force vectors. The length of each side provides the magnitude of the respective forces, which reveals that T is 50 N and R is 86.6 N. The direction of the vectors should be so placed that a tail is attached to the head of the adjacent vector.

▶ **PROBLEM 5–2**

This system may also be solved algebraically by using the first condition of equilibrium ($\Sigma F = 0$). The first step is to draw a free body diagram (Fig. 5–3C) and establish a set of coordinates. We then set up equations for the component forces in the X and Y directions.

$$\Sigma F_x = 0$$
$$\Sigma F_x = W_x + T_x + R_x = 0$$

Since W is vertical, its X component is zero. Thus,

$$T_x + R_x = 0$$

For the Y direction,

$$\Sigma F_y = 0$$

Then,

$$\Sigma F_y = W_y + T_y + R_y = 0$$

Since W, which equals 100 N, is vertical and downward, its Y component (W_y) equals -100 N. Thus,

$$\Sigma F_y = (-100 \text{ N}) + T_y + R_y = 0$$

We now have two equations and four unknown quantities. By using trigonometry, however, we may reduce the four unknown values to two. Thus,

$$T_x = T \cos \phi_1$$
$$T_y = T \sin \phi_1$$
$$R_x = R \cos \phi_2$$
$$R_y = R \sin \phi_2$$

These values may be substituted into the equilibrium formulas, so that if

$$T_x + R_x = 0, \text{ then}$$
$$T \cos \phi_1 + R \cos \phi_2 = 0$$

and if

$$(-100 \text{ N}) + T_y + R_y = 0, \text{ then}$$
$$(-100 \text{ N}) + T \sin \phi_1 + R \sin \phi_2 = 0$$

Hence, we have two equations and two unknowns:

$$\Sigma F_x = T \cos \phi_1 + R \cos \phi_2 = 0$$
$$\Sigma F_y = (-100 \text{ N}) + T \sin \phi_1 + R \sin \phi_2 = 0$$

Further algebraic manipulation of the equation for ΣF_x yields

$$T \cos \phi_1 = -R \cos \phi_2$$
$$T = \frac{-R \cos \phi_2}{\cos \phi_1}$$

This value for T may be substituted in the equation for ΣF_y so that

$$(-100 \text{ N}) + \left(\frac{-R \cos \phi_2}{\cos \phi_1} \right) \sin \phi_1 + R \sin \phi_2 = 0$$

If ϕ_1 equals 30° and $\phi_2 = 120°$, we may obtain their trigonometric values from a calculator or Appendix B and solve for R and T. From trigonometry we find that $\cos 120° = -\cos 60°$ and $\sin 120° = \sin 60°$. Thus,

$$(-100 \text{ N}) + \left(\frac{R \cos 60°}{\cos 30°} \right) \sin 30° + R \sin 60° = 0$$
$$(-100 \text{ N}) + \left(R \frac{0.5}{0.866} \right) 0.5 + R \, 0.866 = 0$$
$$(-100 \text{ N}) + 0.289 \, R + 0.866 \, R = 0$$
$$-100 \text{ N} + 1.15 \, R = 0$$
$$1.15 \, R = 100 \text{ N}$$
$$R = 86.6 \text{ N}$$

The reaction force on the inclined plane equals 86.6 N. We may now solve for T.

$$T = \frac{-R \cos \phi_2}{\cos \phi_1} = -86.6 \left(\frac{-0.5}{0.866} \right)$$
$$T = 50 \text{ N}$$

The tension in the cord is 50 N.
Remember, the only known characteristics for the three forces were as follows:

Force W: magnitude, line of application, and direction.
Force T: line of application and direction.
Force R: point of application and direction.

▶ **PROBLEM 5–3**

The following is an example in which one force is defined and the line of application of the other two concurrent forces is given (Fig. 5–4).

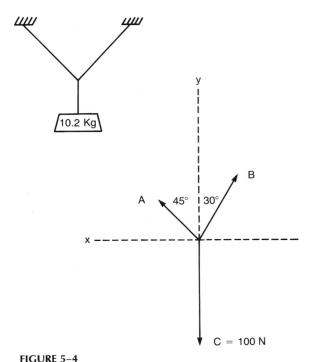

FIGURE 5–4

A 10.2 Kg mass is supported by two cords. Cord A is at a 45° angle with the vertical; cord B is at a 30° angle with the vertical.

Suppose we have 100 N weight (10.2 Kg mass) supported by two cords. One cord (A) makes an angle of 45° with the vertical and the second cord (B) makes an angle of 30° with the vertical. Using the first condition of equilibrium, we have:

$$\Sigma F = 0 \text{ or } \Sigma F_x = 0 \text{ and } \Sigma F_y = 0$$

We can then determine the forces in the X direction:

$$\Sigma F_x = A_x + B_x + C_x = 0$$

Since $A_x/A = \cos 45°$, then $A_x = A \cos 45°$.

Since $B_x/B = \sin 30°$, then $B_x = B \sin 30°$.

Since gravity pulls the weight downward,

$$C_x = 0$$

Substitute these values into the equation ($\Sigma F = 0$). Since A_x is to the left it is given a negative sign. If we used the angle of 135° instead of 45° for A, we would also find that $\cos 135°$ is negative. Therefore,

$$(-A \cos 45°) + (B \sin 30°) + 0 = 0$$
$$\text{or}$$
$$(A \cos 135°) + (B \sin 30°) + 0 = 0$$

We next find the forces in the Y direction.

$$\Sigma F_y = A_y + B_y + C_y = 0$$

Since $A_y/A = \sin 45°$, the $A_y = A \sin 45°$.

Since $B_y/B = \cos 30°$, then $B_y = B \cos 30°$.

$$C_y = 100 \text{ N}$$

Substitute these values into the equation ($\Sigma F_y = 0$):

$$(A \sin 45°) + (B \cos 30°) + (-100 \text{ N}) = 0$$

We now have two equations and two unknown values:

$$-A \cos 45° + B \sin 30° + 0 = 0 \qquad (1)$$
$$A \sin 45° + B \cos 30° - 100 = 0 \qquad (2)$$

We may solve for one value in one equation and then substitute that value into the other equation as follows:

From equation (1) subtract ($-A \cos 45°$) from both sides of the equation. Therefore, $B \sin 30° = A \cos 45°$. Solve for B by dividing both sides of the equation by $\sin 30°$; thus, $B = A \cos 45°/\sin 30°$.

We can now substitute the value for B into equation (2).

$$A \sin 45° + (A \cos 45°/\sin 30°) \cos 30°$$
$$- 100 \text{ N} = 0$$

Add 100 N to each side of the equation.

$$A \sin 45° + (A \cos 45°/\sin 30°) \cos 30° = 100 \text{ N}$$

Substitute all trigonometric values:

$$A (0.707) + A (0.707/0.5)(0.866) = 100 \text{ N}$$

Perform algebraic calculations:

$$0.707 A + 1.22 A = 100 \text{ N}$$

Add the A terms, then

$$1.93 A = 100 \text{ N}$$

Solve for A by dividing both sides by 1.93:

$$A = 100 \text{ N}/1.93 = 51.8 \text{ N}$$

Now substitute this value for A into the solution for B:

$$B = 51.8 (\cos 45° \sin 30°)$$

Substitute for the trigonometric values:

$$B = 51.8 (0.707/0.5)$$

Solve algebraically:

$$B = 73.3 \text{ N}$$

The forces in the cords supporting a 100 N weight are 51.8 N and 73.3 N.

Pulley Systems

Pulleys may be used to set up either linear or concurrent systems. They may be used in a fixed position (Fig. 5–5A) or in a movable position (Fig. 5–5B).

The fixed pulley is used to change the action line of the force without changing its magnitude. An advantage is that although you do not gain force, you may place yourself in a more fa-

vorable position from which to exert the force. Most of us find that it is much easier to pull down than to lift up. Figure 5–5C shows a pulley being used to allow resistive exercise for the shoulder extensors. The tension on the cord is determined by the force of gravity on the weights. In the human body we can find many examples of a fixed pulley. Bony prominences such as the malleoli cause tendons to change direction and gain a more favorable angle of pull (Proctor and Paul, 1982). Surgeons often devise fixed pulley systems for this same purpose (Solonen and Hoyer, 1967).

In the moveable pulley system, one end of the rope is fixed, the pulley moves, and the supporting effort is exerted on the other end of the rope. In this case two strands support the resis-

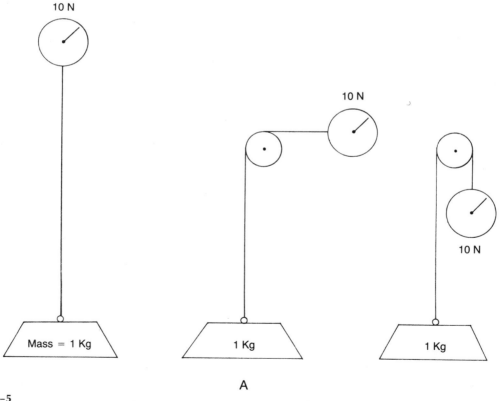

A

FIGURE 5–5

Fixed and moveable pulley systems. *A* and *C* show fixed pulleys, whereas *B* illustrates a moveable pulley. Note load and scale reading for each.

tance attached to the pulley. The force in any strand of the system is equal to that in each of the other strands (Fig. 5–6). In other words, the force in each strand is equivalent to the effort applied to the system. As shown in Figure 5–6,

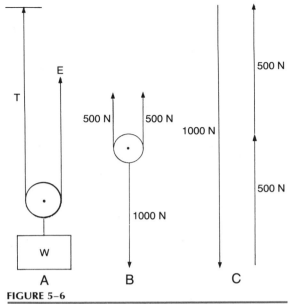

FIGURE 5–6

Moveable pulley system with two supporting strands. *A* through *C* illustrate graphic steps for solution of the forces in the system.

the resistance attached to the pulley is supported by two strands. Thus, if we had a 1000 N resistance, each of the two supporting strands would carry one-half the load, and an effort of 500 N would be needed to support the 1000 N resistance. This system gains in force, but the effort must move twice as far as the resistance.

The movable pulley may be placed in combination with the fixed pulley to gain more force advantage. Figure 5–7 shows a pulley system with four supporting strands. In this case the effort needed to support the resistance is only one-fourth of the resistance. Pulleys or various arrangements of pulleys are used in traction and exercise devices. Figure 5–8 illustrates two types of traction systems, one using a fixed pulley, the other a moveable pulley and two fixed pulleys. Remember that in an exercise pulley system, the effort applied by the patient may not equal the weight being lifted. Check the pulley arrangement.

Various traction devices provide examples of the concurrent arrangement of forces (McRae, 1989). In Figure 5–9, the tension lines converge

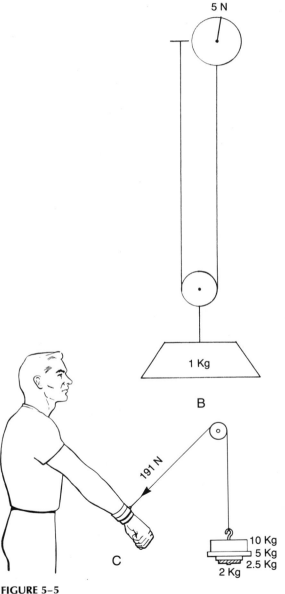

FIGURE 5–5

Continued

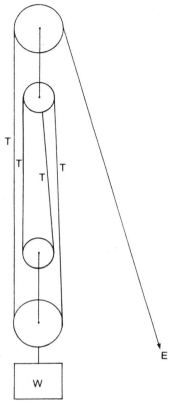

FIGURE 5–7

Moveable pulley system with four supporting strands.

at the sole of the foot, and their combined force is opposed by a force acting cephalad through the leg. Thus, the leg is offering a reaction force against the pulley lines.

To find the resultant of the concurrent force system by the algebraic method, it is necessary to resolve each force acting on the body into rectangular components, that is, to replace each original force by two forces that are at right angles to each other. We select a direction for the X and Y axes, and then take each force in turn and replace it by its X and Y components. Although the X and Y axes may be set up in any direction, for simplicity we usually choose either the X or Y axis to coincide with one of the forces. This will reduce the number of calculations necessary. After all the forces have been replaced by components lying along the X and Y axes, the system has been reduced to two linear systems that are at right angles to each other. For each of these two systems to be in equilibrium, the forces must be equal in magnitude, opposite in direction, and along the same line of action.

As you learned in Chapter 4, the X component is obtained by multiplying the force by the cosine of the angle that the force makes with the X axis. In like manner, the Y component is determined by multiplying the force by the sine of the same angle. Care must be taken to determine the proper algebraic sign for each of these components: remember those extending up and

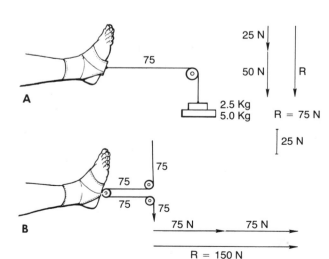

FIGURE 5–8

Fixed (*A*) and moveable (*B*) pulley systems used for traction.

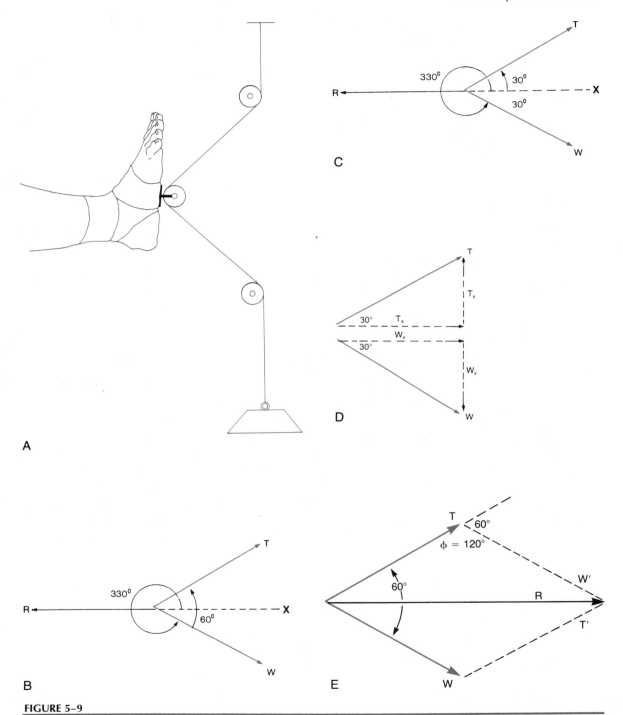

FIGURE 5–9

Leg traction. *B* through *E* illustrate graphic steps for solution of the forces in the system.

to the right are positive, and those directed down and to the left are negative.

▶ **PROBLEM 5–4**

To illustrate this procedure, let's take a look at the traction setup shown in Figure 5–9A. Suppose the weight attached to the traction system is 100 N. One hundred newtons would be acting along W, and 100 N of tension would be acting along T. The angle between W and T is set at 60°.

QUESTIONS:

How much traction force is being placed upon the leg? What is its reaction force?

SOLUTION:

We draw a free body diagram showing all the forces acting on the foot (Fig. 5–9B).

The first step after drawing the free body diagram is to choose coordinates. The problem will be easier if we have the X axis bisect the 60° angle formed by the two traction forces, T and W. This will establish the angles for the action of forces (Fig. 5–9C). Next, we solve each known force into its respective components, as shown in Figure 5–9D. Since the system is in equilibrium, the sum of all the forces equals zero ($\Sigma F = 0$). Thus, the sum of all the forces along the X axis equals zero ($\Sigma F_x = 0$) and the sum of all the forces along the Y axis equals zero ($\Sigma F_y = 0$). To find the components along the X axis, we multiply each force by the cosine of its respective angle with the X axis. Thus,

$$T_x = T \cos 30° \qquad \cos 30° = 0.866$$
$$= 100 \text{ N} \times 0.866$$
$$= 86.6 \text{ N}$$
$$W_x = W \cos 30°$$
$$= 100 \text{ N} \times 0.866$$
$$= 86.6 \text{ N}$$

Similarly, to find the Y components, we multiply each force by the sine of the same angle. Thus,

$$T_y = T \sin 30° \qquad \sin 30° = 0.5$$
$$= 100 \text{ N} \times 0.5$$
$$= 50 \text{ N}$$

Since the angle of W is 30° below the horizontal, its sine is negative ($\sin 330° = -\sin 30°$).

$$W_y = W (-\sin 30°)$$
$$= 100 \text{ N} (-0.5)$$
$$= -50 \text{ N}$$

The magnitude of W_y is 50 N, and since it has a negative sign we know it is directed downward.

To determine the forces acting linearly along the X axis, we can write:

$$\Sigma F_x = 0$$
$$T_x + W_x + R_x = 0$$
$$86.6 \text{ N} + 86.6 \text{ N} + R_x = 0$$

To find R_x, we must subtract R_x from both sides of the equation.

$$86.6 \text{ N} + 86.6 \text{ N} = -R_x$$
$$173.2 \text{ N} = -R_x, \text{ or}$$
$$R_x = -173.2 \text{ N}$$

This answer gives the magnitude for the X component of the leg reaction as 173.2 N and its direction is to the left.

To determine the forces acting along the Y axis, we write:

$$\Sigma F_y = 0$$
$$T_y + W_y + R_y = 0$$
$$50 \text{ N} + (-50 \text{ N}) + R_y = 0$$
$$R_y = 0$$

This shows that the R force has no Y component and lies along the X axis. However, to verify this, we can use the trigonometric function of tangent. Since $\tan \phi = \dfrac{R_y}{R_x}$, $\tan \phi = \dfrac{0}{-173.2}$ and $\tan \phi$ would be equal to 0° with the X axis. This same procedure is used no matter how many forces are involved.

A second method to determine the magnitude of traction force is by using the law of cosines (Fig. 4–9E):

$$R = \sqrt{T^2 + W^2 - 2T W \cos \phi}$$

Substitute the values:

$$R = \sqrt{(100)^2 + (100)^2 - 2(100)(100) \cos 120°}$$

Solve:

$$R = \sqrt{10000 + 10000 + 10000}$$
$$R = \sqrt{30000}$$
$$R = 173.2 \text{ N}$$

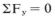

$$\Sigma F_y = 0$$

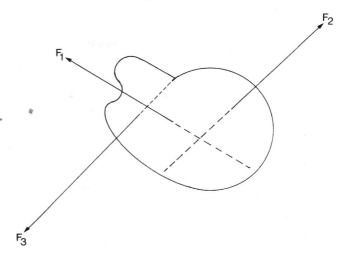

FIGURE 5–10

Noncurrent forces acting on a body.

SECOND CONDITION OF EQUILIBRIUM

In the previous force systems studied, the forces were concurrent. However, in many instances the forces may not all coincide at the same point (Fig. 5–10). In these cases, the forces act to cause rotation around a stationary point.

Parallel Force System

The simplest type of system in which the forces do not coincide may be called the parallel force system, where all the forces are parallel and lie in the same plane but do not have the same line of action (Fig. 5–11).

Two children on a teeter-totter exert downward forces that are parallel to one another. To be in translational equilibrium, the sum of their combined weights must be opposed by the upward force at the axis of the board (Fig. 5–11). In this situation, however, a second condition of equilibrium is introduced. A force acting on a rigid body at a distance from a fixed point tends to cause the body to rotate. In Figure 5–11, we can see that C produces a clockwise (CW) movement around the fixed point A, whereas B pro-

duces a counterclockwise (CCW) rotation. The distance from the point of application of force to the point of rotation is called the moment arm or lever arm. From your experience on a teeter-totter, you probably found that to balance, the heavier person had to sit closer to the axis than the lighter one. This illustrates the importance of the distance from the axis at which the force

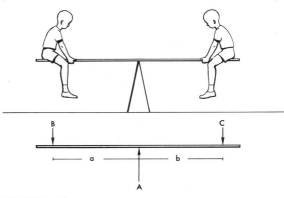

FIGURE 5–11

Here the forces are on opposite sides of the axis; B tends to turn the board in a counterclockwise direction, and C to turn it clockwise. In equilibrium, B + C (downward forces) = A (upward force).

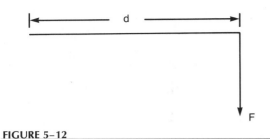

FIGURE 5–12

Application of a force (F) at a distance (d) from an axis. The moment = F × d.

is acting. The effectiveness of a force acting at a distance from the point of pivot depends not only on the magnitude of force but also on its location. An increase in either its magnitude or distance from the point of pivot increases its effectiveness. When you apply force during manual muscle testing, the rotatory effect depends not only on the amount of force you exert but also on the distance you are from the axis of the joints.

MOMENT OF FORCE

The application of force at a distance from the point of pivot provides the concept of *moments*, or *torque*. A moment of force is the tendency of a force to cause rotation about some axis and is equal to the magnitude of the force (F) multiplied by the perpendicular distance from the action line of the force to that point (d). It may also be defined as the product of the force component perpendicular to the lever arm (Fr) (Fig. 5–12) and the distance from the line of this force component to the point of rotation (d) (Fig. 5–13A). Thus, in either case, the moment (M), or torque, equals *force* (F) times *distance* (d), or M = F × d.

Note that in Figure 5–13A and 5–13B the calculations are different. In A, the moment is determined by the distance from the axis to the point of application times Fr, which is the force component of force (F) and is perpendicular to the moment arm (d). The force component, Fr, is calculated as

$$Fr/F = \cos \Theta$$
$$Fr = F \cos \Theta$$

Therefore, the moment is

$$M = Fr \times d, \text{ or}$$
$$M = (F \times \cos \Theta) \times d$$

In B, the moment is determined by the force (F) times d_1. The moment arm d_1 is a line drawn perpendicular to the line of application of force (F) through the axis of the level arm. It would be calculated as

$$d_1/d = \cos \Theta$$
$$d_1 = d \cos \Theta$$

Therefore, the moment is

$$M = F \times d_1, \text{ or}$$
$$M = F \times (\cos \Theta \times d)$$

Note that the factors of F, cos Θ, and d are common to both calculation methods.

Since a moment or torque is the product of a force and a distance, the units of moments are given in Newton meters (Nm), foot-pounds, kilogram-centimeters, or whatever units of

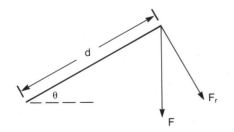

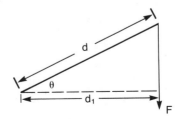

FIGURE 5–13

Two different ways to determine the magnitude of a moment: *A*, Force component (Fr) perpendicular to the force arm (d). *B*, The force (F) times the distance (d_1) perpendicular to the force.

A   B

measurement of distance and force are being used.

For the body to be in rotational equilibrium, the rotational motion must conform to Newton's first law. The body should be either at rest or rotating at a constant velocity. In this chapter we will restrict our study to the body at rest. The second condition of equilibrium states that the sum of moments about a point equals zero ($\Sigma M = 0$). That is, the sum of the clockwise moments (ΣM_{cw}) plus the sum of the counterclockwise moments (ΣM_{ccw}) equals zero. Thus, algebraically, we may write:

$$\Sigma M_{cw} + \Sigma M_{ccw} = 0$$

This is also referred to as the principle of moments. By convention, forces producing clockwise rotation are negative, and those acting to rotate the body counterclockwise are positive. Thus, the clockwise moment magnitude must equal the counterclockwise moment magnitude for no rotation to occur. This concept may be stated in equation form as

$$\Sigma M_{cw} = \Sigma M_{ccw}$$

Examples of various arrangements of moments of force are shown in Figure 5–14. Each of these arrangements illustrates how a clockwise moment set by 200 N and 25 cm is bal-

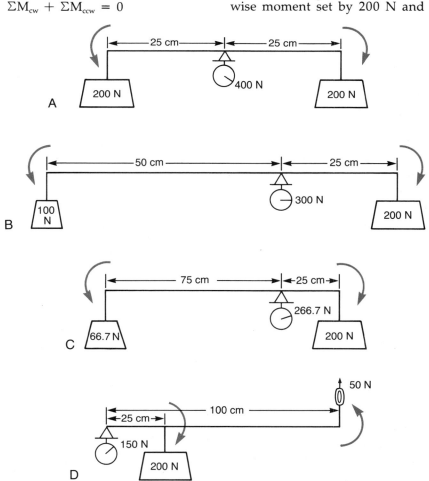

FIGURE 5–14

Various arrangements of moments to balance clockwise moment of a 200 N (20.4 Kg mass) at a distance of 25 cm.

anced by a counterclockwise moment. Note that force is located at the point of rotation (fulcrum) as well.

Lever System

Moments developed by coplanar forces can be seen in lever systems. A lever is one of the simplest machines known. Basically, it consists of two forces, an effort force and a resisting force, acting around a supporting force that provides for a point of pivot (Fig. 5–15). This axis or point of pivot is often called the *fulcrum*. The distance from the effort force to the fulcrum is the force arm (df) while the distance from the resisting force or resistance to the fulcrum is the resistance arm (dr). We may determine the mechanical advantage (MA) of the lever by dividing the force arm distance by the resistance arm dis-

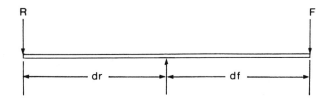

A

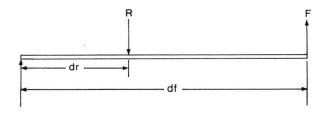

FIGURE 5–15

Three classes of levers: *A*, First class lever. *B*, Second class lever. *C*, Third class lever.

B

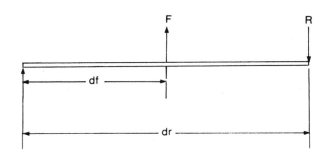

C

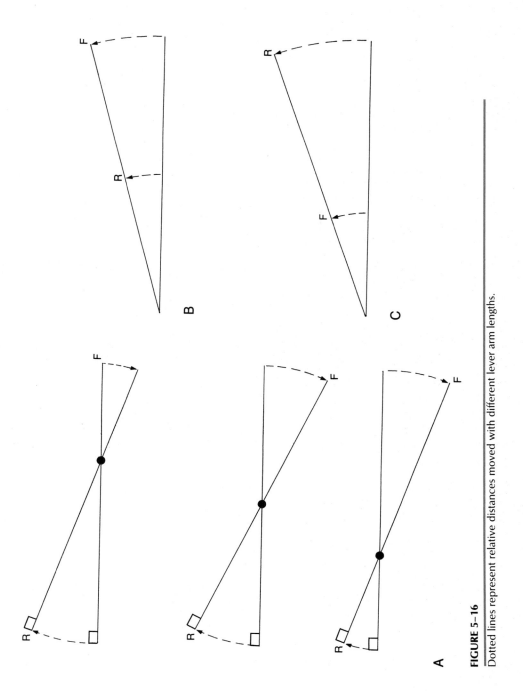

FIGURE 5-16

Dotted lines represent relative distances moved with different lever arm lengths.

tance $\left(\text{MA} = \dfrac{df}{dr} \right)$. Thus, the mechanical advantage of a lever depends upon where the forces are located. Knowledge of the MA provides a good estimate of the forces acting on the lever system. A lever may be used to increase force, change the effective direction of the effort force, or gain distance. It may be one of three types, depending upon the location of the two forces with respect to the fulcrum.

The *first class lever* has the fulcrum located between the effort and resistance. It is the most versatile of the lever systems. Depending upon the relative distances of the effort and resistance arms, it may take a small effort to lift a large resistance (Fig. 5–15A), or the effort may act at a small distance to move the resistance a greater distance (Fig. 5–16A). Its mechanical advantage can be either greater or less than one. The direction of force with the first class lever is always changed. That is, if the effort moves down, the resistance will move upward, and vice versa (Fig. 5–16A). The teeter-totter and a pair of scissors are good examples of the first class lever. Anatomical examples are the triceps muscle action on the ulna when the arm is held over the head (Fig. 5–17) and the splenius muscles, acting to extend the head across the atlanto-occipital joints (Fig. 5–18).

In the *second class lever*, the resistance is located between the effort and the fulcrum (Fig. 5–15B). Since the resistance arm is always less than the force arm, its mechanical advantage is always greater than one. The effort will be less than the resistance. However, in this arrangement, the effort must always move a greater distance than the resistance (Fig. 5–16B). The direction of movement is such that if the effort moves upward, the resistance moves upward, and if the effort moves downward, the resistance will go downward. Examples of the second class lever are the wheelbarrow and the nutcracker.

The *third class lever* arrangement has the effort located between the fulcrum and the resistance (Fig. 5–15C). In this situation, the effort arm is always less than the resistance arm. The mechanical advantage is always less than one. To support the resistance, effort must be of greater magnitude than the resistance, but the effort moves less distance than the resistance (Fig. 5–16C). Hence, we lose in effort but gain in distance. The third class lever system is seen in tweezers and fishing poles. Anatomically, many bony lever arrangements are of the third class type—for example, the biceps muscle action on the forearm (Fig. 5–19).

Based upon the preceding ideas, let's look at a few examples.

▶ PROBLEM 5–5

Consider three parallel forces acting vertically downward whose magnitudes from left to right are 320, 120, and 240 N. The distance between the 320 and 120 N forces is 0.6 m, and the distance between the 120 and 240 N forces is 0.4 m (Fig. 5–20).

QUESTION:

Find the resultant of the three forces—the single force that would have the same effect as all three.

SOLUTION:

As in the linear system, the magnitude of the resultant is equal to the sum of the forces ($R = \Sigma F$). Thus,

$$R = 320\,\text{N} + 120\,\text{N} + 240\,\text{N}$$
$$= 680\,\text{N}$$

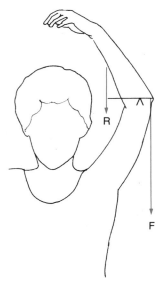

FIGURE 5–17

The forearm as a first class lever.

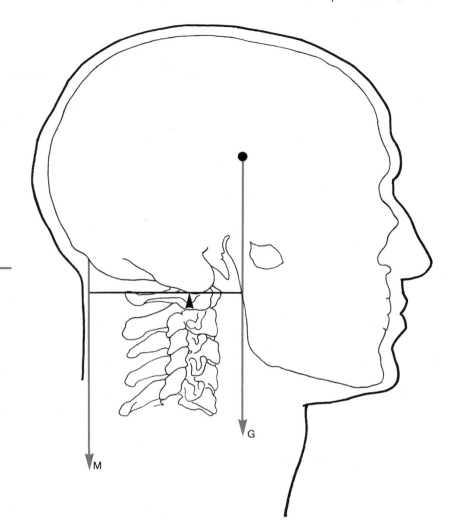

FIGURE 5–18

The head as a first class lever.

We now know the magnitude of the resultant. In this problem all the forces are acting in the same direction, so the resultant also must be acting in that direction, which in this case is downward. The remaining unknown term is the location of the resultant. We must apply the principle of moments to determine its position, and the first step is to choose a point from which to compute moments.

Selection of the point to be used as the moment center, or fulcrum, is most desirable on the action line of one of the forces. This eliminates one term from the equation, since the distance from that force to the selected point is zero. By selecting a moment center on the action line of the 320 N force, we will designate as X the distance from this point to the action line of the resultant (R). Then, according to the law of moments, R times X must be equal to the sum of the moments of the original forces about the moment center, and X will be equal to the sum of those moments divided by R, the magnitude of the resultant (Fig. 5–20).

$$RX = (120 \text{ N} \times 0.6 \text{ m}) + (240 \text{ N} \times 1.0 \text{ m})$$
$$= 72 \text{ Nm} + 240 \text{ Nm}$$
$$= 312 \text{ Nm}$$

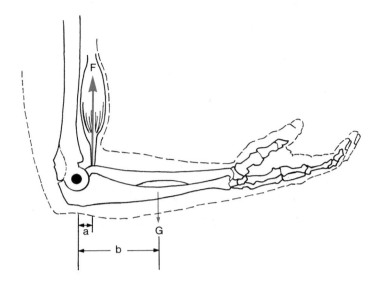

FIGURE 5–19

The forearm as a third class lever.

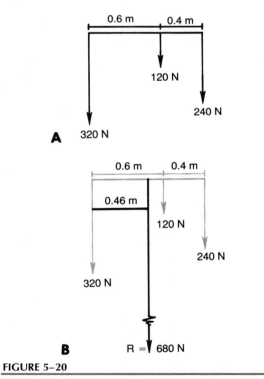

A

B

R = ▼ 680 N

FIGURE 5–20

A, Diagram of force system, problem 5–5. *B*, Location and magnitude of resultant.

We have already determined that R = 680 N hence

$$680 \text{ N X} = 312 \text{ Nm}$$

$$X = \frac{312 \text{ Nm}}{680 \text{ N}}$$

$$X = 0.46 \text{ m}$$

Since the two original forces both tend to rotate in a clockwise direction about the chosen moment center, the resultant force must also tend to rotate in the clockwise direction. The resultant is acting downward so the X distance, 0.46 m, must be measured to the right of the moment center in order to locate the action line of the resultant properly (i.e., a downward force rotating clockwise). An upward force with a magnitude of 680 N acting at this point would be an equilibrant, or reaction force, to place the system in equilibrium.

To illustrate that the center about which moments are taken can be selected arbitrarily at any point, let us repeat the computation by taking the action line of the 240 N force as the moment center (Fig. 5–21).

$$680X = (320 \text{ N} \times 1.0 \text{ m}) + (120 \text{ N} \times 0.4 \text{ m})$$

$$X = \frac{320 \text{ Nm} + 48 \text{ Nm}}{680 \text{ N}}$$

$$X = \frac{368 \text{ Nm}}{680 \text{ N}}$$

$$X = 0.54 \text{ m}$$

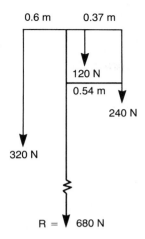

0.6 m   0.37 m

120 N

0.54 m

240 N

320 N

R = 680 N

FIGURE 5–21

Second solution to problem 5–5.

Here the forces are acting in a counterclockwise direction about the selected moment center; therefore, the resultant must be located 0.54 m to the left of this point, or at precisely the location arrived at in the previous solution.

▶ **PROBLEM 5–6**

In Problem 5–5 we found the resultant of forces acting on a lever. In this problem we will solve for a reaction force when the system is in equilibrium. Suppose that boy B weighs 330 N and is 1.5 m from the center of the teeter-totter, A, and that boy C weighs 260 N (Fig. 5–11).

QUESTION:

How much force is reacting to their body weight? How far from the center of the teeter-totter must C be in order to balance the system?

SOLUTION:

The first step after drawing the free body diagram is to solve for the reaction force at A using the first condition of equilibrium ($\Sigma F = 0$). All the forces in this case are vertical. Since B and C are acting downward, they are assigned negative values. Thus,

$$A + (-330 \text{ N}) + (-260 \text{ N}) = 0$$
$$A - 330 \text{ N} - 260 \text{ N} = 0$$
$$A - 590 \text{ N} = 0$$
$$A = 590 \text{ N}$$

Therefore, A is reacting upward with a force of 590 N.

The next step is to use the second condition of equilibrium ($\Sigma M = 0$) to solve for the location of C. Since B is acting counterclockwise and C is acting clockwise, B would be assigned a positive value. Thus,

$$\Sigma M = 0; \ \Sigma M = F \times d$$
$$\Sigma M_{cw} + \Sigma M_{ccw} = 0$$
$$(330 \text{ N} \times 1.5 \text{ m}) + (-260 \text{ N} \times C) = 0$$
$$(495 \text{ Nm}) + (-260 \text{ N} \times C) = 0$$
$$495 \text{ Nm} = 260 \text{ N} \times C$$
$$1.9 \text{ m} = C$$

The smaller boy (C) must sit 1.9 m from the axis of the board to balance the heavier boy (B).

Another example of parallel forces appears when the forearm is flexed to horizontal, gravity pulls downward on the forearm, and the biceps muscle pulls upward (Fig. 5–22). Since the lever arm of G is greater than that of B, the force B must be larger to counterbalance the moment exerted by the force G.

With the biceps muscle supporting the forearm at 90° of elbow flexion, the lever arm may be considered as the perpendicular distance from the tendon to the axis of the elbow joint. In this instance, the lever arm is anatomically fixed, but the magnitude of the muscle force can be varied to alter the moment.

The clockwise (CW) or counterclockwise (CCW) rotation of forces about the axis is indicated by means of a negative or positive sign (Fig. 5–23), or we can designate the actual direction of rotation by small curved arrows. In the example shown, the biceps muscle pull is a counterclockwise force opposed by the clockwise force of gravity, both acting about an axis or fulcrum at the elbow joint. These two opposing forces acting on the forearm follow exactly the same rule in regard to moments as do the children on the teeter-totter, even though here they are both on the same side of the fulcrum. When the forearm is in equilibrium, B × d must equal G × d'.

▶ **PROBLEM 5–7**

We may calculate the force needed by the muscle to maintain the forearm in the horizontal position and the joint force developed in the elbow. Suppose the forearm weighs 20 N and its center of mass is 15 cm from the elbow joint. The biceps muscle has a lever arm of 5 cm.

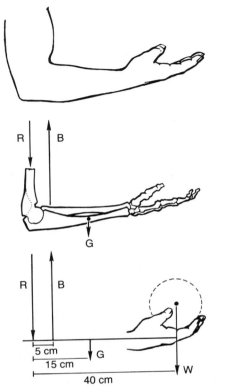

FIGURE 5–22

A parallel force system acting on the forearm in which W = weight in the hand; G = gravitational pull on the forearm; B = upward force of biceps muscle; and R = reaction force, shown as pressure of humerus against ulna. (A pressure equal and opposite to R is applied by the ulna against the humerus.)

We know the location of each force in the lever system. We do not know the magnitude of two of the three forces.

The first step to solve this problem is to use an equation with one unknown. Using the second condition of equilibrium will provide the needed equation.

By setting the moment axis at the elbow joint, one of the unknown forces (R) created no moment around that point (R × 0 = 0). Its lever arm equals zero. Therefore:

$$\Sigma M = 0$$

$$(B \times 5 \text{ cm}) + (-G \times d_G) = 0$$

Substitute the known values into the equation:

$$(B \times 5 \text{ cm}) + (-20 \text{ N} \times 15 \text{ cm}) = 0$$

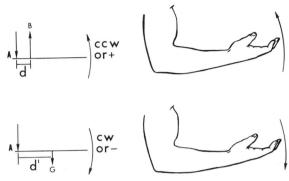

FIGURE 5–23

Designation of clockwise (CW) and counterclockwise (CCW) turning forces. The choice of signs to denote these is arbitrary but once selected must be used consistently throughout the problem. B × d = moment of biceps pull; G × d′ = moment of gravitational force. Force at joint = A.

Perform algebraic manipulations:

$$(5B \text{ Ncm}) + (-300 \text{ Ncm}) = 0$$

Add (300 Ncm) to each side of the equation:

$$300 \text{ Ncm} = 5B \text{ Ncm}$$

Divide both sides by 5:

$$300 \text{ Ncm}/5 \text{ cm} = B$$

Thus, B = 60 N.

The muscle must therefore pull with a force of 60 N in order for the clockwise moment to equal the counterclockwise moment.

A weight (W) of 45 N in the hand 40 cm from the elbow adds still another parallel force to the system, and the reacting force (R) on the distal humerus should also be included in our problem. Figure 5–22 shows the added turning effect, or moment of the weight in the hand about the elbow.

With the addition of a second clockwise moment, the muscle force acting in the previous example is increased.

QUESTION:
What muscle force is necessary to maintain the position of the forearm and weight? What is the reaction force at the elbow?

SOLUTION:
The free body diagram is shown in Figure 5–22. Obviously in this case the elbow joint is the axis of motion and the joint force would produce no moment, since its distance from the axis is zero (R × 0 = 0). The moments produced by each force separately

need to be calculated, and then these moments are added algebraically. We may write:

$$(-20 \text{ N} \times 15 \text{ cm}) +$$
$$(-45 \text{ N} \times 40 \text{ cm}) + (B \times 5 \text{ cm}) = 0$$
$$(-300 \text{ Ncm}) +$$
$$(-1800 \text{ Ncm}) + (B \times 5 \text{ cm}) = 0$$
$$(-2100 \text{ Ncm}) +$$
$$(B \times 5 \text{ cm}) = 0$$
$$B \times 5 \text{ cm} = 2100 \text{ Ncm}$$
$$B = \frac{2100 \text{ Ncm}}{5 \text{ cm}}$$
$$B = 420 \text{ N}$$

The plus sign for the moment indicates that the 420 N muscle force is acting counterclockwise.

After determining the muscle force, we may find the joint force using the first condition of equilibrium ($\Sigma F = 0$). Since the forces are parallel and vertical, there is no force acting in the X direction. Thus, for the Y direction: $\Sigma F_y = 0$. Since G and W are acting downward, they are given negative signs. The direction of R will be determined with the solution of the problem:

$$420 + (-20) + (-45) + R = 0$$
$$420 - 20 - 45 + R = 0$$
$$420 - 65 + R = 0$$
$$355 + R = 0$$
$$R = -355 \text{ N}$$

Therefore, the magnitude of the reaction force is 355 N acting downward.

It is important to note that if the total force on the rigid body is zero, and the total moment about a point in the body is zero, then the total moment about any point on the body will also be zero. By beginning with the second condition of equilibrium, we may set the turning point at the point of application of one of the unknown forces. This reduces the moment of that force to zero, since its distance from the turning point is zero.

▶ **PROBLEM 5–8**

We may then check the previous problem by taking the point of muscle insertion as the point of pivot. The distances of each force must be changed accordingly (Fig. 5–24). The 45 N weight and forearm still produce a clockwise motion, so the joint force probably acts counterclockwise. We may write:

$$(-20 \text{ N} \times 10 \text{ cm}) +$$
$$(-45 \text{ N} \times 35 \text{ cm}) + (R \times 5 \text{ cm}) = 0$$
$$(-200 \text{ Ncm}) + (-1575 \text{ Ncm}) +$$
$$(R \times 5 \text{ cm}) = 0$$
$$(-1775 \text{ Ncm}) + (R \times 5 \text{ cm}) = 0$$
$$R \times 5 \text{ cm} = 1775 \text{ Ncm}$$
$$R = \frac{1775 \text{ Ncm}}{5 \text{ cm}}$$
$$R = 355 \text{ N}$$

The positive value for R indicates that it is acting counterclockwise. Using the first condition of equilibrium, we may determine B as follows:

$$B + (-355) + (-20) + (-45) = 0$$
$$B + (-420) = 0$$
$$B = 420 \text{ N}$$

The muscle force has a magnitude of 420 N acting upward. These answers are the same as those found in the first procedure. This second procedure serves as a check for the first and also illustrates that for a body in equilibrium, any point may be selected as the axis. However, it is more convenient to choose the moment center at one of the unknown forces.

Often forces on a body reduce to a parallel force system in which there are two noncolinear parallel forces equal in magnitude and opposite in direction. Since the forces are equal in magnitude and opposite in direction, the sum of forces equals zero ($\Sigma F = 0$), and no linear motion will occur. In this situation, however, these forces combine to produce a turning effect on the body. The axis of motion is midway between the two forces. This pair of forces is called a *couple*. An example of a couple is two hands on a steering wheel (Fig. 5–25A). We can draw a free body diagram (Fig. 5–25B) and algebraically determine the general formula for force couples. In this case, F represents the magnitude of force, which is the same applied by each hand, r represents the radius of the wheel, and d is the diameter of the wheel. If we take the axis of the wheel as the center of rotation, we may write the equation for the clockwise moments:

$$C \text{ (couple)} = (F \times r) + (F \times r)$$
$$= 2 (F \times r)$$
$$= 2Fr$$
$$C = Fd, \text{ since } d = 2r$$

Thus, the resultant moment of a couple is $C = Fd$, where F is the magnitude of one of the forces, and d is the distance between them.

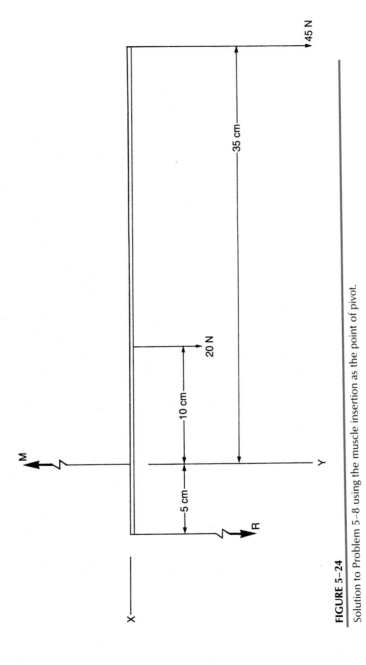

FIGURE 5–24

Solution to Problem 5–8 using the muscle insertion as the point of pivot.

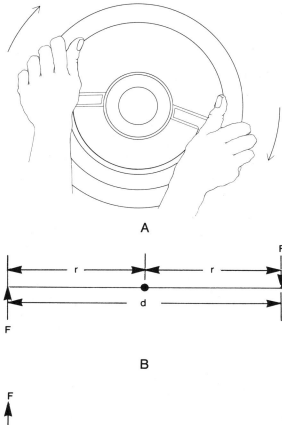

A

B

C

FIGURE 5–25

Force couple. *A*, Steering wheel. *B*, Moments around axis. *C*, Fd equivalent to 2 Fr.

Note that this formula is the same as if we used one of the forces for the axis (Fig. 5–25C) but not as a couple.

The clockwise moment is the force (F) times the distance (d) from the axis, or

$$M = Fd$$

Suppose nurses N and S in Figure 5–26 wish to turn a bed around. Each pushes with a force of 100

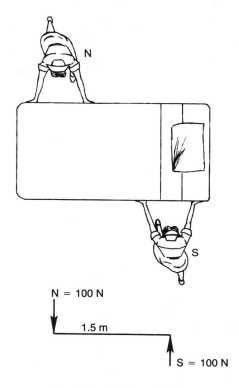

N = 100 N

1.5 m

S = 100 N

C = 1.5 × 100 N = 150 Nm

FIGURE 5–26

Example of a couple (C) in which equal and opposite forces are applied to either end of a bed to turn it around. C = the product of one of the forces and the distance between them.

N at opposite ends of the bed in opposing directions. The forces are applied 1.5 m feet apart, thus exerting a moment of 150 Nm in a counterclockwise direction. In this case the sum of the forces in the force system is zero; however, the sum of the moments is not zero, but equal to the magnitude of the couple. The equations for the resultant become

$$R = \Sigma F, \text{ and } C = \Sigma M$$

▶ **PROBLEM 5–9**

Consider the parallel force system shown in Figure 5–27.

QUESTION:
Find the resultant of the system.

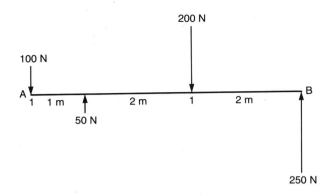

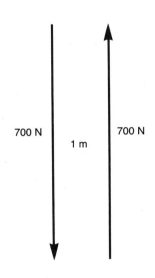

FIGURE 5–27

Force system in which the resultant is a couple. C = 700 Nm.

SOLUTION:

With the upward forces positive, then

$$\Sigma F = (-100) + (-200) + (250) + (50) = 0$$

Taking moments about point A (CW moments are negative)

$$C = \Sigma M_A$$
$$= (50 \text{ N} \times 1 \text{ m}) + (-200 \text{ N} \times 3 \text{ m})$$
$$+ (250 \text{ N} \times 5 \text{ m})$$
$$= 700 \text{ Nm}$$

The resultant is a counterclockwise couple of 700 Nm. If we select another center about which to take moments, for example, point B on the 250 N force, the answer will be the same:

$$C = (200 \text{ N} \times 2 \text{ m}) + (-50 \text{ N} \times 4 \text{ m})$$
$$+ (100 \text{ N} \times 5 \text{ m})$$
$$C = 700 \text{ Nm}$$

The magnitude of the forces in the couple is unimportant so long as the product of one force and the intervening distance is 700 Nm. Note that the forces in the couple must be directed to give counterclockwise rotation, since the answer is positive.

It is apparent that if all the forces in a force system extend in the same direction, the resultant cannot be a couple. Pure rotation cannot take place unless there is a couple. If nurse N or nurse S in Figure 5–26 pushed alone, the bed would move sideways in addition to rotating about a central point.

Examples of arrangements of muscles that suggest the action of a couple include those bringing about axial rotation of segments as follows:

1. Sternocleidomastoid and contralateral splenius capitis muscles act together to rotate the head about the axis between the first and second cervical vertebrae.

2. External oblique and contralateral latissimus dorsi muscles rotate the thorax on the pelvis or vice versa. (The large central portion of the external oblique muscle depends on the pull of the opposite internal oblique muscle to accomplish axial rotation.)

3. The horizontal component of the upper trapezius muscle pulls together with the serratus anterior (Fig. 5–28) to rotate the scapula upward in arm elevation and control its downward rotation. When the serratus anterior is paralyzed, the arm cannot be lifted above shoulder level.

Another example is rotation of the pelvis in the sagittal plane around the frontal axis. Anterior tilting is accomplished by hip flexors and lumbar extensor muscles, and posterior tilting by anterior abdominal muscles and hip extensors.

When assisting a patient in walking, the physical therapist may apply manual guiding forces to rotate the thorax or pelvis in the manner of a couple, with one hand on each side of the part. Some manual stretches for scoliosis involve vigorous twisting forces applied to the trunk in opposite directions.

Since the turning effect of a couple is measured by the product of one of the forces and the distance between them, a couple composed of small forces with a large distance between them is just as effective in producing turning as one in which the forces are large and the distance between them is small. For example, nurses N and S in Figure 5–26 would have to push twice as hard if they were only 0.75 m apart to produce the same effect on the bed. Turning forces applied to the large steering wheel of a bus or truck provide a greater moment for a given effort than would the same forces applied to the smaller wheel of an automobile. A large doorknob is easier to turn than a small bolt.

When the arm is rotated about its longitudinal axis, the total forces producing the rotation must constitute a couple; these forces must be acting at the glenohumeral joint, since rotation takes place here. The forearm or thigh can also be rotated by muscle forces, which produce a couple. The fact that muscle forces provide a couple to produce rotation can be demonstrated readily. Suppose the hand grasps a stick held at right angles to the forearm. If a single force is applied to one end of the stick, it will not prevent rotation of the forearm. Rotation can be prevented only if two forces of equal magnitude and opposite direction (a couple) are applied to the stick.

A couple acting on a body will always cause rotation of the body, or will tend to make the body rotate if it is being held at rest by opposing forces. The only method of maintaining equilibrium of an object on which a couple is acting is by means of another couple acting in the opposite direction and having the same magni-

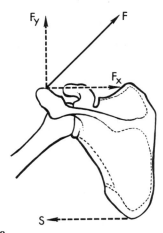

FIGURE 5–28

Resolution of upper trapezius force (F) into supporting component (F_y) and adductory component (F_x). Abductor force (S) of serratus anterior muscle is shown below. (Adapted from Inman VT, Saunders JB, Abbott LC: The function of the shoulder joint. J Bone Joint Surg 26A:1–30, 1944.)

tude. A couple cannot be held in equilibrium by means of a single force. The points of application of the forces that constitute a couple are immaterial in regard to the production of rotation. That is, the body will rotate regardless of where the couple is applied to it.

The free body diagram shown in Figure 5–29 was used by Radcliffe (1957) to illustrate the force system acting at mid-stance when an amputee walks on a Canadian-type hip-disarticulation prosthesis. The forces acting on the amputee are exerted by gravity and by the prosthesis at this point in the gait cycle, since the normal foot is off the ground. The four forces acting on the torso form two sets of force couples that act in opposite directions. The body weight (W) acting through the center of gravity and the upward supporting force (I) of the prosthesis form a clockwise couple. This would cause the pelvis to tilt downward on the side of the upraised normal foot if it were not opposed by a second couple acting in a counterclockwise

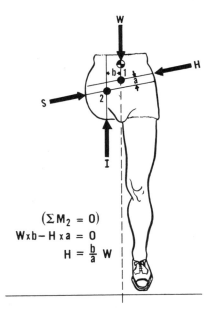

$$(\Sigma M_2 = 0)$$
$$W \times b - H \times a = 0$$
$$H = \frac{b}{a} W$$

FIGURE 5–29

Force analysis of Canadian-type hip-disarticulation prosthesis. W (body weight) and I (prosthesis) acting at distance b are opposed by H and S (waist band tension and reaction of the opposite hip) acting at distance a.

direction. This is provided by tension in the waist band and by reaction against the normal hip. The four forces shown are of the same order of magnitude, since the dimensions a and b are approximately equal.

General Force System

The parallel system is simply a special system in which all forces are parallel. In many situations the forces acting on a body are neither parallel nor linear nor concurrent. If we encounter a system of forces in a plane that does not fit into any of the previous categories—linear, concurrent, or parallel—we are dealing with a general force system. A general force system in equilibrium always includes at least four forces. A system of three forces in equilibrium must fall into one of the categories already considered. For examples of general force systems, we may return to previous problems in which the weight of the part was omitted. For instance, consider again the Russell traction apparatus shown in Figure 4–12 with a resultant force in line with the femur. Suppose we add the weight of the leg and foot (36 N) to the computation of the resultant force. We find that the force system does not fit into any of our previous classifications. As before, in problems involving the general force system we may be required to find the resultant of a number of forces, or we may be dealing with an object known to be in equilibrium.

▶ **PROBLEM 5–10**

Let's take the example of the biceps muscle acting on the forearm when the elbow is not at a 90° angle, but when the forearm is 30° below the horizontal and the biceps inserts at an angle of 45° with the forearm. The muscle insertion is 5 cm from the elbow joint, the 20 N forearm weight is centered 15 cm from the elbow, and a 40 N weight is held in the hand 30 cm from the joint center (Fig. 5–30). With the forearm position other than horizontal, gravity cannot act at 90° to the limb. However, a component of its force will act perpendicular to the limb. Similarly, with the change in position, the biceps muscle will not pull at 90° to the forearm, but, as shown in Chapter 4, a component of its force will.

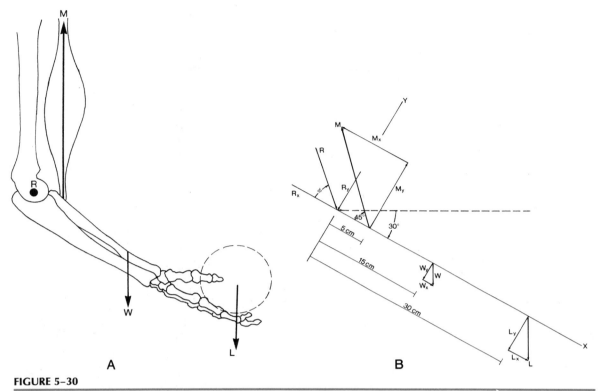

FIGURE 5–30

Static forces about the elbow joint when the forearm is 30° below the horizontal.

QUESTIONS:

What is the muscle force needed to maintain the forearm position 30° below the horizontal? What are the elbow joint forces?

SOLUTION:

Again we draw a free body diagram as shown in Figure 5–30B. Since the pull of gravity and the muscle insertion are not perpendicular to the forearm, we must find their perpendicular components. From the principle of supplementary angles, we find that the weight components, perpendicular to the forearm (W_y and L_y) form 30° angles with the force of gravity (W) and the load (L). Thus, $W_y = W \cos 30°$ and $L_y = L \cos 30°$. The muscle force is 45° with the forearm, so $M_y = M \sin 45°$. After setting the X axis along the forearm, we use the elbow joint as the axis of motion and solve for the sum of moments around this point ($R_y \times 0 = 0$).

$$\Sigma M = 0$$

$$(M_y \times 5 \text{ cm}) + (W_y \times 15 \text{ cm}) + L_y \times 30 \text{ cm}) = 0$$

Substitute for y values:

$$(M_y \times 5 \text{ cm}) + (W \cos 30° \times 15 \text{ cm})$$
$$+ (L \cos 30° \times 30 \text{ cm}) = 0$$

Substitute in values:

$$(M_y \times 5 \text{ cm}) + (-20 \text{ N} \times 0.866 \times 15 \text{ cm})$$
$$+ (-40 \text{ N} \times 0.866 \times 30 \text{ cm}) = 0$$

Solve:

$$(M_y \times 5 \text{ cm}) + (-259.8 \text{ Ncm}) + (-1039.2 \text{ Ncm}) = 0$$
$$(M_y \times 5 \text{ cm}) + (-1299 \text{ Ncm}) = 0$$

Add 1299 to both sides:

$$(M_y \times 5 \text{ cm}) = 1299 \text{ Ncm}$$

Divide by 5 cm:

$$M_y = 1299 \text{ Ncm/5 cm}$$
$$M_y = 259.8 \text{ N (CCW)}$$

Solve for M:

$$M_y = M \sin 45°$$

$$M_y/\sin 45° = M$$

Substitute values:

$$259.8/0.707 = M$$

Divide by 0.707:

$$M = 367.5 \text{ N}$$

The rotatory component of the muscle has a magnitude of 259.8 N, producing a counterclockwise moment. Since M_y is acting upward, it is given a positive sign.

$$M_y = M \sin 45°$$

$$259.8 \text{ N} = M \times 0.707$$

$$M = 367.5 \text{ N}$$

For the joint force, we use the sum of the force components acting along the forearm, and the sum of the rotatory components, where $\Sigma F_x = 0$ and $\Sigma F_y = 0$:

$$\Sigma F_x = M_x + W_x + L_x + R_x = 0$$

$$M_x = M \cos 45°$$
$$= 367.5 \text{ N} \times 0.707$$
$$= -259.8 \text{ N to the left}$$

$$W_x = W \sin 30°$$
$$= 20 \text{ N} \times 0.5$$
$$= 10 \text{ N to the right}$$

$$L_x = L \sin 30°$$
$$= 40 \text{ N} \times 0.5$$
$$= 20 \text{ N}$$

$$(-259.8 \text{ N}) + (10 \text{ N}) + (20 \text{ N}) + R_x = 0$$

$$(-229.8 \text{ N}) + R_x = 0$$

$$R_x = 229.8 \text{ N}$$
to the right

$$\Sigma F_y = M_y + W_y + L_y + R_y = 0$$

$$(259.8 \text{ N}) + (-17.32 \text{ N}) +$$
$$(-34.64 \text{ N}) + R_y = 0$$

$$(207.84 \text{ N}) + R_y = 0$$

$$R_y = -207.84 \text{ N}$$
downward

The magnitude of the joint force (R) is found using the Pythagorean theorem:

$$R = \sqrt{R_x^2 + R_y^2}$$
$$= \sqrt{52808.04 + 43197.46}$$
$$= \sqrt{96005.5}$$
$$= 309.85 \text{ N}$$

We determine the direction using any one of the trigonometric functions:

$$\tan \phi = \frac{R_y}{R_x}$$
$$= \frac{207.84}{229.84}$$
$$= 0.904$$
$$\phi = 42°$$

The direction is to the right and downward at a 42° angle with the X axis.

In the previous problem the moment of a force may be found by multiplying the total force by the perpendicular distance from its action line to the moment center (Fig. 5–31). This product will be the same as that obtained by taking the rotatory component and multiplying by the perpendicular distance from its action line to the moment center.

The choice of method in finding moments is a matter of convenience. For example, in Figure 5–32 it would be difficult to measure accurately distances 1 and 1′, and the method used in the previous problem would be preferable. Replacing vectors by equivalent components enables us to change the force diagram to a form that will permit us to solve problems. For more practice, solve the forearm problem as previously presented except for a change in its position to 30° above the horizontal, and 15°, 45°, and 60° above and below the horizontal.

EXAMPLES FROM THE LITERATURE

An example of the linear system of forces has been developed by Ilizarov (1990). Ilizarov has designed an external skeletal fixation system for the management of orthopedic problems including limb-length discrepancies, fracture healing, nonunions, bone deformities, and bone infections (Schwartsman et al., 1989; Ilizarov,

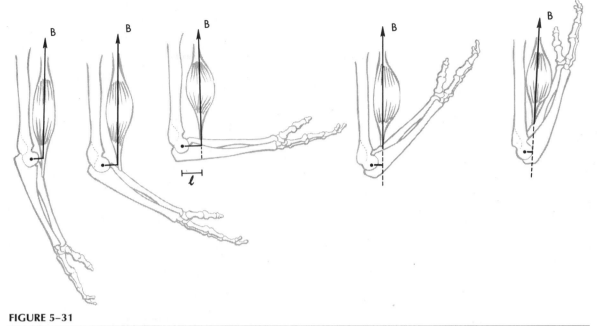

FIGURE 5–31

The biceps (B) at various points of elbow flexion, showing variations in the lever arm (l = perpendicular distance from action of tendon to elbow axis).

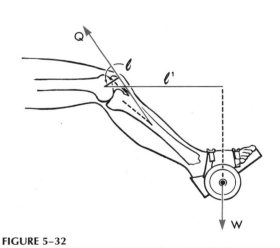

FIGURE 5–32

Alternate method of computing moments which does not involve finding rectangular components. Q × l = moment of quadriceps muscle; W × l¹ = moment of exercise load (W).

1990). The basis of this method is the principle of tension-stress, which states that living tissue, when placed under a constant low-magnitude force, begins to proliferate. In general, the linear force should allow 1.0 mm distraction per day at about 60-step intervals. If the apparatus is incorrectly applied and the forces are not directed properly, lateral, rotational, or a combination displacement may occur. A second linear force, compression, is needed to activate earlier mineralization. During the fixation treatment time, weight-bearing and range of motion are essential.

A similar application of linear forces across the epiphyseal plate has been reported by Kenwright and co-workers (1990). They state that distraction of the epiphysis is regularly being used to correct leg-length inequality and to lengthen limbs of achondroplastic patients. Small daily loads below 20 N were used successfully in their experiments.

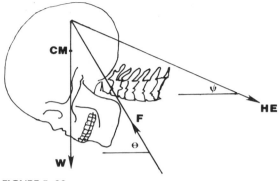

FIGURE 5–33

Free body diagram used to calculate the force of the extensor muscles needed to maintain the neck in extension. W = weight of the head; CM = center of mass; HE = force of the extensor muscles; F = joint reaction force; θ = angle at which the joint reaction forces bisect the line of extensor pull, and ψ = angle of inclination of the cervical spine. (From Nolan Jr., JP, Sherk HH: Biomechanical evaluation of the extensor musculature of the cervical spine. Spine *13*:9–11, 1988.)

The concurrent forces system was used to validate an experimental model by Nolan and Sherk (1988) to determine the force needed by the extensor muscles of the cervical spine to balance the weight of head and neck while in the prone position (Fig. 5–33). Their calculated value of 13.56 Kg-force (133 N) was 94.5 percent of the experimental results of 14.38 Kg-force (141 N). From these calculations, the joint force in the cervical area can be determined. You must remember that errors in placement of the center of mass and muscle line of application could have been reasons for part of the discrepancy in the comparison.

The concurrent forces system has also been used to illustrate the forces at the patellofemoral joint (Fig. 5–34) by Reilley and Martens (1972), Maquet (1976), and Ferguson and co-workers (1979). The values of the quadriceps muscle force and patellar tendon force must first be established by using the second condition of equilibrium. The patellofemoral joint forces have been studied under various conditions including lifting weights, deep knee bends, going up and down stairs, level walking, and following certain surgical procedures. They determined that the patellofemoral joint force depends both on the contraction force of the quadriceps and the angle of the knee. The more the knee is flexed, the greater the joint force will be. (This result supports what you learned in Chapter 4.) The greatest value of the patellofemoral joint force (7.5 times the body weight) was found during deep knee bends (Reilly and Martens, 1972). The joint force was shown to be reduced following anterior tibial tubercle elevation (Ferguson et al., 1979).

A university applied clinical example of the parallel force system is the so-called three-point pressure principle of brace design. The supporting forces of the brace are so arranged that two

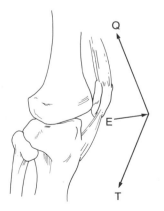

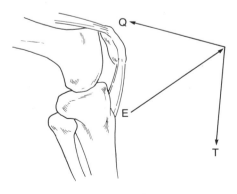

FIGURE 5–34

Concurrent force system at the patellofemoral joint. Q = quadriceps muscle force; T = patellar tendon force; E = equilibrant of the two forces that occurs at the patellofemoral joint. Note that the magnitude of E changes as the knee angle and muscle force change.

A

B

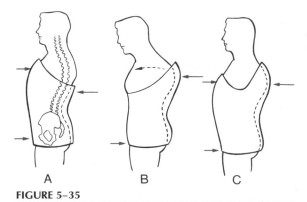

FIGURE 5–35

A, Basic principle of three-point pressure in bracing, applied to control of vertebral column alignment. B, Stabilization inadequate because brace is too low in front, allowing upper trunk to move forward. C, Stabilization inadequate because brace is too high in back, obtaining compression but not correction of alignment.

forces pressing against the trunk or limb are opposed by a third force, which is located between the other two, Jordan (1939) has explained this principle as follows:

"Three main forces . . . should be distributed over adequate surfaces or divided into a number of single units, the sum of which is equal in degree and direction to the desired or main force." The force per unit area is an important factor, as are the "give" or yield of the material in the brace parts, and the nature of the body tissues sustaining the pressure. Jordan emphasized that brace forces "must be active." In other words, the brace must fit well and do its job of immobilization or support of the body.

In a discussion of proper application of three-point pressure in bracing, Thomas (1952) stated that the single opposing force is equal in magnitude to the two forces acting in the same direction. This is an important factor in skin pressure. Figure 5–35, redrawn from Jordan (1939), illustrates the desired three-point application of forces in spinal bracing: thrusts in the posterior direction against the pelvis and upper thorax are opposed by an anterior thrust against the spine. A poorly designed brace or cast will fail to provide the necessary forces at the proper levels. In B the brace is too low in front and the upper force is absent. In C the brace is too high in back.

The treatment of scoliosis may also be approached using the three-point principle or parallel force system (Radin et al., 1979; Schijvens et al., 1982). Schijvens and associates (1982) described a method in which lateral force applied

FIGURE 5–36

A, Transverse forces needed to correct scoliosis. B, Graphic representation of the bending-moment variation needed to correct scoliosis. C, Bending moment caused by the transverse forces. (From Schijvens AWM, Snijders CJ, Seroo JM, et al.: Mechanics of the spine: Analysis of its flexibility and rigidity, postural control and correction of the pathological spine. *In* Ghista DN (Ed): Osteoarthromechanics. Washington, DC, Hemisphere Publishing, 1982, pp 263–314.)

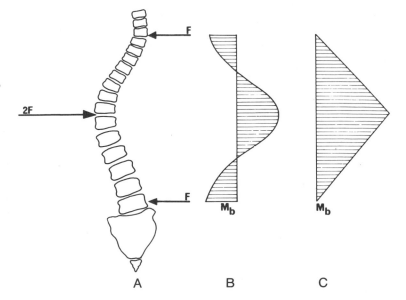

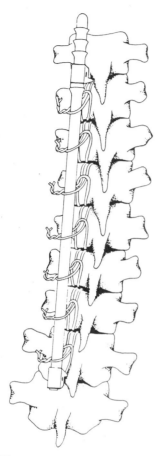

FIGURE 5–37

Schematic of scoliotic spine with distracted Harrington rod (Moe type) secured in place by twisted wires. (From Silverman BJ, Greenbarg PE: Idiopathic scoliosis posterior spine fusion with Harrington rod and sublaminar wiring. Orthop Clin North Am *19*:269–279, 1988.)

directly to the vertebrae is used to correct scoliosis (Fig. 5–36). The correction is followed by linear force from an internal fixator such as the Harrington distraction rod (Fig. 5–37). Ghista and associates (1988) presented a similar approach for surgical correction of scoliosis. They described a system of combined lateral wires and a distraction rod, either in conjunction with a Luque rod or without it (Fig. 5–38). Radin and associates (1979) have indicated that such a

curved rod or a straight rod in a curved bone will provide three-point fixation.

Another treatment option was described by Radin and co-workers (1979). In this case a body jacket and serial casting apply the transverse forces. However, as Jordon warned in 1939, Watts (1979) admonished that the placement of the pads for the three-point forces must be done with extreme care. Pads placed as little as one vertebral segment too high above the apex of the curve may increase the curve (Fig. 5–39).

Axial loading using linear force may be combined with the body jacket. Axial loading may be applied using halopelvic or halofemoral traction (Fig. 5–40). The use of combined parallel and linear forces appears to be particularly suitable for the treatment of scoliosis (White and Panjabi, 1976; Silverman and Greenbarg, 1988; Moe et al., 1984; Ghista et al., 1988; Mielke et al., 1989; Jayaraman et al., 1989; Winter and Lonstein, 1989).

The same basic design is applied in leg bracing. In describing a leg brace for genu valgum, Trosclair (1959) stated, "There are in use today various types of leg braces, but practically all types use the same basic three-point principle." These may have double or single uprights. In the brace shown in Figure 5–41, straps attach to the upright above and below the knee and buckle to the contoured medial knee cup. Pressure in this brace

is present at some of the most permissible places . . . at the thigh from below greater trochanter to just above the knee; at the lateral portion of the calf (. . . not enough to place excessive pressure on the peroneal nerve); at the ankle (where some patients will require a pressure button); and last on the medial condyles of the knee where we do not have nerve or blood supply of superficial position.

Forces necessary for the correction of foot deformity are shown in Figure 5–42. The same principle of three-point pressure is utilized for this purpose. Plaster casts are applied for the correction of various types of clubfeet (Fig. 5–42B). T-straps on foot braces may be used to exert force in the control of foot or ankle alignment. Figure 5–42C shows a brace designed to

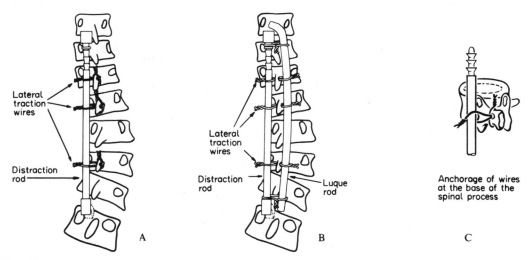

FIGURE 5–38

Combined distraction and lateral traction application systems: *A*, Without Luque rod. *B*, With Luque rod (on *right*). *C*, Attachment of wires to the base of the spinous processes. (From Ghista DN, Vivani GR, Subbaraj K, et al.: Biomechanical basis of optimal scoliosis surgical correction. J Biomech *21*:77–88, 1988.)

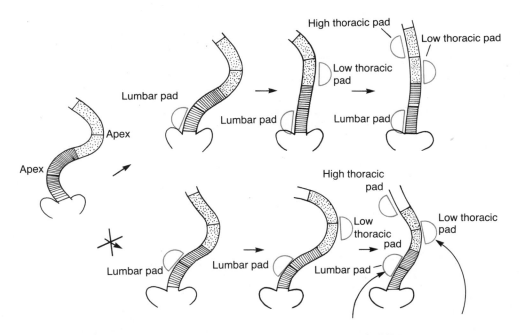

PAD TOO HIGH PREVENTS SPINE FROM CORRECTING AND INCREASES CURVE ABOVE

FIGURE 5–39

Pads applied for correction of lateral spinal curve. (From Watts HG: Bracing spinal deformities. Orthop Clin North Am *10*:769–785, 1979.)

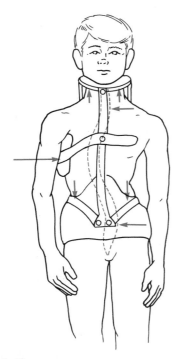

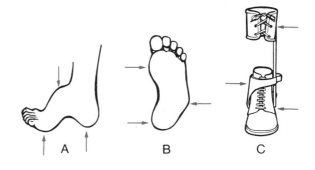

Three-point pressure in correction of foot deformity. *A*, Sites of corrective forces in treatment of pes cavus. *B*, Forefoot adduction. *C*, Short leg brace with ankle T-strap to correct foot pronation on the left side.

FIGURE 5–40

The Milwaukee brace showing the three-point and traction forces. Note that this is a combined loading system that should allow for maximum control or alteration of the scoliosis. (From Radin EL, Simon SR, Rose RM, et al.: Practical Biomechanics for the Orthopedic Surgeon. © 1979 by John Wiley and Sons. Reprinted by permission of John Wiley and Sons, Inc.)

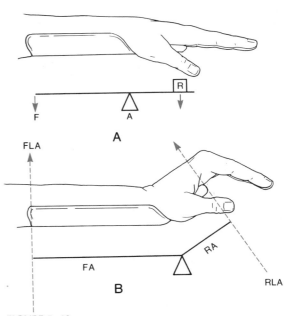

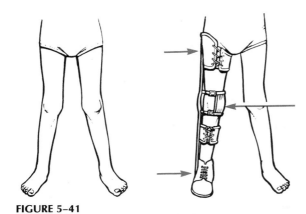

FIGURE 5–41

Three-point pressure in bracing for genu valgum (knock-knee) deformity.

FIGURE 5–43

A, Many splints may be functionally classified as first class levers. F = force; A = axis; R = resistance. *B*, With the wrist bar placed in extension, the splint continues to act as a first class lever, but the direction of the resistance line of action is altered. FLA = force line of action; FA = force arm; RA = resistance arm; RLA = resistance line of action. (From Fess EE, Phillips CA: Hand Splinting Principles and Methods, 2nd Ed. St Louis, CV Mosby, 1987.)

correct foot pronation. In varus deformity of the foot, the arrangement is reversed, with the upright inside and the T-strap outside.

Several authors (Kiel, 1983; Fess and Philips, 1987; Duncan, 1989) have discussed the lever system for hand splinting. They present the simple wrist cock-up splint as a first-class lever. The basic device with the wrist in the neutral position has a three-point parallel force system (Fig. 5–43) with the central axis point (W) always being exactly over the wrist joint (Kiel, 1983). The hand (R) may be considered the resistance, while the forearm trough (F) provides the force or effort.

Fess and Philips (1987) describe another configuration in which the wrist bar is placed in extension so that the three forces are no longer parallel (Fig. 5–44). The forces in this example may be solved by either the general or concurrent forces system if the magnitude of one of the forces is known and the location of the forces is determined.

Soeur (1982) and Gozna (1982) describe the effect of parallel forces causing a fracture (Fig. 5–44A). In a child this loading situation would result in a greenstick fracture (McRae, 1989).

Tomford (1987) advocated the use of three-point fixation to align the fracture as the cast is applied (Fig. 5–45B). An intramedullary rod

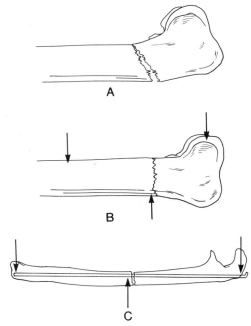

FIGURE 5–45

Application of fixation should provide a three-point system for correction: *A*, Fracture. *B*, Casting results. *C*, Intramedullary rod fixation by three-point contact with a precurved rod (or a straight rod in a curved long bone). Flexibility is necessary for such a fixation. (From Radin EL, Simon SR, Rose RM, et al.: Biomechanics for the Orthopedic Surgeon. New York, Wiley & Sons, 1979.)

may also provide three-point contact (Radin et al., 1979). Either the rod or the bone must be curved to provide such forces. In such a case the forces are in the opposite direction of the forces that caused the fracture (Harrington, 1982).

An interesting application of parallel forces was used by Arkin (1949) in advancing the hypothesis that deformity in idiopathic scoliosis is related to asymmetric pressure on the vertebra, leading to arrest of epiphyseal growth. In the example cited, the vertebra at the apex of the curve is considered to be five vertebral diameters distant from the action of gravity (Fig. 5–46). The edge of the disk acts as a pivot point or fulcrum, a compression point. The distance from this point to the gravity line is X, and Y is the distance to the "ligament or supporting

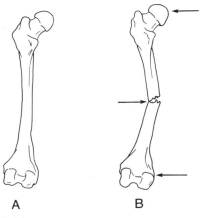

FIGURE 5–44

Bending load causing transverse fracture. (Modified from Gozna ER: Biomechanics of Musculoskeletal Injury. © 1982, The Williams & Wilkins Company, Baltimore.)

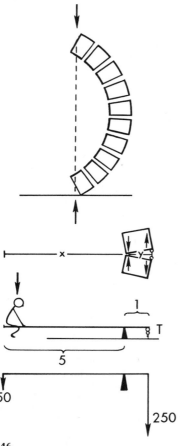

FIGURE 5–46

Analysis of spinal deformity involving a parallel force system. (Adapted from Arkin AM: The mechanism of structural changes in scoliosis. J Bone Joint Surg (Am) *31*:519–528, 1949.)

structure" on the convexity of the column, which is under tension. The seated figure represents the superincumbent weight, considered to be 250 N. The ratio of distances involved is 5:1. Then,

$$\Sigma M = 0$$
$$(T \times 2.5 \text{ cm}) + (250 \text{ N} \times 12.5 \text{ cm}) = 0$$
$$2.5 \text{ T} + (3125 \text{ Ncm}) = 0$$
$$T = -1250 \text{ N}$$

and

$$\Sigma F = 0$$
$$(-250 \text{ N}) + (-1250) + F = 0$$
$$F = 1500 \text{ N}$$

Both the superincumbent weight and the tension (T) developed in the ligamentous structures on the convexity of the curve exert a compression force on the edge of the vertebral body, which now becomes a fulcrum. This tremendous concentration of pressure, Arkin proposes, leads to arrest of vertebral epiphyseal growth and consequent wedging of the vertebral body.

Distribution of forces in cadaver feet was investigated by Manter (1946), who utilized a parallel force system in loading the specimens (Fig. 5–47). A metal bar was placed on the middle of the upper surface of the talus. It was attached to the calcaneus posteriorly. The bar was positioned over the space between the second and third toes, forming a longitudinal "loading axis." A weight of 100 N was suspended on the

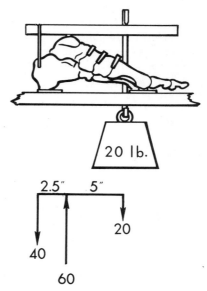

FIGURE 5–47

Manter's method of loading cadaver feet for experimental determination of articular pressures. (Adapted from Manter JR: Distribution of compression forces in the joints of the human foot. Anat Rec 96:313–321, 1946.)

bar "at a distance giving it a mechanical advantage of 3 at the point of contact with the talus." In other words, the weight was hung twice as far anterior to the talus as the distance from the talus to the calcaneus attachment posteriorly. The forces along the bar were then 100 N, 300 N, and 200 N, respectively. Is there a parallel between this example and the static force acting on the hip joint in the frontal plane? Might the direction of each vector as shown in Figure 5–47 be reversed? How would you "read" the figure in this case?

The determination of muscle and joint forces has been performed by many researchers (Williams and Stutzman, 1959; Haffajee et al., 1972; Olson et al., 1972; Reilly and Martens, 1972; Smidt, 1973; Ghista and Roaf, 1981a and 1981b). These determinations are based upon the use of the general force system. Williams and Stutzman (1959) studied the forces through the range of motion of various muscle groups including elbow flexion, knee flexion and exten-

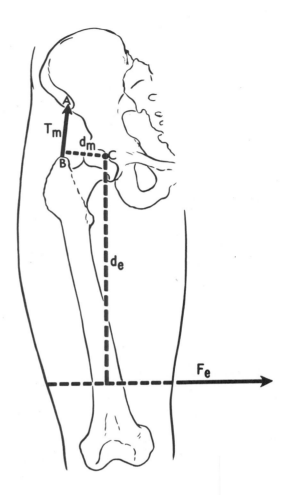

$$T_m \times d_m = F_e \times d_e$$

FIGURE 5–49

Diagram of the right hip: *A*, Anterior superior iliac spine. *B*, Greater trochanter. *C*, Center of rotation of femoral head; d_m = moment arm for the abductor muscles; T_m = line of action of the abductor muscles; d_e = moment arm for external force; F_e = line of action for external force. (From Olson VL, Smidt GL, Johnston RC: The maximum torque generated by the eccentric, isometric and concentric contractions of the hip abductor muscles. Phys Ther 52:149–158, 1972. Reprinted from PHYSICAL THERAPY with the permission of the American Physical Therapy Association.)

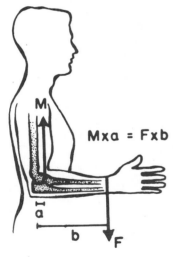

$$M \times a = F \times b$$

FIGURE 5–48

Principal forces in test: counterclockwise torque, muscle pull (M) times lever arm (a), equals clockwise torque, tensiometer sling (F) times lever arm (b). (From Williams M, Stutzman L: Strength variations through the range of motion. Phys Ther Rev 39:145–152, 1956. Reprinted from PHYSICAL THERAPY with the permission of the American Physical Therapy Association.)

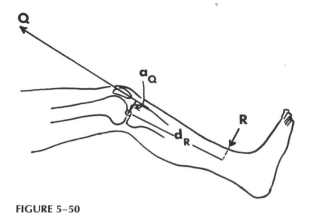

FIGURE 5–50

Rotatory equilibrium around the knee joint: Forces necessary for translatory equilibrium are not considered. R = external resisting force; d_R = lever of R; Q = quadriceps contraction force; a_Q = lever of Q; M_{ext} and M_{int} = external and internal moments, respectively. (From Haffajee D, Moritz U, Svantesson G: Isometric knee extension strength as a function of joint angle, muscle length and motor unit activity. Acta Orthop Scand *43*:138–147, 1972.)

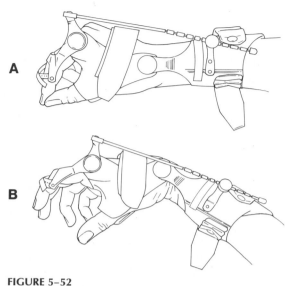

FIGURE 5–52

Digital grasp and release patterns are controlled by active wrist extension (*A*) and gravity-assisted flexion (*B*) in this tenodesis splint. (From Fess EE, Philips CA: Hand Splinting Principles and Methods, 2nd ed. St. Louis, Mosby, 1987.)

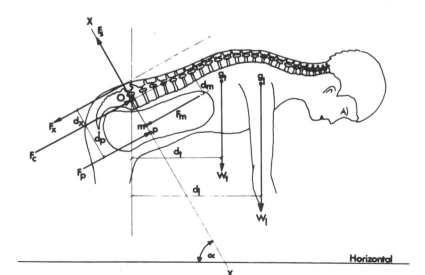

FIGURE 5–51

Free body diagram showing the forces acting across and along a plane X-X through the lumbosacral disc when in the flexed posture. Point O is the instantaneous center of rotation within the disc. (From Stott JRR, Cyron BM, Hutton WC, et al.: The mechanics of spondylolysis. *In* Ghista DN, Roaf R (Eds): Orthopedic Mechanics: Procedures and Devices, vol 3. New York, Academic Press, 1981.)

sion, shoulder flexion and extension, shoulder horizontal adduction, hip abduction, and hip flexion. They graphed the results for each activity. Haffajee and co-workers (1972) and Smidt (1973) studied the torque through the range of motion for the knee; Olsen and associates (1972) studied the torque during the range of motion of hip abductor muscles; and Ghista and Roaf (1981a and 1981b) evaluated models of the back during trunk flexion. Figures 5–48 through 5–51 show the diagrams used for these evaluations.

The source of force for control splints and terminal devices of upper limb prostheses provides examples of the general force system (Fess and Philips, 1987; Vitali et al., 1978; Banerjee, 1982). For a splint the driving rod or cable provides the force that opens or closes the device. The axis of the splint is placed at the joint of the part being moved. The body part moved provides the resistance to the lever system (Fig. 5–52). For the voluntary opening terminal device, a cable provides the force and a spring or rubber band offers the resistance (Fig. 5–53A). For the voluntary closing device the rubber band provides the force, while the cable offers the resistance along with any object placed between the jaws (Fig. 5–53B). In mechanical hands, the cable will provide a force that acts through a first class lever system with the resistance often

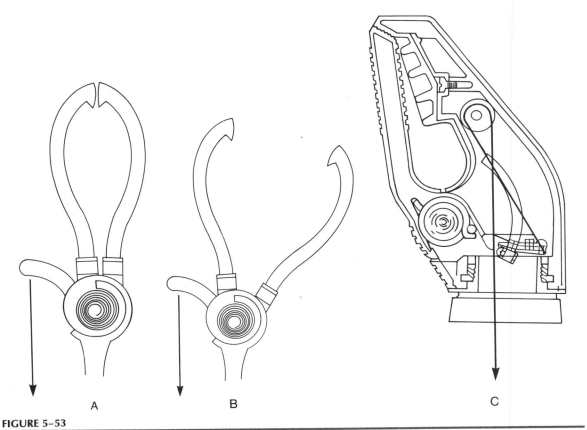

FIGURE 5–53

Lever systems used for terminal devices: *A*, Voluntary opening device. *B*, Voluntary closing device. *C*, Child Amputee Prosthetic Project (CAPP) device (from Shaperman J, Setoguchi Y: The CAPP terminal device, size 2: A new alternative for adolescents and adults. Prosth Orthot Int *13*:25–28, 1989).

provided by a spring that regulates the operation of the terminal device (Fig. 5–53C). Shaperman and Setoguchi (1989) have described the Children's Amputee Prosthetic Program (CAPP) terminal device, which operates on such a principle.

Many additional examples of force systems can be found in the literature and in clinical situations. They are not difficult to analyze if the two conditions of equilibrium are understood.

SUMMARY

When an object is known to be at rest, the equations of equilibrium may be applied. In this case one, two, or three unknown values may be determined. Facility with the free body diagram is essential. In the free body diagram, forces must be shown acting at all points at which the free body makes contact with another member. These forces must be represented as vectors (showing their direction), with letters being assigned to them to represent their magnitudes. If we are to arrive at the correct solution, all forces pertinent to the problem must be included, and none that are not involved may be included. Steps in the solution of the equilibrium problem are as follows:

1. Select the free body appropriate to the solution of the problem.
2. Draw the free body diagram.
3. Choose coordinate axes and moment centers.
4. Substitute the forces from the free body diagram into the pertinent equations of equilibrium ($\Sigma F = 0$; $\Sigma M = 0$).
5. Select the necessary force components.
6. Solve the equations of equilibrium to obtain the unknown values.

QUESTIONS

1. No moment of force is present if the forces are concurrent. Explain why.
2. Define concurrent, colinear, coplanar, and concentric.

3. What are the two conditions of equilibrium?
4. Draw and label the three classes of levers.
5. What is the resisting tension force in Codman's pendulum exercise for the shoulder when the 700 N patient holds a 25 N weight?
6. Assume your body weight to be 550 N; you are standing and holding a load of books weighing 55 N. What is the total force between your feet and the ground? Between each foot and the ground? Is this tension or compression force?
7. Your forearm weighs 20 N and you are carrying a portable diathermy machine weighing 100 N. (Your elbow is extended.) What is the force in the joint structures and muscles crossing the elbow joint counterbalancing this load? Is this tension or compression force? What is the magnitude of the tension force at the shoulder? (Assume your upper arm weighs 15 N.)
8. A patient exercising on wall pulleys pulls on the rope with a force of 300 N; the load on the weights is also 300 N. What force exists in the rope as a result of these forces that are applied to its ends? Is the arm moving?
9. A Sayre sling has a single supporting strand of rope to which is applied a force of 100 N. What magnitude of tension is produced in the structures of the neck when traction is applied to a 900 N patient in a sitting position? What would the answer be if the sling were suspended by a pulley system with three supporting strands instead of one? (Ignore the weight of the apparatus.)
10. A patient weighing 600 N hangs by both hands from the top rung of the stall bars. What force is produced between each hand and the bar? What is this force if he stands on a scale and supports 130 N of his weight on his feet instead of hanging free?
11. A pole 2 m high serving as a weight rack for storing exercise weights has five pegs along its length at 1 ft. intervals. Starting at the bottom the weights are 350 N, 350 N, 250 N, and 150 N with 100 N at the top.
   (a) What is the maximum total force at the bottom of the pole?

(b) Find the compression force in the pole between the 250 N and 150 N weights.

(c) Compare the relative compression forces on the intervertebral disks at various levels of the vertebral column; the relative superincumbent weight supported by the ankle, knee, and hip joints in standing; and the tension forces in the shoulder, elbow, and wrist joint structures when the arm is hanging at the side.

12. An 800 N man has a walking cast on one leg that weighs 55 N. What is the total tension in the joint structures crossing the hip joint and supporting his load and the limb when the foot is elevated off the floor? What is the total tension in the joint structures crossing the knee?

13. A physical therapist wants to apply 65 N of tension to the muscles and ligaments of a patient's neck with cervical traction. Assuming the head weighs 45 N and the traction cord is pulling on the seated patient at a 70° angle for neck flexion, how much force must be applied by the traction device? How much force is needed to relieve the weight of the head? Would more or less force be needed if the traction were applied with the patient supine? Explain.

14. A physician wishes to apply a vertical force of 45 N downward on a special splint on a patient's shoulder. To avoid the patient's shoulder and ribs, the physician uses two cords, one slanting forward and downward and the other backward and downward from the patient's shoulder. What is the tension in each cord if each makes a 30° angle with the vertical?

15. Solve the problems in Figure 5–54 using the laws of equilibrium.

16. Which muscle has a greater effect in producing rotatory motion, one that pulls along the shaft or one that pulls at right angles to the bone?

17. Most muscle attachments are of what class of lever? What are the advantages and disadvantages of this anatomic arrangement?

18. A weight of 45 N is being supported by two cords that make angles of 60° and 75°, respectively, with the horizontal. Find the tension on each cord.

19. If a head traction apparatus has two vertical strands and a third strand making an angle of 50° with the horizontal plane, what force is applied to the head sling when a load of 25 N is placed on the end of the rope?

20. How might you set up a traction apparatus for stretching the cervical spine so that a force equal to 1.5 times head weight could be applied to a 700 N patient? Mention at least three possible arrangements.

21. Is an object in equilibrium always stationary? What is the definition of a state of equilibrium in mechanics?

22. Explain in your own words the principle of moments. Why is this so important in analysis of body movement?

23. How does the procedure of finding the resultant differ in the linear and in the parallel force systems? Between parallel and general force systems?

24. What are the two requirements of equilibrium in a parallel force system? Explain them in your own words.

25. Give an example of decreasing or increasing an exercise load by changing the position of a body segment. Explain.

26. How does the lever arm of the brachialis muscle vary through the range of elbow flexion as compared with the variation in lever arm of the triceps in elbow extension? (Do they vary equally?)

27. Is there more variation in lever length of the hamstrings during knee flexion than of the Achilles tendon during plantar flexion? At which joint positions are these lever arms maximal? Minimal?

28. For the following, visualize and estimate the lever arm and its variation through the range of motion:

(a) The semimembranosus in hip extension or in knee flexion.

(b) The gluteus medius in hip abduction.

(c) The wrist and ankle flexors.

(d) Other muscles and movements.

29. A 270 N boy (A) sits 1.6 m from the axis of a teeter-totter facing a 220 N boy (B) on the other end of the board. How far from the axis must B sit to balance A? Where would B have to sit if A weighed 180 N?

30. Let us say that your own elbow is flexed to 90° with the forearm horizontal. Estimate the

25 N ←————————●————————→ F

(a) F = _____

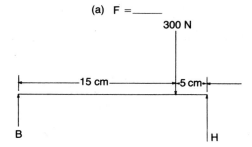

(c) B = _____
     H = _____

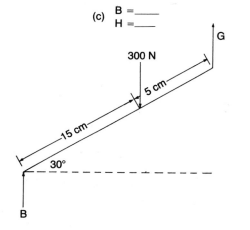

(e) B = _____
     G = _____

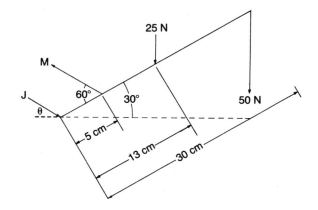

(g) M = _____
     J = _____
     θ = _____

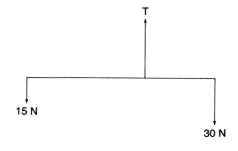

(b) T = _____

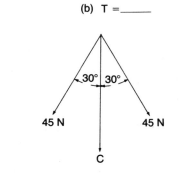

(d) C = _____

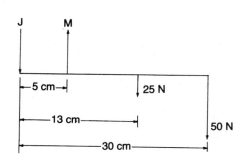

(f) M = _____
     J = _____

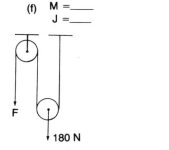

(h) F = _____

FIGURE 5–54

Problem 15—equilibrium problems.

weight of the forearm and hand and the distance from its center of mass to the elbow axis. (See Appendix A.)

(a) What is the moment of the gravitational force tending to extend the forearm?

(b) If the biceps tendon is 5 cm from the elbow axis, what force must this muscle, inserted at 90°, exert to maintain the forearm in a horizontal position?

31. Give an example of a muscle that pulls at an angle of 90° to the long axis of the part at some point in the range of motion. Are there many such muscles? Give an example of a muscle force in which the lever arm has little variation through the range of joint motion.

32. When you stand at the end of a diving board 4 m from where it is anchored to the ground, what moment do you exert about the fixed point of the board? Where would a person 1¼ times your weight stand in order to exert the same moment about this fixed point?

33. Why is it more difficult to do a sit-up exercise with the arms above the head than with them at the side of the trunk? (Draw a free body diagram.)

34. A shoulder wheel has a handle that may be adjusted at various distances from the center or axis. Compare the effort required by the patient to turn the wheel when the handle is 15 cm and when it is 40 cm from the center point.

35. From the point of view of resistance offered by the weight of the limb, is it easier when lying supine to perform a "leg raising exercise" with the knee extended than with it flexed? Why?

36. At what point during a leg-raising exercise (subject supine) is lumbar hyperextension most likely to occur? Why?

37. When two physical therapists are lifting a patient to a wheelchair, therapist A takes the legs and therapist B carries the trunk. If the center of mass of a 700 N patient is 65 cm from therapist A and 20 cm from therapist B, how much weight will each therapist be supporting?

38. A person performs bent knee sit-ups with hands behind the head. The head, trunk, and arms weigh 450 N and the combined center of mass of these segments is located 40 cm from the hip joint. Calculate the moment of force caused by the upper body weight about the hip

joint when the trunk is at 0°, 30°, 45°, 60°, and 90° with the horizontal. What is the most difficult part of the sit-up? Why would the exercise increase in difficulty if it were performed on a 30° inclined board with the head down?

39. Set up and solve some concurrent, parallel, and general force systems of your own. If possible, think of an equilibrium problem that may be analyzed first as a concurrent force system and then, by adding the weight of the part, as a general force system. Compare answers obtained by each method.

REFERENCES

Arkin AM: The mechanism of the structural changes in scoliosis. J Bone Joint Surg (Am) *31*:519–528, 1949.

Banerjee SN: Rehabilitation Management of Amputees. Baltimore, Williams & Wilkins, 1982.

Duncan RM: Basic principles of splinting the hand. Phys Ther *69*:1104–1116, 1989.

Ferguson AB, Jr, Brown TD, Fu FH, et al.: Relief of patellofemoral contact stress by anterior displacement of the tibial tubercle. J Bone Joint Surg (Am) *61*:159–166, 1979.

Fess EE, Philips CA: Hand Splinting Principles and Methods, 2nd ed. St. Louis, C. V. Mosby, 1987.

Ghista DN, Roaf R: Orthopaedic Mechanics: Procedures and Devices, vol. 2. New York, Academic Press, 1981a.

Ghista DN, Roaf R: Orthopedic Mechanics: Procedures and Devices, vol. 3. New York, Academic Press, 1981b.

Ghista DN, Vivani GR, Subbaraj K, et al.: Biomechanical basis of optimal scoliosis surgical correction. J Biomech *21*:77–88, 1988.

Gozna ER: Biomechanics of Musculoskeletal Injury. Baltimore, Williams & Wilkins, 1982.

Haffajee D, Moritz U, Svantesson G: Isometric knee extension strength as a function of joint angle, muscle length and motor unit activity. Acta Orthop Scand *43*:138–147, 1972.

Harrington IJ: Biomechanics of joint injuries. *In* Gozna ER (Ed): Biomechanics of Musculoskeletal Injury. Baltimore, Williams & Wilkins, 1982, pp 31–84.

Ilizarov GA: Clinical application of the tension-stress effect for limb lengthening. Clin Orthop *250*:8–26, 1990.

Inman VT, Saunders JB, Abbott LC: The function of the shoulder joint. J Bone Joint Surg (Am) *26*:1–30, 1944.

Jayaraman G, Zbib HM, Jacobs RR: Biomechanical analysis of surgical correction techniques in idiopathic scoliosis: Significance of bi-planar characteristics of scoliotic spines. J Biomech *22*:427–437, 1989.

Jordan HH: Orthopedic Appliances. New York, Oxford University Press, 1939.

Kenwright J, Spriggins AJ, Cunningham JL: Response of the growth plate to distraction close to skeletal maturity. Clin Orthop *250*:61–72, 1990.

Kiel JH: Basic Hand Splinting: A Pattern-Designing Approach. Boston, Little, Brown and Company, 1983.

McRae R: Practical Fracture Treatment, 2nd ed. New York, Churchill Livingstone, 1989.

Manter JR: Distribution of compression forces in the joints of the human foot. Anat Rec 96:313–321, 1946.

Maquet P: Biomechanics of the Knee: With application to the pathogenisis and surgical treatment of osteoarthritis. New York, Springer-Verlag, 1976.

Mielke CH, Lonstein JE, Fennis F, et al.: Surgical treatment of adolescent idiopathic scoliosis. J Bone Joint Surg (Am) 71:1170–1177, 1989.

Moe JH, Kharrat K, Winter RB, et al.: Harrington instrumentation without fusion, plus external orthotic support for the treatment of difficult curvature problems in young children. Clin Orthop 185:35–45, 1984.

Moore JR: Clubfoot braces. In Alldrege RF (Ed): Orthopedic Appliances Atlas, vol. 1. Ann Arbor, MI, JW Edwards, 1952, pp 472–495.

Nolan JP, Jr, Sherk HH: Biomechanical evaluation of the extensor musculature of the cervical spine. Spine 13:9–11, 1988.

Olson VL, Smidt GL, Johnston RC: The maximum torque generated by the eccentric, isometric and concentric contractions of the hip abductor muscles. Phys Ther 52:149–158, 1972.

Phelps WM: Bracing in the cerebral palsies. In Alldrege RF (Ed): Orthopedic Appliances Atlas, vol 1. Ann Arbor, MI, JW Edwards, 1952, pp 521–536.

Procter P, Paul JP: Ankle joint biomechanics. J Biomech 15:627–634, 1982.

Radcliffe CW: The biomechanics of the Canadian-type hip-disarticulation prosthesis. Artificial Limbs 4(2):29–32, 1957.

Radin EL, Simon SR, Rose, RM, et al.: Practical Biomechanics for the Orthopedic Surgeon. New York, John Wiley & Sons, 1979.

Reilly DT, Martens M: Experimental analysis of the quadriceps muscle force and patello-femoral joint reaction force for various activities. Acta Orthop Scand 43:126–137, 1972.

Schijvens AWM, Snijders CJ, Seroo JM, et al.: Mechanics of the spine: Analysis of its flexibility and rigidity, postural control and correction of the pathological spine. In Ghista DN (Ed): Osteoarthromechanics. Washington, DC, Hemisphere Publishing, 1982, pp 263–314.

Schwartsman V, McMurray MR, Martin SN: The Ilizarov methods—the basics. Contemp Orthop 19:628–638, 1989.

Scott JRR, Cyron BM, Hutton WC, et al.: The mechanics of spondylolysis. In Ghista DN, Roaf R (Eds): Orthopedic Mechanics: Procedures and Devices, vol. 3. New York, Academic Press, 1981, pp 65–93.

Shaperman J, Setoguchi Y: The CAPP terminal device, size 2: A new alternative for adolescents and adults. Prosth Orthot Int 13:25–28, 1989.

Silverman BJ, Greenbarg PE: Idiopathic scoliosis posterior spine fusion with Harrington rod and sublaminar wiring. Orthop Clin North Am 19:269–279, 1988.

Smidt GL: Biomechanical analysis of knee flexion and extension. J Biomech 6:79–92, 1973.

Solonen KA, Hoyer P: Positioning of the pulley mechanism when reconstructing deep flexor tendons of the fingers. Acta Orthop Scand 38:321–328, 1967.

Soeur R: Fractures of the Limbs: The Relationships Between Mechanism and Treatment. Springfield, IL, Charles C Thomas, 1982.

Tomford W: Basics of broken bones for the nonorthopedist: 1. The fundamental principles. Emergency Medicine 19(15):26–33, 1987.

Trosclair MJ: Corrective braces in knee curvatures. Braces Today, December 1959, Newsletter of the Pope Foundation Inc. (reprinted from the Orthopaedic and Prosthetic Appliance Journal, June 1959).

Vitali M, Robinson KP, Andrews BG, et al.: Amputations and Prostheses. London, Baillière Tindall, 1978.

Watts HG: Bracing spinal deformities. Orthop Clin North Am 10:769–785, 1979.

White AA, Panjabi MM: The clinical biomechanics of scoliosis. Clin Orthop 118:100–111, 1976.

Williams M, Stutzman L: Strength variations through the range of motion. Phys Ther Rev 39:145–152, 1959.

Winter RB, Lonstein JE: Adult idiopathic scoliosis treated with Luque or Harrington rods and sublaminar wiring. J Bone Joint Surg (Am) 71:1308–1313, 1989.

6

Friction

INTRODUCTION

Friction is a contact force that has a major effect on motion. Walking requires adequate friction between the sole of the foot and the floor, so that the foot will not slip forward or backward and the effect of limb extension can be imparted to the trunk. Lack of friction on icy surfaces is compensated for by hobnails on boots or chains on tires. Friction is necessary to the operation of a self-propelled vehicle, not only to start it and keep it going but to stop it as well. A wheelchair can be pushed only because of the friction developed between the pusher's shoes and the floor, and friction must likewise be developed between the wheels and the floor so they will turn and not slide. Crutches and canes are stable as a result of friction between their tips and the floor. The stability is often increased by use of a rubber tip, which has a high coefficient of friction with the floor.

Many friction devices are used in exercise equipment to grade resistance to movement, as with a shoulder wheel or stationary bicycle. Brakes on wheelchairs and locks on bed casters utilize the principles of friction. Application of cervical or lumbar traction to a bed patient depends on adequate opposing frictional forces developed between the patient's body and the bed.

In the operation of machines, sliding friction wastes energy. This energy is transformed into heat, which may have a harmful effect on the machine, as with burned-out bearings. To reduce friction, materials having a very smooth or polished surface are used for contacting parts, or a lubricant, such as oil or grease, is placed between the moving parts. Frictional effects are than absorbed between the layers of the lubricant rather than by the surfaces in contact. Friction also exists within the human body. Normally ample lubrication is present as tendons slide within synovial sheaths at sites of wear, and the articulating surfaces of joints are bathed in synovial fluid.

DEFINITION

Frictional Force

When two surfaces are pressed together, as shown in Figure 6–1, a force in the lateral direction is required to make one surface slide over the other. The resistance to this force developed at the surface of contact is termed the *frictional force*. The magnitude of the force required to produce motion of one surface with respect to the other depends on (1) how tightly the two surfaces are pressed together and (2) the kinds of materials in contact with each other, including the roughness of their surfaces.

Coefficient of Friction

A factor called the *coefficient of friction*, designated by the symbol μ (mu), is used to describe the effect of different materials and the roughness of the contact surfaces. Different types of materials have different coefficients of friction; these can be determined approximately by a simple experiment, since

$$F_{max} = \mu N$$

where F_{max} is the maximum possible friction force, μ is the coefficient of friction, and N is the "normal" force, or force perpendicular to the surfaces in contact, pressing the surfaces together. If the force necessary to start an object sliding along a horizontal surface can be carefully measured, it will approximate (be slightly more than) the maximum force of friction between the contacting surfaces. Some common coefficients of friction are listed in Table 6–1.

▶ **PROBLEM 6–1**

A force of 200 N is needed to start a 1000 N box sliding across a wooden table.
   QUESTION:
What is the coefficient of friction between the box and the table?
   SOLUTION:
Filling in the known values in our equation, we have

$$200 = \mu 1000$$
$$\mu = \frac{200}{1000}$$
$$\mu = 0.2$$

Notice that the area of contact is not important. A given force pressing the contacting surfaces together will produce a frictional effect regardless of whether the contacting surface is large or small.

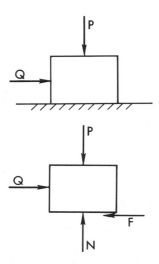

FIGURE 6–1

Force Q pushes horizontally against a box of weight, P. The weight of the box is opposed by the normal force, N, perpendicular to the surface. The force of friction (F) opposes horizontal force (Q). Note that force N cannot actually be in line with P, since the couple produced by Q and F must be balanced by a couple consisting of P and N.

TABLE 6–1. COEFFICIENTS OF FRICTION (μ)

Surfaces	μ
Wood on wood, dry	0.23–0.50
Metal on metal, dry	0.15–0.20
Metal on tile	0.10–0.15
Metal on metal, greased	0.03–0.05
Rubber on concrete, dry	0.60–0.70
Rubber crutch tip on clean tile	0.30–0.40
Hard rubber cane tip on clean tile	0.18–0.22
Rubber crutch tip on rough wood	0.70–0.75
Hard rubber cane tip on rough wood	0.38–0.44

Another important point is that it takes more force to set an object in motion than to keep it moving. As long as the surfaces in contact with each other are at rest, the value of μ is constant. When motion takes place between the surfaces, μ always has a lower value than when the surfaces are at rest. It takes more force to start a sled moving than to keep it moving.

If frictional forces are equal to the applied forces that tend to make an object slide, it will remain at rest. As we have seen, the use of the coefficient of friction permits us to express mathematically the maximum frictional force that can be developed in terms of the pressure existing between surfaces in contact. All the equations of equilibrium that have previously been developed apply in problems where frictional forces are involved. An important factor that has not appeared previously is that frictional force may have any magnitude from zero to the F_{max} value. The direction of frictional force is dependent on the direction in which the object tends to move; the frictional force always acts to oppose motion, or potential motion, as shown in Figure 6–1.

Example

Suppose a gymnasium mat rests on the floor with a child sitting on the mat (Fig. 6–2). The child and mat together weigh 150 N. If the coefficient of friction between the mat and floor is 0.15, the maximum frictional force that can be developed will be

$$F_{max} = \mu N$$
$$= 0.15 \times 150 \text{ N}$$
$$= 22.5 \text{ N}$$

If we push on the mat with a force of 20 N to the right, our equations of equilibrium show that the frictional force developed will be 20 N acting to the left. If we push on the mat toward the left with a force of 10 N, the opposing frictional force developed will be 10 N to the right, and so on. The magnitude of the frictional force is always obtained by the equations of equilibrium, but its maximum value can never exceed F_{max}. If a 50 N force were to be applied to the mat, only a 22.5 N frictional force could be developed. In this case the mat would no longer

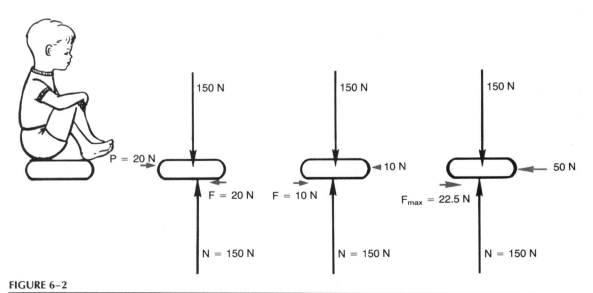

FIGURE 6–2

The magnitude and direction of frictional force is determined by the external force applied, but it can never exceed F_{max}, which in this case is 22.5 N. The figure on the right will slide, as F_{max} has been exceeded.

be in equilibrium but would slide in the direction of the applied force.

APPLICATION

General

Many instances of application of friction can be seen in physical therapy. As friction plates on exercise apparatus wear smooth, they have to be pushed together more tightly and eventually replaced. (N must increase as μ decreases to maintain F_{max}.) Setscrews on knobs and handles work loose and must be tightened, as do bolts and nuts. In raising and lowering infrared and ultraviolet lamps, one must be certain that the friction applied by the knob and screw is adequate to maintain the weight of the lamp head in the desired position. Very heavy lamps are usually counterbalanced to reduce the friction required to support the equipment safely at various heights. Grasping a knob with the hand to turn it makes use of the friction developed between the fingers and the knob. Grasping more tightly, if the knob fails to turn, increases F_{max}. Foam rubber also grips the skin firmly when applied beneath an elastic bandage (Knockne and Knockne, 1945), the bandage providing the necessary normal force.

While there are many instances in which friction is applied clinically to good purpose, at other times we try to minimize its effects. A lubricant is used in massage so that the hands will slide smoothly over the patient's skin. An exercise board with powder sprinkled on the surface makes bed exercise easier. Surface friction is eliminated entirely in exercises in a pool or with sling suspension. In functional and assistive apparatus, swivel joints and ball bearing and roller bearing joints minimize frictional drag, so that the patient can utilize his strength to best advantage in movement. In braces and prostheses the requirements for free motion at joints must be balanced against requirements for stability and ruggedness of the apparatus. One of the most common means of reducing friction, of course, is by lubricating the joints. This also helps to eliminate squeaks in noisy joints.

In the solution of problems involving friction, care must be taken to obtain the correct value of the normal force or pressure between the contact surfaces. This is not always equal to the weight of the part, as will be shown in the next two problems.

Traction

Cervical and pelvic traction are examples of treatment involving friction.

▶ **PROBLEM 6–2**

Consider a patient with neck traction applied by calipers or tongs attached to the skull (Fig. 6–3). Let us say the head weighs 50 N and the coefficient of friction between the back of the head and the bed is 0.17. The action line of the pulley force is parallel to the bed surface.

QUESTION:

Find the maximum frictional force that must be overcome before the traction pull will be effective in stretching the cervical structures.

SOLUTION:

The force of pulley rope, T, weight of the head, W, and the normal reacting force, N, are shown in Figure 6–3A. We know that maximum frictional force is acting in this case since motion of the head is impending, and that F_{max} must act in a direction to oppose impending motion. The equations of equilibrium can be applied, since we know that the head is at rest and not moving.

Substituting into the equation $F_{max} = \mu N$, and solving for F_{max}, we obtain

$$F_{max} = 0.17 \times 50 \text{ N}$$
$$= 8.5 \text{ N}$$

A force of 8.5 N on rope, T, is necessary to overcome the friction between the head and bed in this case.

▶ **PROBLEM 6–3**

Now consider a similar traction system in which the pulley rope forms an angle of 10° with the horizontal plane, a technique sometimes used to stretch the posterior neck structures (Fig. 6–3B). The pulley rope applies a force, T.

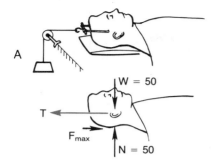

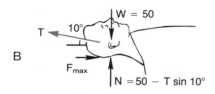

FIGURE 6–3

A, Application of cervical traction through skull calipers. Head weight (W) is opposed by N, the force normal to the supporting surface; traction load T is opposed by F_{max}. *B,* When the traction rope is slanted upward 10°, the value of N depends on T as well as W. C represents tension on cervical structures.

QUESTION:

Find the force T required to start the head moving upward toward the end of the bed.

SOLUTION:

The same conditions apply as in the previous problem. Substituting into the equation $\Sigma F_y = 0$, and solving for N we obtain

$$(-50) + T \sin 10° + N = 0$$
$$N = 50 - T \sin 10°$$

From this equation we see that in this case N is not equal to the weight of the head but is also dependent on the force T and the angle at which it is applied. When the pulley rope is slanted upward, the maximum frictional force between the head and bed is decreased.

Suppose T, the traction load, is 60 N. Then

$$\Sigma F_y = 0$$
$$(-50) + (60 \sin 10°) + N = 0$$
$$N = 50 - 60(0.174)$$
$$= 39.6 \text{ N}$$

Now we can determine F_{max} and the stretching force, C, applied to the cervical structures in this case.

$$F_{max} = \mu N$$
$$= 0.17 \times 39.6$$
$$= 6.7 \text{ N}$$

Of the total traction load applied, a horizontal component of 6.7 N will be used up in overcoming the maximum force of friction developed between the head and the bed. To determine the cervical tension (C) we will substitute in the formula $\Sigma F_x = 0$:

$$T \cos 10° - F_{max} - C = 0$$
$$60(0.985) - 6.7 = C$$
$$C = 52.4 \text{ N}$$

A traction load of 52.4 N under these circumstances applies a tension of 52.4 N to the cervical structures. It is evident that the magnitude of the normal force will decrease with larger angles of force application (increased upward slant of the traction line) and with larger upward traction loads. This same solution can be used for the situation of sliding a box by pulling on a rope (Fig. 6–4).

In solving problems, if a proper free body diagram is drawn, showing all the forces acting, and these forces are inserted into the equations of equilibrium, the correct value of the normal force (N) can be obtained. Also, the frictional force (F) must be shown acting in the proper direction, if the direction can be ascertained from the setup of the problem. It is also important to recognize when the maximum friction force (F_{max}) is developed; this will be the case whenever motion is about to take place.

An interesting clinical use of friction in a cervical traction pulley system has been suggested by Jackson (1958). With the patient in the upright position, she demonstrated by radiographs of the cervical spine that "the conventional amount of weight of 5 to 10 pounds [20 to 45 N

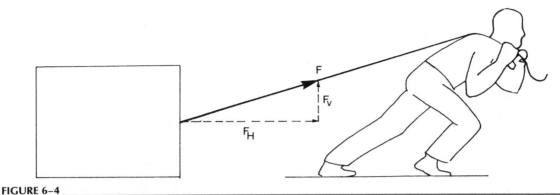

FIGURE 6–4

Forces acting to slide a box along the floor.

traction force] does nothing more than lift the weight of the head from the neck." However, 20 to 25 pounds (90 to 100 N) resulted in distraction between the cervical vertebrae, and this was more marked with 35 pounds (155 N). For home treatment she advocated an overhead pulley system, such as that shown in Figure 6–5. When a 20 pound (90 N) load is suspended from the end of the rope, according to Jackson, traction on the head halter is about 15 pounds (67 N). The discrepancy is said to be due to friction developed between the rope and the pulleys. Then "if the patient slumps or slides down in the chair, the actual pull may be increased to 25 or 30 pounds (110 to 135 N) without altering the position of the weights." This would indicate that the maximum force of friction in the pulley system was reversed in direction because the head was now pulling on the system of weights. As additional force is added by the shift in posture to oppose the traction weights, F_{max} is approached until eventually the weights would move upward. The shift in posture without movement of the weights provides a simple way for the patient himself to control the magnitude of neck traction and to grade it over a small range.

In tests of apparatus, a scale for monitoring traction forces applied through a pulley system is always placed between the patient and the first pulley to rule out the effects of friction in the system.

Commercially available power-spring traction reels attached to the bed eliminate the use of pulleys and traction weights. In these devices a revolving drum adjusts the tension in the rope to movements of the patient and maintains a constant pre-set force in the line attached to the part. Traction forces are applied by such devices, assuming that adequate counterforce is available to stabilize the patient so that he will

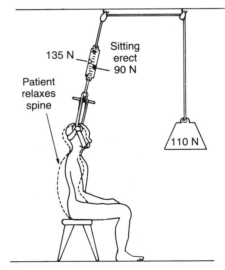

FIGURE 6–5

Pulley system for applying cervical traction with the patient in the upright position. (Adapted from Jackson R: The Cervical Syndrome, 2nd ed. Springfield, IL, Charles C Thomas, 1958.)

not be moved along in the direction of the traction line. In other words, the friction developed between the patient's body and the bed must never be exceeded by the traction force applied. If the patient tends to slide in the direction of the traction force, the bed may be tilted up to oppose this movement. This adds a component of the body weight to the maximum available force of friction stabilizing the patient.

Judovich (1955) investigated the friction forces associated with pelvic traction and concluded that the usual application of 10 to 15 pounds (45 to 67 N) on each side is completely neutralized by "surface traction resistance" or friction of the lower limbs. He experimented with a cadaver and three living subjects, applying weights until surface friction was exceeded. By sectioning the cadaver between lumbar vertebrae 3 and 4 and disarticulating the hips and knees, he determined that the average force necessary to overcome frictional resistance was 54 percent of the weight of the parts or of the entire body. Judovich estimated the portion of the body distal to the lumbar 3–4 interspace to be 49 percent of total body weight; 54 percent of this amount is about 26 percent of body weight, a figure that he suggested can be used to estimate frictional resistance to pelvic traction due to the weight of the lower limbs. Intermittent pelvic traction in the range of 60 to 80 pounds (270 to 350 N) was recommended, "of which 40 to 50 pounds [180 to 225 N] are lost in dissipating surface resistance." In the cervical region the dissipating force due to head-bed friction was said to be 6 pounds (25 N).

On the basis of these figures, the coefficient of friction developed between a 750 N patient and the bed can be determined. If the lower segments weigh 368 N (49 percent × 750 N) and 54 percent of this value (198 N) is the maximum force of friction, then

$$F_{max} = \mu N$$
$$198 = \mu 368$$
$$\mu = 0.54$$

In the case of cervical traction, if the dissipating force due to friction is 25 N and $\mu = 0.54$, we can compute the weight of the head as follows:

$$F_{max} = \mu N$$
$$25 = 0.54 \, N$$
$$N = \frac{25}{0.54}$$
$$= 46 \, N$$

This coefficient of friction is high in relation to those for other materials. The firmness of the mattress and the materials in contact with the body would be important factors affecting this value.

Judovich devised a bed with upper and lower sections, each with a separate mattress. The patient lay with his or her lumbar region over the division. The lower section of the bed was placed on rollers and a motor-driven mechanism moved it rhythmically back and forth in relation to the upper segment. Here the surface friction between the patient and the bed served to stabilize the upper and lower segments on the divided sections, so that the lumbar region could be stretched. If traction forces greater than maximum friction values were desired, a pelvic belt and shoulder harness could be applied (Judovich, 1955).

Moving an Object

As another example, consider a friction problem involving an infrared lamp (Fig. 6–6).

▶ **PROBLEM 6–4**

The coefficient of friction between the floor and the lamp base is 0.22. A therapist attempts to move the lamp by pushing against the upright with force (P). The distance between the floor and the center of mass of the lamp is 75 cm, and between the floor and the therapist's hand is 95 cm (dp). The distance from a vertical line through the center of mass of the lamp to the edge of the base is 15 cm (dn).

QUESTION:
As the therapist pushes, will the lamp slide as intended or tip over?

SOLUTION:
We must solve the problem twice. First, we will assume the lamp will slide and solve for F_{max} and P to satisfy this condition (Fig. 6–6A). From $\Sigma F_y = 0$, we have W = N.

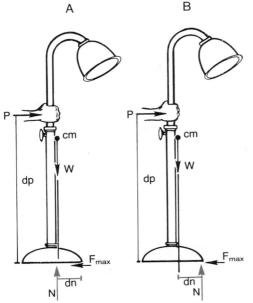

FIGURE 6–6

A, Method of moving an infrared lamp, where N = normal force, P = push by therapist attempting to slide the lamp, and μ = 0.22. It is assumed here that the lamp will slide. *B,* Here it is assumed that the lamp will tip over as a result of force P, so N acts at the edge of the base on the side opposite the push.

From our assumption of sliding

$$F_{max} = \mu N$$
$$= 0.22 \, N$$
$$= 0.22 \, W$$
$$\Sigma F_x = 0, P = F_{max}$$
$$= 0.22 \, W$$

For our next solution we will assume that the lamp is about to tip over (Fig. 6–6B). The force (N) in this case will have to act at the edge of the lamp base. Taking moments about this point we have

$$\Sigma M = 0$$
(W × 15) acts counterclockwise
$$(-P \times 95) + (W \times 15) = 0$$
$$P \times 95 = W \times 15$$
$$P = \frac{15 \, W}{95}$$
$$= 0.16 \, W$$

Looking at both solutions, we see that a force of 0.16 W is required to tip the lamp over, while a force of 0.22 W is necessary to make it slide. Therefore, if the original plan is carried through, the lamp will tip.

What should the therapist do to prevent this mishap? Repeat the above computation with push (P) exerted 60 cm from the floor instead of 95 cm. Where along the upright of the lamp will the effect of P change from a tip to a slide? What effect has the size of the lamp base on this problem? Would a larger lamp base (with the same lamp weight) increase the coefficient of friction between the base and the floor? What difference would it make if the lamp head were directed toward instead of away from the pusher as shown in Figure 6–6? What difference would it make if the coefficient of friction were 0.12 between the lamp and the floor instead of 0.22?

To determine the distance above the floor below which the lamp will slide and not tip, we can replace P with the friction force (0.22 W) and replace 95 cm with dp:

$$\Sigma M = 0$$
$$(0.22 \, W \times dp) + (-W \times 15) = 0$$
$$0.22 \, W \times dp = W \times 15$$
$$dp = 15 \, W/0.22 \, W$$
$$dp = 68.2 \, cm$$

Therefore if the therapist pushed above 68.2 cm, the lamp will tip. Pushing below 68.2 cm will cause the lamp to slide.

Notice in the case of the infrared lamp that a high center of mass will cause the lamp to tip more easily than a lower center of mass. The moment arm for the high center of mass becomes very small as the lamp begins to tip (center of mass moves rapidly toward edge of base). When the center of mass is lower, its moment arm decreases very little with tipping, which tends to keep the lamp upright. For this reason some physical therapists make it a habit to lower all lamp heads before moving equipment around the department.

Locomotion

We are able to walk or run only because of the frictional force at the ground acting on the foot in the direction in which we want to move (Fig. 6–7). The importance of frictional force developed between the shoe and the ground during walking, especially at heel strike and toe-off,

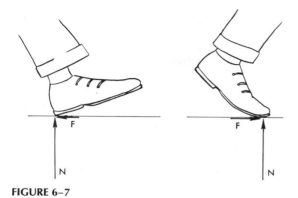

FIGURE 6–7

Horizontal (shear) force at heel strike and toe-off in walking. The vertical force of ground reaction (N) is more than body weight at these points in the gait cycle.

was mentioned earlier. Force plate studies indicate that the horizontal component of foot force at heel strike is about 15 percent of body weight, and at toe-off, 20 percent of body weight (Klopsteg and Wilson, 1954). F_{max} must exceed these values if the foot is not to slip. The value of the normal force at these points in the gait cycle is more than body weight, owing to the momentum of the body at heel strike and the thrust of plantar flexion before the toe-off. This increase in normal force helps to provide adequate stabilization for the foot. The friction developed in walking is generally less than the F_{max} value, but it may reach the F_{max} value on slippery surfaces, where the coefficient of friction is reduced.

Heel strike is a more hazardous point than toe-off for a foot to slip. Fundamental gait studies have shown also that there are lateral shear forces and torques exerted against the ground by the supporting foot, which must be opposed by friction (Klopsteg and Wilson, 1954).

Graphic Solution of Friction Problems

In some friction problems a graphic solution will be the easiest to use. In this procedure, F_{max} and N are combined into a single resultant force (R) (Fig. 6–8). Now, from the equation $F_{max} = \mu N$, we can write $\mu = F_{max}/N$.

From the relationship of the forces N and F_{max}

in Figure 6–8, we see that the tan $\phi = F_{max}/N$ also, where ϕ is the angle between the normal force and the resultant (R) of the normal and maximum frictional force. Therefore $\mu = \tan \phi$, where ϕ is called the *angle of friction*. Whenever the maximum frictional force is developed, the tangent of the angle between the resultant force and the normal is equal to the coefficient of friction. For example, in Figure 6–9, suppose we are to find the minimum force (P) and the angle alpha (α) at which it must act in order to start the block of weight (W) moving if the coefficient of friction is μ. In a free body diagram we can show R, the resultant of N and F_{max}, acting at the angle of friction ϕ with the vertical. If we draw a force polygon starting with W, whose magnitude and direction are known, and R, whose direction is known, we can complete the triangle by drawing the shortest line possible from the beginning of W to the action line of R. This line will have to be at right angles to the action line of R and so will define the magnitude of P and R and the direction of P. This latter direction obviously makes an angle ϕ with the horizontal. We now have the necessary characteristics of P needed for our answer.

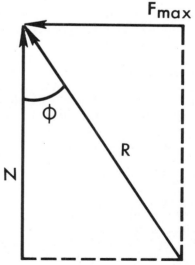

FIGURE 6–8

Graphic solution of friction problem in which F_{max} and N are shown as a single resultant force (R).

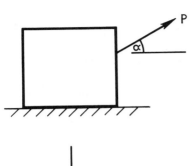

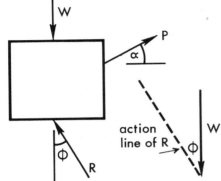

FIGURE 6–9

Determination by a force polygon of the minimum force (P) necessary to move block W; P acts at angle α with the horizontal.

Inclined Plane

Consider the block resting on a plane making an angle α with the horizontal, as shown in Figure 6–10A. The reaction (R), which is the resultant of F and N, must be in line with W for equilibrium to exist, and from the geometry of the figure it is apparent that the angle between R and N will be equal to the slope of the inclined plane α. From this we can see that as the slope of the plane increases until the angle of inclination reaches the value of ϕ (the angle of friction), the angle between N and R will also increase to ϕ where F_{max} will be developed (Fig. 6–10B). Now if we attempt to increase the slope of the plane further, it will be impossible to increase the angle between R and N since this angle is limited by the coefficient of friction (μ). Therefore, if the angle were increased, R would no longer line up with W, equilibrium could not exist, and the block would slide down the plane.

Another way to view the angle of friction is by calculating the forces on a box resting on an inclined plane (Fig. 6–11A).

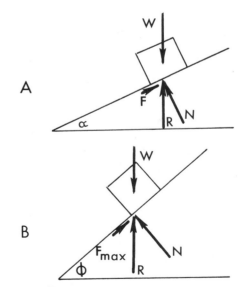

FIGURE 6–10

A, Behavior of friction forces on an inclined plane, where α is the angle formed by the plane with the horizontal. N is perpendicular to the plane and W and R are colinear. *B*, The slope is increased until the angle of inclination reaches ϕ, the angle of friction.

FIGURE 6-11

A, The forces on a box resting on an inclined plane. *B,* The forces on a box as a force (P) is used to begin sliding it up an inclined plane.

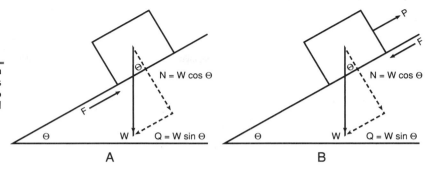

$N = W \cos \Theta$

$Q = W \sin \Theta$

A

$N = W \cos \Theta$

$Q = W \sin \Theta$

B

As a box rests on an inclined plane, the weight of the box (W) is directed vertically. Its components are the normal force (N), which is perpendicular to the supporting surface, and the force (Q) which is parallel to the supporting surface tending to cause the box to slide down the incline. The frictional force (F) resists the box from sliding down the incline until Q is greater than F_{max}. The box will begin to slide just as Q becomes greater than F_{max}. Thus, the greatest force Q may have without sliding occurs when Q is equal to F_{max}. Note that as Θ increases, N will decrease and Q will increase. In this situation W can be considered the resultant of N and Q. The angle Θ is the angle between W and N and is equal to the slope of the incline. (The equality of these angles can be easily seen by using geometric principles related to congruent triangles.)

The following manipulation of equations will show how the coefficient of friction relates to the angle of friction and the slope of an inclined plane.

$$F_{max} = \mu N$$

Using $\Sigma F = 0$ with Q directed left

$$-Q + F_{max} = 0$$

Therefore

$$-Q + \mu N = 0$$
$$\mu N = Q$$
$$\mu = Q/N$$
$$Q/N = \tan \Theta$$

Therefore

$$\mu = \tan \Theta$$

By knowing the coefficient of friction between two objects, you can determine the angle of an inclined plane above which friction will no longer resist sliding between the two objects.

This concept is important for constructing outside ramps for wheelchairs and patients who are using crutches. A wet ramp has a decreased coefficient of friction. If the coefficient of friction is low and the ramp is steep, a wheelchair may not be able to go up the ramp. The wheelchair or patient with crutches will not be able to descend the ramp safely. Can you think of other examples where this concept is important?

▶ **PROBLEM 6-5**

Suppose we wish to slide a 100 N box up a 30° inclined plane (Fig. 6-11B). What magnitude of force (P) will be needed to begin upward sliding of the box if $\mu = 0.3$?

$$F_{max} = \mu N$$
$$\frac{N}{W} = \cos \Theta$$
$$N = W \cos \Theta$$
$$Q/W = \sin \Theta$$
$$Q = W \sin \Theta$$

Set the X coordinate along the surface of the inclined plane

$$\Sigma F_x = 0$$
$$P + F_{max} + Q = 0$$

F_{max} and Q act to the left

$$P - \mu N - Q = 0$$
$$P - \mu W \cos \Theta - W \sin \Theta = 0$$
$$P = \mu W \cos \Theta + W \sin \Theta$$
$$P = W(\mu \cos \Theta + \sin \Theta)$$
$$P = 100[(0.3)(0.866)$$
$$+ (0.5)]$$
$$P = 100(0.76)$$
$$P = 76 \text{ N}$$

Tendon Friction

Friction also acts between flexible and rigid members. Thus, frictional forces may exist between a tendon and a bony prominence over which it passes or between a rope and a pole that it encircles. It is a matter of everyday experience that taking a turn of rope around a pole or capstan makes it much easier to resist a force pulling on the other end. If the greater force in the rope is designated as T_{max} and the lesser force as T_{min}, the relationship between them is given by the equation

$$T_{max} = T_{min} \cdot e^{\mu\alpha}$$

where e is 2.718 (the base of the natural system of logarithms), μ is the coefficient of friction between the surfaces of contact, and α is the angle of contact between the surfaces. This angle contact must be expressed in radians. (There are 2 π radians and 360° in a circle, so one radian equals 57.3°. Figure 6–12 illustrates the forces acting on a rope passing over a pole. The free body diagram of the rope shows that a whole series of normal and frictional forces exist along the contact area between the rope and the pole.

Since it will be necessary to employ logarithms to obtain a solution to tendon friction problems, a brief review of the basic principles will be given. Consider the expression

$$B^L = N$$

L is called the logarithm of N to the base B, and an equivalent expression can be written thus:

$$L = \text{Log}_B N$$

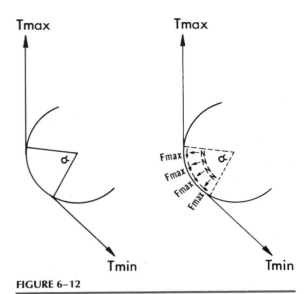

FIGURE 6–12

Effect of friction on the forces in a rope or tendon passing over a surface which changes its direction.

By definition, the logarithm of a number is the exponent to which the base must be raised in order to obtain the desired number. The common system of logarithms always uses 10 as the base, and the natural system uses the base 2.718. For the common system, the equivalent expressions are shown in Table 6–2.

The logarithms of the numbers in Table 6–2 are very easily obtained, but suppose the logarithm of a number between 10 and 100, say 20, is desired. It is obvious that it will be somewhere between 1 and 2, and the fractional part of the

TABLE 6–2. COMMON LOGARITHMS

$10^1 = 10$	or	$\text{Log}_{10} 10 = 1$
$10^2 = 100$		$\text{Log}_{10} 100 = 2$
$10^3 = 1000$		$\text{Log}_{10} 1000 = 3$
$10^0 = 1$		$\text{Log}_{10} 1 = 0$
$10^{-1} = \dfrac{1}{10^1} = 0.1$		$\text{Log}_{10} 0.1 = -1$
$10^{-2} = \dfrac{1}{10^2} = 0.01$		$\text{Log}_{10} 0.01 = -2$
$10^{-3} = \dfrac{1}{10^3} = 0.001$		$\text{Log}_{10} 0.001 = -3$

value required can be obtained from a table of logarithms (Appendix B) or from a calculator. The integral part of the logarithm, called the characteristic, is always obtained by inspection and is one less than the number of digits to the left of the decimal point, or a negative one more than the number of zeros to the right of the decimal point. This may be seen by inspection of Table 6–2. The fractional part is independent of the position of the decimal point, and in our example, this value is 0.3010. The fractional part would be the same if the original number were 2, 20, 200, etc. The complete logarithm is the sum of the characteristic and the fractional part (called the mantissa) and, for our example, is 1.3010. (The logarithm of 200 would be 2.3010.)

Since the following laws exist,

$$10^n \times 10^m = 10^{n+m}$$

$$\frac{10^n}{10^m} = 10^{n-m}$$

$$(10^n)^m = 10^{n \cdot m}$$

we see that the product of two numbers can be obtained by adding their logarithms, the quotient of two numbers can be obtained by subtracting their logarithms, and a number can be raised to a power by multiplying its logarithm by the power.

Using these definitions and the following relationships between the natural and common system of logarithms:

$$Log_{10} 2.718 = 0.4343$$

$$\text{and } Log_e 10 = 2.3026$$

we can write the basic tendon friction equation:

$$e^{\mu\alpha} = \frac{T_{max}}{T_{min}}$$

$$Log_e \frac{T_{max}}{T_{min}} = \mu\alpha$$

$$\text{or } Log_e T_{max} - Log_e T_{min} = \mu\alpha$$

In terms of logs to the base 10, this equation is

$$Log_{10} T_{max} - Log_{10} T_{min} = 0.4343 \, \mu\alpha$$

▶ **PROBLEM 6–6**

As an example, suppose we were to lower a patient in a wheelchair down a 30° ramp. The total weight of patient and wheelchair is 1000 N. A rope tied to the wheelchair takes a half turn around a pipe at the top of the ramp, the coefficient of friction between the rope and the pipe being 0.2.

QUESTION:
What force must be applied to the rope to control the motion of the chair and patient?

SOLUTION:
From a free body diagram of the wheelchair, we find the force in the rope to be 500 N. Since the rope takes a half turn around the pipe, α is π radians. Substituting in the basic equations

$$Log_{10} T_{max} - Log_{10} T_{min} = 0.4343 \, \mu\alpha$$

$$Log_{10} 500 - Log_{10} T_{min} = 0.4343 \times 0.2 \times \pi$$

$$Log_{10} T_{min} = Log_{10} 500 - 0.4343 \times 0.2 \times \pi$$

$$Log_{10} T_{min} = 2.6990 - 0.2726 = 2.4264$$

Looking up the mantissa 0.4264 in the log table gives 267, and the characteristic of 2 indicates that three digits are to the left of the decimal point so

$$T_{min} = 267 \text{ N}$$

Friction Within the Body

Friction within the body exists between joint surfaces, between layers of tissues, and around structures that slide on one another. Indeed, frictional effects are present down to the microscopic level in the complex body systems.

Sacs filled with fluid are frequently located at sites of wear. These are called bursae and are found between layers of muscle tissue and tendon, between connective tissue structures, such as fascia, fat, and bone, and beneath skin that moves across bony prominences, such as the olecranon. Bursae are flattened structures with smooth mucosal linings, and they serve to decrease friction occurring between moving surfaces. Important examples are the large subacromial bursa, which allows the humeral head to slip underneath the acromial process when the arm is elevated, the trochanteric bursa beneath the abductor tendons at the hip, and bursae around the patellar ligament and tendon of Achilles insertion. A bursa may develop at a site subjected to wear where none was present originally.

Tendons passing through bony grooves are supplied with synovial sheaths, which reduce friction and wear. The long head of the biceps brachii, and the flexor and extensor tendons at the wrist and ankle are examples. Relationships between forces in the tendon and the friction between the tendon and its sheath where it passes around a bony prominence may be investigated by the same method used in the preceding problem.

▶ **PROBLEM 6–7**

Suppose we are attempting to find the coefficient of friction existing between the peroneus longus tendon and its sheath as it passes around the lateral malleolus.

QUESTION:
Find the value of μ.

SOLUTION:
By measurement we might find that T_{max} is 330 N and T_{min} is 327 N. We also note that the direction of the tendon changes as it turns around the malleolus by an angle of 45° (see Fig. 6–12), which is equivalent to $\pi/4$ radians. Substituting in our basic equation,

$$Log_{10}\ T_{max} - Log_{10}\ T_{min} - 0.4343\ \mu\alpha$$

$$Log_{10}\ 330 - Log_{10}\ 327 = 0.4343\ \mu\ \frac{\pi}{4}$$

$$\mu = \frac{Log_{10}\ 330 - Log_{10}\ 327}{0.4343\ \frac{\pi}{4}}$$

$$\mu = \frac{2.5185 - 2.5145}{0.4343\ \frac{\pi}{4}}$$

$$\mu = 0.012$$

The articular surfaces of the joints glide and pivot during movement and, as we saw earlier, sustain tremendous compression forces. Fortunately, the coefficient of friction of articular cartilage is extremely low. On the basis of experiments with human knee joint cartilage, Charnley (1959) estimated the coefficient of kinetic friction to be about 0.013; Fung (1981) reported the values from 0.003 to 0.004, while others have given a figure of 0.02 (Jones, 1934; Tanner, 1959; Collins and Kingsbury, 1982) for normal animal joints. These values are very much lower than the values for engineering materials, such as 0.041 for Co-Cr alloy/polyester, 0.044 for Co-Cr alloy/high-density polyethylene, and 0.034 for stainless steel/polytetrafluoroethylene (Mears, 1979). This is one of the difficulties in producing an artificial hip prosthesis to substitute for the natural joint. Different types of metal and plastic materials have been used for this purpose with varying degrees of success. A roller-bearing design has been suggested as necessary to duplicate the natural low friction mechanism (Tanner, 1959).

The next problem suggests an approach to calculation of frictional effects in joints of the human body. The coefficient of friction between articular surfaces is assumed to be 0.015, based on experimental tests cited previously (Charnley, 1959; Jones, 1934; Tanner, 1959; Fung, 1981; Collins and Kingsbury, 1981). Measurements of the radius of joint curvature were taken from x-ray films.

Joint Friction

We will examine the problem of friction with regard to the curved surface shown in Figure 6–13A. With the applied load centered over the center of curvature (O), the reaction (R) is normal to the surface and no friction exists. If a force (P) is added as shown in Figure 6–13B, the resultant of the applied load moves to the left, as shown, and for equilibrium to exist the reaction (R) must also move to the left to coincide with it. This reaction is the resultant of a normal force that passes through the center of curvature and a frictional force that is tangent to the curve at the point of load application. As shown in Figure 6–12C, this is analogous to the inclined plane problem described earlier. As the resultant moves farther from the center of curvature, the slope of the plane increases, and the angle between R and N will increase until the angle of ϕ (the angle of friction) is reached. With further movement of the resultant, equilibrium will be destroyed and motion will occur. The following

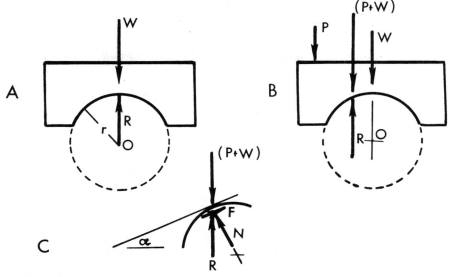

FIGURE 6–13

Analysis of friction in relation to a curved surface (see text).

problem will be used to illustrate these principles.

▶ PROBLEM 6–8

Consider the tibiotalar joint with the weight of the body of a 1000 N man centered over the center of curvature of the talus surface (Fig. 6–14A). A 500 N force will be acting on each ankle (neglecting the weight of the foot) and all muscle forces will be zero.
  QUESTION:
What force must be exerted through the Achilles tendon by the leg muscles before the joint starts to move?
  SOLUTION:
With the addition of a force, T (Fig. 6–14B), in the tendon acting at a distance a from the vertical axis through the center of curvature, the first step is to find the distance x to the resultant of W and T. Taking moments about W

$$Ta = x(W + T) \quad \text{or} \quad x = \frac{Ta}{W + T}$$

With motion impending, the angle between N and R (and between N and the vertical also) will be the angle of friction (ϕ). We have previously determined

the relationship between the coefficient of friction and ϕ to be

$$\mu = \tan \phi$$

From the figure

$$\sin \phi = \frac{x}{r}$$

where r is the radius of curvature, and for small angles, such as occur in joint friction, the sine of the angle is approximately equal to the tangent. Then we can write

$$\sin \phi \approx \tan \phi = \mu = \frac{x}{r}$$

Substituting the previously obtained expression for x we have

$$\mu = \frac{Ta}{r(W + T)}$$

and solving this for the maximum value of T that can be developed before motion occurs, we obtain

$$T = \frac{\mu r W}{a - \mu r}$$

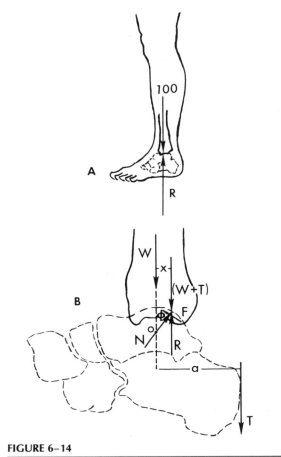

FIGURE 6–14

Calculation of friction at the tibiotalar joint (see text).

were increased under pathologic conditions, these relationships would change.

The role of synovial fluid in joint lubrication is under investigation. The accepted theory has been that synovial fluid is necessary for proper function of joints and has special viscous properties owing to a complex mucopolysaccharide it contains—hyaluronic acid. A fluid film between the joint surfaces is believed to absorb the frictional effects of motion and protect the articular cartilage from wear. Lack of fluid in a "dry joint" has been observed clinically to cause pain and to hinder normal function. On the other hand, some investigators contend that the synovial fluid in a joint has little or no importance to movement. When tested in an artificial joint, synovial fluid was found by Ropes and associates (1947) to have questionable lubricating properties. It has been claimed that after synovial fluid was wiped from the articular surfaces of joints, the coefficient of friction was not significantly altered (Charnley, 1959). The concept of a "synovial sponge" has been advanced in which synovial fluid is believed to be extruded from the cartilaginous surfaces as the articular cartilage is compressed. "It thus becomes impossible to decide whether the smear of synovial fluid which may be present on the joint surfaces derives from the joint cavity and is laid on the sliding surfaces, or whether the sliding surfaces generate the synovial fluid" (Jones, 1934). If the latter is the case, synovial fluid can be considered merely a byproduct of function.

Friction in the joints is of help in stabilizing the body when one is standing still. Since the synovial fluid is believed to be squeezed out from between the articular surfaces when they are under load for some time, the frictional force in the joint, which always acts to oppose motion, acts to hold the body in equilibrium. The frictional forces are, of course, augmented by muscle and ligamentous forces to maintain balance, but balance is not provided by these structures alone. Another factor in joint stability is the deformation of the articular cartilages as they are placed under load.

The many divergent views regarding joint function indicate that a great deal more experimental work must be done before normal and pathologic articular mechanisms are well under-

If we assume the coefficient of friction to be 0.015, and measure r and a and obtain 2.8 and 6 cm, respectively, we can substitute these values in this equation and solve for T:

$$T = \frac{0.015 \times 2.8 \times 500}{6 - 0.015 \times 2.8}$$

$$T = 3.5 \, N$$

EXAMPLES FROM THE LITERATURE

It appears from our calculations that frictional effects at the joint are small in relation to articular compression forces (Wright and Johns, 1960). However, if the coefficient of friction

stood. Indeed, this can be said also of the many areas of biomechanics as the subject is applied to musculoskeletal function of the human body and to the useful application of this knowledge in patient care.

QUESTIONS

1. Upon what does the frictional force between two objects depend?

2. What is the coefficient of friction between a 50 N box and the floor if a force of 15 N is needed to slide the box horizontally along the floor?

3. Suppose a child is pulling a 50 N box along a floor ($\mu = 0.5$) with a rope, making a 50° angle with the horizontal. What force must she be exerting on the rope? Assume the velocity is constant. What would happen if the rope were longer?

4. A 50 N box is resting on a tilt table ($\mu = 0.45$). As the table it tilted, at what angle will the box begin to slide?

5. What force is necessary to slide a 250 N box along a surface if the coefficient of friction between their surfaces is 0.6? What force would be necessary to pull the box up the incline if the surface were inclined to 30° with the horizontal? Would it require more force to lift the box or to slide it, if the incline is greater than 35°? At what degree of incline would it start to slide down the surface if the coefficient of friction were 0.36?

6. A therapist attempts to slide a box 1.3 m tall and 200 N in weight along the floor ($\mu = 0.3$). The base of the box is 0.6 m by 0.6 m with its mass evenly distributed. How much force is needed to slide the box? What will happen if she pushes horizontally at the top of the box? Where must she push on the box to slide it without having it tip over? Compare this example with a diathermy machine with poorly lubricated wheel axles.

7. Crutch tips have a greater tendency to slip as the angle with the supporting surface decreases. Explain.

8. Explain the reaction of crutch tips as a patient goes up and down a ramp.

9. If the coefficient of friction between the wheels and ramp surface is 0.3, what is the steepest angle the ramp may be and yet prevent a wheelchair from slipping?

10. A slippery ramp (m = 0.125) has an angle of 8° with the horizontal. Can a patient wheel his wheelchair up the ramp?

11. List at least ten different instances in which friction is a help or hindrance in physical therapy.

REFERENCES

Chaffin D, Andersson GBJ: Occupational Biomechanics. New York, John Wiley & Sons, 1984.

Charnley J: The lubrication of animal joints. Symposium on Biomechanics. London, Institution of Mechanical Engineers, 1959, pp 12–19.

Collins R, Kingsbury HB: Lubrication mechanism of articular joints. *In* Ghista DB (Ed): Osteoarthro Mechanics. Washington, DC, Hemisphere Publishing, 1982.

Fung YC: Biomechanics. New York, Springer-Verlag, 1981, pp 406–412.

Jackson R: The Cervical Syndrome, 2nd ed. Springfield, IL, Charles C Thomas, 1958.

Jones ED: Joint lubrication. Lancet 1:1426, 1934.

Judovich BD: Lumbar traction therapy—elimination of physical factors that prevent lumbar stretch. JAMA 159:549–550, 1955.

Klopsteg PE, Wilson PD: Human Limbs and Their Substitutes. New York, McGraw-Hill, 1954.

Knocke FJ, Knocke LS: Orthopaedic Nursing. Philadelphia, FA Davis, 1945.

Mears DC: Materials and Orthopedic Surgery. Baltimore, Williams & Wilkins, 1979.

Ropes MW, Robertson WB, Rossmeisl EC, et al.: Synovial fluid mucin. Acta Med Scand (Suppl) 196:700–734, 1947.

Tanner RI: The lubricating properties of synovial fluid. Symposium on Biomechanics. London, Institution of Mechanical Engineers, 1959.

Wright V, Johns RJ: Physical factors concerned with stiffness of normal and diseased joints. Bull Johns Hopkins Hosp 106:215–231, 1960.

7

Dynamics

INTRODUCTION

The previous chapters have been concerned with objects in static positions. To analyze movement of the human body we must study the principles of *dynamics*. Dynamics is the study of motion. This science is further subdivided into the areas of *kinematics*, the study of the characteristics of motion, and *kinetics*, the study of the forces that affect motion. Kinematics allows us to describe precisely the motion characteristics of position, velocity, and acceleration. For example, in the analysis of gait patterns we are concerned with the change in position of the center of mass of the body, the range of motion of the various segments, and the speed and direction of their motion. Kinematics is not concerned with the forces that cause the motion or the changes in motion. That is the province of kinetics. Gravity, friction, water and air resistance, muscle contraction, and elastic components are examples of forces that affect the motion of a body. By observing the characteristics of motion and by applying Newton's laws of motion, the characteristics of the forces involved may be more precisely determined. The study of dynamics is invaluable in the fields of medicine and physical education. Biomechanical investigations have played major roles in the analysis of gait patterns, development of prosthetics and orthotics, analysis of muscle function in a variety of skills, the effect of water and air resistance on the moving body, and the analysis of sports injuries. The basic principles of dynamics, along with a few examples, will be presented in this chapter. However, many problems dealing with dynamics are beyond the scope of this book.

TIME

The analysis of temporal factors is the first approach to the study of human movement. Factors related to time include cadence, duration of a movement phase, and the temporal pattern. The analysis of gait, for example, includes the number of steps per minute and is divided into the stance phase, in which the limb is in contact with the ground, and the swing phase, in which the limb is swinging free of the ground. The phases of double support, in walking, and of nonsupport, in running, may also be analyzed. The relationship of these various phases describes the temporal patterns of the movement. Knowledge of the time factor is essential in kinematic and kinetic analysis of motion since changes of position are always intimately connected with changes in time.

KINEMATICS

Motion is defined as a continuous change of position. Thus, when we consider motion we are concerned with *displacement*, that is, the change in position of a body. This change may be *translational*, whereby every point of the body is displaced along parallel lines (Fig. 7–1A), it may be *rotational*, with the points of the body describing concentric circles around an axis (Fig. 7–1B), or it may be a combination of the two (Fig. 7–1C). For example, the general movement of the human body during locomotion is translatory. However, to obtain this end result, the limbs act with rotatory motion around many joints (Fig. 7–2).

Translation

DISPLACEMENT

Let's look first at translation and its special case of linear motion. When a point is moved from one position (S_1) to another position (S_2) displacement occurs (Fig. 7–3). The straight line

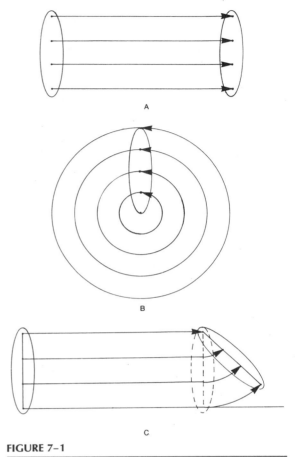

FIGURE 7–1

Types of motion: *A*, Translational. *B*, Rotational. *C*, Combination of translational and rotational motion.

distance (measured in units of length) between these two points is the magnitude of the displacement. Since we have stated that the point was moved from one location to another in a straight line, we must assign a direction to the movement. Thus, displacement is a vector quantity, with magnitude and direction, while distance is a scalar quantity, providing the magnitude without the direction. Figure 7–3 shows the displacement of a point at position S_1 to another position, S_2. By establishing a coordinate system, we may define the locations of S_1 and S_2 in terms of X and Y coordinates. We may then

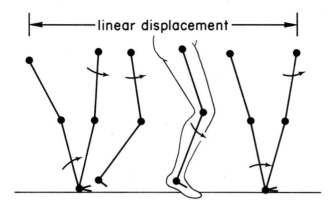

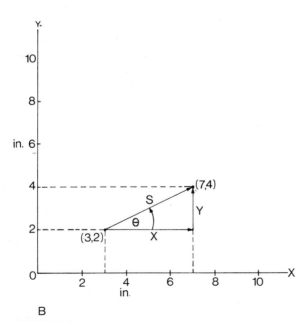

FIGURE 7-2

Rotation of the limbs to obtain translation of the body.

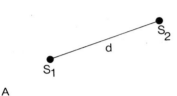

A

B

FIGURE 7-3

Linear displacement from point S_1 to point S_2.

determine the magnitude of displacement, or distance, between the two positions by using the Pythagorean theorem (a special case of the law of cosines). The direction of the displacement can be calculated by using one of the trigonometric functions.

▶ PROBLEM 7-1

QUESTION:
Suppose we moved a point from S_1 ($X_1 = 3$ m; $Y_1 = 2$ m) to S_2 ($X_2 = 7$ m; $Y_2 = 4$ m). What is the magnitude and direction of the displacement of the point?

SOLUTION:
We have established a coordinate system and defined the location of the points. The distance from S_1 to S_2 is unknown, but we can set up a right triangle with the magnitude of the displacement as its hypotenuse, and the X and Y displacements as its sides. The magnitude of the sides of the triangle may be determined by subtraction. For the X magnitude, $X_2 - X_1 = X$; for the Y magnitude, $Y_2 - Y_1 = Y$. Thus, for X, 4 m − 2 m = 2 m, and for Y, 7m − 3m = 4 m. The resulting displacement (S) may now be found by the Pythagorean theorem:

$$S = \sqrt{(4)^2 + (2)^2}$$
$$= \sqrt{16 + 4}$$
$$= \sqrt{20}$$
$$= 4.47 \text{ m}$$

Its direction with the X axis can be found using one of the trigonometric functions as follows.

$$\text{Tan } \theta = \frac{Y}{X}$$

$$= \frac{2 \text{ m}}{4 \text{ m}}$$

$$= 0.5$$

$$\theta = 26.5°$$

The point was moved 4.47 m to the right and upward at a 26.5° angle with the X axis.

VELOCITY

The change in position, however, provides us with only a minimum of information. We are often concerned with the amount of time that was needed to move the body from the initial position to the final position. Displacement per unit of time gives us the rate of displacement, or *velocity*. Similarly, speed is the distance per unit of time. Thus, velocity is a vector quantity, and speed, the magnitude of velocity, is a scalar quantity. The average linear velocity of an object is calculated by dividing the displacement (S) by the change in time taken to move from the first position to the final position. The symbol $\bar{v}$ will be used to represent average velocity. Thus,

$$\bar{v} = \frac{\text{displacement}}{\text{elapsed time}} = \frac{S_2 - S_1}{t_2 - t_1}$$

Often in literature the Greek letter delta (Δ) is used to represent change. Thus, instead of writing $S_2 - S_1$, we may write ΔS, meaning change in position. Instead of $t_2 - t_1$, Δt would mean change in time. The equation for average velocity then becomes

$$\bar{v} = \frac{\Delta S}{\Delta t}$$

This equation may be algebraically rearranged to become

$$S = \bar{v}t$$

The difference between speed and velocity is the direction factor of velocity. The algebraic equations may reveal nothing of the direction. The terms may be used interchangeably when the direction of motion is of no concern or is obvious.

▶ PROBLEM 7–2

QUESTION:
Suppose the displacement in the preceding problem took 0.2 sec. What would be the average velocity of the movement?
SOLUTION:
The distance moved was 4.47 m in a time of 0.2 sec.

Using the formula $\bar{v} = \frac{S}{t}$, we find that

$$\bar{v} = \frac{4.47 \text{ m}}{0.2 \text{ sec.}} = 22.35 \text{ m/sec.}$$

Notice that the equation provides only the magnitude of the velocity and not its direction.

The velocity of an object at a specific instant of time or at a certain point on its path is called its instantaneous velocity. Average velocity calculated over a short period of time will approach the value for instantaneous velocity.

The average velocity is $\Delta x / \Delta t$. However, as Δx decreases, the average velocity is computed over shorter time intervals. We may then define the instantaneous velocity as the limiting value of the average velocity as the change in displacement gets smaller and smaller. Thus, as the time interval (Δt) approaches 0,

$$v(t) = \lim_{\Delta t \to 0} \frac{\Delta x}{\Delta t} = \frac{dx}{dt}$$

This is the derivative of the displacement with respect to the time. The instantaneous velocity at any point on a displacement-time graph equals the slope of the tangent to the graph at that point.

ACCELERATION

As an object moves from one location to another, its velocity may not be constant over the entire distance. The magnitude of velocity may increase or decrease relative to its straight line of displacement, or the direction of velocity may change. These phenomena are known commonly as *acceleration* and *deceleration*. Deceleration is essentially negative acceleration. Therefore, mathematically, only the term acceleration needs to be dealt with. Acceleration occurs when there is a change in velocity. Since this change in velocity takes place over a certain time interval, we can say that acceleration is the rate of change in velocity. Mathematically, the average acceleration (ā) is the change in velocity from initial to final values ($v_f - v_i$) divided by the time taken for change to occur ($t_f - t_i$) or

$$\bar{a} = \frac{v_f - v_i}{t_f - t_i} = \frac{\Delta v}{\Delta t}$$

If v_f is greater than v_i, the object is accelerating, or has positive acceleration. If v_f is less than v_i, the object is decelerating or has negative acceleration.

▶ **PROBLEM 7–3**

Suppose a runner starting from a standstill reached his maximum velocity of 5 m/sec. in 4 sec.
  QUESTION:
What was his average acceleration from standing to his final velocity?
  SOLUTION:
The runner's movement is illustrated in Figure 7–4. His initial velocity (v_i) was 0 m/sec.; his final velocity (v_f) was 5 m/sec.; and the change in time was 4 sec. Substituting in the equation

$$\bar{a} = \frac{\Delta v}{\Delta t}$$
$$= \frac{5 \text{ m/sec.} - 0 \text{ m/sec.}}{4 \text{ sec.}}$$
$$= 1.25 \text{ m/sec.}^2$$

The average acceleration of the runner over a period of 4 sec. was 1.25 m/sec.² If we would analyze his motion in smaller time periods, we would see that his acceleration was greater or less than this value at certain intervals. Very small time intervals approach his instantaneous acceleration values.

Instantaneous acceleration at a specific point in time or at a specific location is defined in the same way as instantaneous velocity. It is the rate at which changes in velocity occur. As the time interval, Δt, approaches 0,

$$\bar{a}(t) = \lim_{\Delta t = 0} \frac{\Delta v}{\Delta t} = \frac{dv}{dt} = \frac{ddx}{dtdt} = \frac{d^2x}{dt^2}$$

Instantaneous velocity is the first derivative of the distance with respect to time, while acceleration is the second derivative of the distance with respect to time.

The instantaneous acceleration at any point on a velocity-time graph equals the slope of the tangent to the graph at that point.

To determine the acceleration in terms of displacement, we may perform the following:

$$\bar{a} = \frac{dv}{dt}\frac{dx}{dx} = \frac{dx}{dt}\frac{dv}{dx} v \frac{dv}{dx}$$

If the linear acceleration is given, the velocity and position can be found by methods of integral calculus. To find velocity (v):

$$dv/dt = a(t)$$
$$dv = a(t) \, dt$$
$$\int dv = \int a(t)dt$$
$$v = \int a(t)dt + C_1$$

C_1 can be determined if v is known at any time. Often C_1 is expressed in terms of Vo when t = 0. To find position (x):

$$dx/dt = v(t)$$
$$dx = v(t)dt$$
$$\int dx = \int v(t)dt$$
$$x = \int v(t)dt + C_2$$

If a is given as a function of x, then

$$v \, dv/dx = a(x); \quad \int vdv = \int a(x)dx;$$
$$v2/2 = \int a(x)dx + C_3$$

The change in velocity in any time interval is equal to the area between the acceleration-time graph and the time axis.

$$v_2 - v_1 = \int_{T_1}^{T_2} vdt$$

The displacement in any time interval is therefore equal to the area between a velocity-time graph and the time axis.

$$x_2 - x_1 = \int_{T_1}^{T_2} adt$$

Rotation

DISPLACEMENT

Rotational motion, which is often called angular motion, occurs about a fixed axis. As we study rotational motion, we will see that many of the equations describing the angular movement about a fixed axis are analogous to those describing linear motion. In rotation of a rigid body, all lines on the body rotate through the same angle at the same time. Every particle on

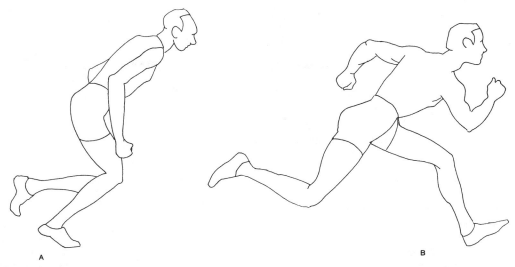

FIGURE 7–4

Acceleration of a runner.

the body travels in an arc with the same angular displacement. Thus, instead of being measured in terms of length, rotational displacement is measured as angular change in terms of degrees or radians. A *radian* is defined as the ratio of an arc (s) to the radius (r) of a circle (Fig. 7–5).

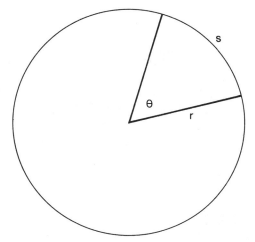

FIGURE 7–5

A radian $\theta = \dfrac{s}{r} = 1$.

Thus, θ (in radians) = s/r. Since the length units of the arc divided by the length units of the radius cancel one another, the radian measure is unitless.

One radian equals the angle (θ) formed at the center of the circle by an arc (s) of a length equal to the radius (r) of the circle. The relationship between the measurement of radians and degrees is shown as follows.

We know that the circumference of the circle equals 2π times the radius (r) and a circle equals 360°, or c = $2\pi r$ = 360°. The length of the arc (s) is a portion of the circumference (c); and the central angle (θ) is the same portion of 360°. Thus:

$$\frac{s}{c} = \frac{s}{2\pi r} = \frac{\theta}{360}$$

For 1 radian, s = r, then

$$\frac{1}{2\pi} = \frac{\theta}{360°}$$

and $\qquad 2\pi\theta = 360°$

Then $\qquad \theta = \dfrac{360°}{2\pi}$

and $\qquad \theta = 57.3°$

Thus, the angle formed when the length of the arc (s) equals the radius of the circle (r) is 57.3°. Mathematically, radians are easier to work with than degrees.

Angular displacement is probably the most common kinematic measurement taken for human motion. Because of the structure of the human body as a linked system of rigid segments moving about joint axes, the kinematics of the body is often approached by analysis of rotational motion.

Similar to linear displacement, rotational displacement refers to change in position. However, in the case of rotation, the change is angular, with the rotational displacement of the body specified by an angle in relation to a reference line. The magnitude of the change in position can be found by subtracting the initial position, θ_1, from the final position, θ_2 ($\theta_2 - \theta_1 = \Delta\theta$).

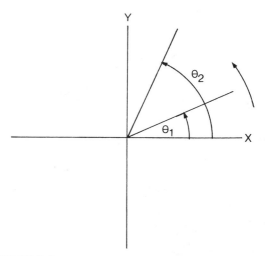

FIGURE 7–6

Rotational or angular displacement.

▶ **PROBLEM 7–4**

QUESTION:
Suppose a body shown in Figure 7–6 forming an angle θ_1 of 25° with the X axis is rotated to a position θ_2, which is at an angle of 68° with the X axis. What is the angular displacement of the body?

SOLUTION:
The angular displacement is the change in position from θ_1 to θ_2. Its direction, determined from Figure 7–6, is counterclockwise. The change in position is found by

$$\Delta\theta = \theta_2 - \theta_1$$
then
$$\Delta\theta = 68° - 25°$$
$$= 43°$$
in radians
$$\theta = \frac{43°}{57.3°} = 0.75 \text{ rad.}$$

The angular displacement of the body is 43 degrees or 0.75 radian.

VELOCITY

Angular velocity or rate of change of angular displacement is another important concern in the study of human motion. It is determined in a manner similar to that of finding linear veloc-ity. Thus, the change of angular displacement ($\theta_f - \theta_i$), divided by the change in time ($t_f - t_i$) in which the displacement occurs, reveals the average angular velocity ($\overline{\omega}$). We write

$$\overline{\omega} = \frac{\theta_f - \theta_i}{t_f - t_i} = \frac{\Delta\theta}{\Delta t}$$

▶ **PROBLEM 7–5**

QUESTION:
If the change in position in the previous problem occurred in 0.3 sec., what is the average angular velocity of the body?

SOLUTION:
Using the equation $\overline{\omega} = \frac{\Delta\theta}{\Delta t}$, we substitute in the known values

$$\overline{\omega} = \frac{0.75 \text{ rad.}}{0.3 \text{ sec.}} = 2.5 \text{ rad./sec.}$$

As was stated for linear motion, the magnitude of the velocity or speed is our major concern. Hence, we will be using the terms *angular velocity* and *angular speed* interchangeably.

Instantaneous angular velocity may be determined in the same way instantaneous linear velocity was calculated. As the time interval becomes smaller and smaller, the average velocity approaches an instantaneous value. The instantaneous angular velocity may be defined as the ratio of the very small change in the angular position at a very small time interval. As the change in time (Δt) approaches 0,

$$\omega(t) = \lim_{\Delta t \to 0} \frac{\Delta \theta}{\Delta t} = \frac{d\theta}{dt}$$

This is the derivative of the displacement with respect to time.

ACCELERATION

A change in the magnitude of angular velocity over a given time interval is called the average angular acceleration ($\overline{\alpha}$). This corresponds to the change in the magnitude of velocity in linear motion and is determined by the general equation

$$\overline{\alpha} = \frac{\omega_f - \omega_i}{t_f - t_i} = \frac{\Delta \omega}{\Delta t}$$

where ω_i is the initial angular velocity, and ω_f is the final angular velocity. If ω_f is greater than ω_i, the acceleration is positive; if it is less, the acceleration is negative.

▶ **PROBLEM 7–6**

QUESTION:
If a body starting from rest had a final velocity of 15 rad./sec. after a period of 2 sec., what would be the average acceleration of that body?
SOLUTION:
Figure 7–7A illustrates the movement of the body. By using the formula

$$\overline{\alpha} = \frac{\Delta \omega}{\Delta t},$$

then $\dfrac{15 \text{ rad./sec.} - 0 \text{ rad./sec.}}{2 \text{ sec.}} = 7.5 \text{ rad./sec.}^2$

The body would have a positive average acceleration of 7.5 rad./sec.^{2}

▶ **PROBLEM 7–7**

QUESTION:
What is the average angular acceleration of a body if after rotating with an angular velocity of 6.2 rad./sec., it comes to a stop within 0.2 sec.?
SOLUTION:
The body's movement is shown in Figure 7–7B. Again we use the formula

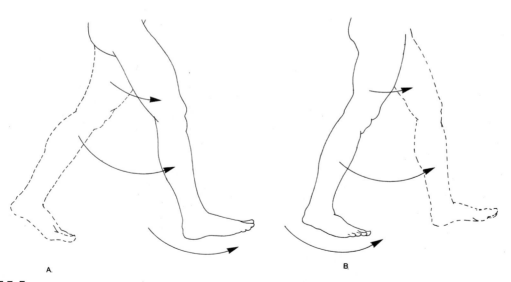

A.   B.

FIGURE 7–7

Angular acceleration: A, Positive. B, Negative.

$$\overline{\alpha} = \frac{\Delta\omega}{\Delta t}$$

$$= \frac{0 \text{ rad./sec.} - 6.2 \text{ rad./sec.}}{0.2 \text{ sec.}} = -31 \text{ rad./sec}^2$$

The rotating object brought to a halt has a negative acceleration, or deceleration, of 31 rad./sec.²

The instantaneous angular acceleration, as for linear acceleration is the second derivative of angular displacement with respect to time, or

$$\alpha = \lim_{\Delta t \to 0} \frac{\Delta\omega}{\Delta t} = \frac{d\omega}{dt} = \frac{dd\theta}{dtdt} = \frac{d^2\theta}{dt^2}$$

Another useful way to determine instantaneous angular acceleration is to calculate it in terms of change of position as follows:

$$\alpha = \frac{d\omega}{dt}\frac{d\theta}{d\theta} = \frac{d\theta d\omega}{dt d\theta} = \frac{wd\omega}{d\theta}$$

Relationship Between Linear and Angular Motion

Often we may need to know the linear parameters of various points on a body that is rotating. For example, the linear motion of the foot depends upon the angular motion of the lower limb. When we defined the radian, a relationship between the length of an arc (s) subtended by an angle (θ) measured in radians, and the radius (r) of the circle was presented as $\theta = \frac{s}{r}$ or s = rθ (see Fig. 7–5). The distance Δs that any point moves on a rotating body can be determined from the angular displacement Δθ through which the body has rotated, and the distance the point lies from the axis of rotation. Note from Figure 7–8 that a point having a greater radius (r_2) also travels a greater distance (Δs_2) although the angular displacement is exactly the same. If we assume that the particular point on a rotating body moves in a straight line between successive positions, a small point revolving in a circular path has an approximate displacement of Δs (Fig. 7–9). With a sufficiently high sampling rate, the approximation is fairly accurate. Thus, to calculate the linear distance traveled by a point rotating about an axis, we use the formula s = rθ. By algebraic manipu-

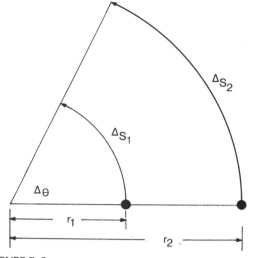

FIGURE 7–8

Relationship between angular and linear motion.

lation, we can determine the equation relating linear and angular velocity. We write

$$\omega = \frac{\theta}{t}, \text{ v} = \frac{s}{t}, \text{ and s} = \theta r$$

then $$v = \frac{\theta r}{t}$$

and $$v = \omega r$$

Although a particle on a rotating body is following a curved path, at any particular instant its velocity is tangent to the path, and it has a linear velocity.

This linear velocity relationship may also be found in the following manner:

$$S = r\theta$$

Differentiate both sides of the equation with respect to time:

$$dx/dt = r \, d\theta/dt$$

Since dx/dt is the magnitude of the linear velocity (v) of the point on the rotating body, then

$$v = rW$$

The linear acceleration related to the angular acceleration in this case is tangential to the circle

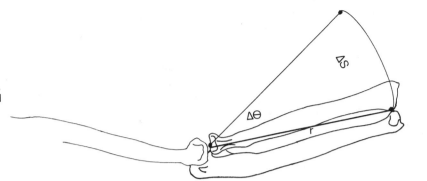

FIGURE 7–9

Relationship between angular and linear displacement.

and is related to the magnitude of the angular acceleration. We write

$$\alpha = \frac{\omega}{t}, \; a = \frac{v}{t}, \text{ and } v = \omega r$$

then $\quad a_T = \dfrac{\omega r}{t}$

and $\quad a_T = \alpha r$

As the time approaches 0, by differentiating both sides of the equation $v = \omega r$ with respect to time we have:

$$dv/dt = r \, dw/dt$$
$$\text{or } a_T = r\alpha$$

Since v is the linear magnitude of the angular velocity, a_T would represent the tangential component of the angular acceleration.

Another component of angular acceleration is related to its constant change in direction. Since the linear velocity of a particle in rotational motion is tangent to the circle, the direction of the velocity (v) is always changing. Thus, acceleration is always present. The change in direction points toward the center of the circle, along its radius. Hence, it is called radial acceleration, a_R.

If the magnitude of velocity is constant for a point on a body with angular motion, and t is the time to complete one revolution ($2 \pi r$), then this magnitude of velocity would be

$$v = 2\pi r/t$$

The average acceleration, when the magnitude of velocity is constant, must be related to the change in direction of the velocity. The average acceleration ($\Delta v/\Delta t$) in this case must be in the direction of the vector (v) which always points toward the center of rotation.

Derivations beyond the scope of this book reveal that

$$a_R = \frac{\Delta v}{\Delta t} = \frac{v}{r} \frac{\Delta s}{\Delta t} = \frac{v^2}{r}$$

The instantaneous radial acceleration would be

$$a_R = \lim_{\Delta t \to 0} \frac{v}{r} \frac{\Delta s}{\Delta t} = \frac{v}{r} \lim_{\Delta t \to 0} \frac{\Delta s}{\Delta t} = \frac{v}{r} v$$

or

$$a_R = \frac{v^2}{r}$$

Mathematical principles beyond the scope of this book derive the formula for the radial acceleration as

$$a_R = r\omega^2 = \frac{v^2}{r}$$

The tangential acceleration component and the radial acceleration component of the particle are perpendicular to each other (Fig. 7–10). Hence, the resulting acceleration (a) of a particle rotating around an axis can be calculated using the Pythagorean theorem. Thus,

$$a = \sqrt{a_T^2 + a_R^2}$$

The importance of observing the radial acceleration is related to part of Newton's first law.

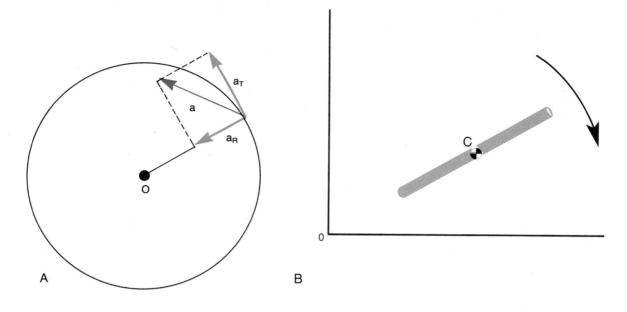

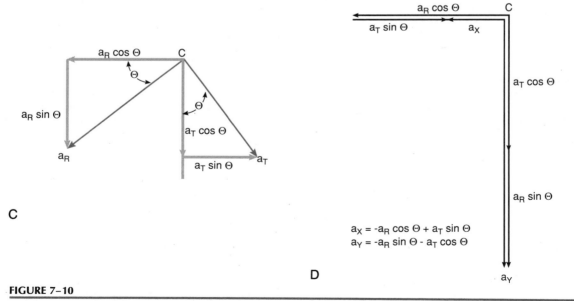

FIGURE 7–10

A, Components of angular acceleration. *B*, Rod turning around point O. *C*, X and Y components of a_R and a_T. *D*, Summation of X and Y components. *E*, Relationship between linear and angular acceleration components.

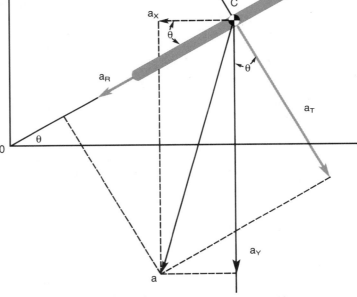

FIGURE 7–10

Continued E, Relationship between linear and angular acceleration components.

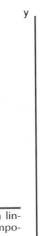

If you remember, a body tends to move in a straight line unless acted upon by an outside force. The radial acceleration directed toward the center of the circle is a result of an outside force (centripetal force) acting on the particle.

If the angular acceleration is given, the velocity and position can be found by methods of integral calculus, as was done in the linear situation. To find velocity (w):

$$d\omega/dt = \alpha(t)$$
$$d\omega = \alpha(t)dt$$
$$\int d\omega = \int \alpha(t)dt$$
$$\omega = \int \alpha(t)dt + c_1$$

c_1 can be determined if v is known at any time. Often c_1 is expressed in terms of ωo when $t = 0$.

To find position (Θ):

$$dx/dt = v(t)$$
$$dx = v(t)dt$$
$$\int dx = \int v(t)dt$$
$$X = \int v(t)dt + c_2$$

If α is given as a function of Θ, then

$$\omega d\omega/d\Theta = \alpha(\Theta); \int \omega d\omega = \int \alpha(\Theta)d\Theta;$$
$$\omega^2/2 = \int \alpha(\Theta)d\Theta + c_3$$

▶ PROBLEM 7–8

Note that when converting angular to linear parameters, or vice versa, the radius from the point involved to the axis of motion is the relating factor (that is, $s = \Theta r$, $v = \omega r$, $a_T = \alpha r$). For example, a rigid

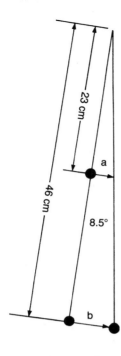

t = 0.2 second

FIGURE 7–11

Linear motion of a point on a rotating rigid body in time interval (t) of 0.2 seconds.

body 46 cm long moves with a uniform angular velocity through a range of motion of 8.5° counterclockwise (Fig. 7–11) in 0.2 sec.

QUESTIONS:

What is the angular velocity of the body? What is the distance moved by a point (*a*) 23 cm from the axis? What is the linear velocity of point *a*? What is the distance moved by a point (*b*) at the end of the rigid body 46 cm from the axis? What is the linear velocity of point *b*? What is the acceleration of point *b*?

SOLUTION:

To determine the angular velocity, we convert the 8.5° to radians and divide by the elapsed time.

$$\frac{\theta}{57.3} = \text{rad.}; \frac{8.5°}{57.3°} = 0.148 \text{ rad.}$$

$$\omega = \frac{\theta}{5} = \frac{0.148 \text{ rad.}}{0.2 \text{ sec.}}$$

$$\omega = 0.74 \text{ rad./sec.}$$

The angular velocity of the rigid body is 0.74 rad./sec. To find the distance traveled by point *a* 23 cm

from the axis and for point *b* 46 cm from the axis, we use the formula s = rθ. Thus, for point *a*

$$s_a = 23 \text{ cm} \times 0.148 \text{ rad.}$$

$$= 3.4 \text{ cm}$$

and for point *b*

$$s_b = 46 \text{ cm} \times 0.148 \text{ rad.}$$

$$= 6.8 \text{ cm}$$

Thus, point *a* travels an arc of 3.4 cm, while point *b* moves 6.8 cm. The linear velocity is found by the equation

$$(1) \ v = r\omega, \text{ or } (2) \ v = s/t$$

Then, for point *a*

$$(1) \ v = 23 \text{ cm} \times 0.74 \text{ rad./sec.}$$

$$= 17 \text{ cm/sec.}$$

or

$$(2) \ v = 3.4 \text{ cm/0.2 sec.}$$

$$= 17 \text{ cm/sec.}$$

and for point *b*

$$(1) \ v = 46 \text{ cm} \times 0.74 \text{ rad./sec.}$$

$$= 34 \text{ cm/sec.}$$

or

$$(2) \ v = 6.8 \text{ cm/0.2 sec.}$$

$$= 34 \text{ cm/sec.}$$

Point *b*, which is twice the distance from the axis of motion as point *a*, traveled twice the distance with twice the magnitude of velocity as point *a*. Thus, although both points are on a rigid body traversing the same angle, their linear velocities are different.

Since the angular velocity has a constant magnitude, there would be no angular acceleration and, hence, no tangential acceleration of point *b*.

$$\alpha = \frac{\Delta\omega}{\Delta t} = \frac{0}{0.2} = 0$$

$$a_T = \alpha r = 0 \times 46 \text{ cm} = 0$$

The direction of the tangential velocity, however, has been changed, resulting in radial acceleration.

$$a_R = \frac{v^2}{r}$$

$$= \frac{34 \text{ cm/sec.}^2}{46 \text{ cm}}$$

$$= \frac{1156 \text{ cm}^2/\text{sec.}^2}{46 \text{ cm}}$$

$$= 25 \text{ cm/sec.}^2$$

The resulting acceleration, using the Pythagorean theorem, is

$$a = \sqrt{(a_T)^2 + (a_R)^2} = \sqrt{0 + (25)^2}$$
$$= 25 \text{ cm/sec.}^2$$

Point *b* on the body is being accelerated toward the axis of rotation at a magnitude of 25 cm/sec.^{2} If the point had both radial and tangential acceleration, one of the trigonometric functions could be used to calculate its resultant direction. Thus, in the previous problem, if we considered the radius as the X axis and the tangent as the Y axis, the angle of the resultant acceleration with the radius would be

$$\tan \theta = \frac{a_T}{a_R} = \frac{0}{25} = 0$$

$$\theta = 0° \text{ with the radius}$$

Correlation of Acceleration Components

The values of a_R and a_T represent the radial and tangential components of acceleration (Fig. 7–10A). We may need a_T sometime to relate these components of a point moving in a curved path to their rectangular components a_X and a_Y. The correlation between the radial and tangential components and the rectangular components is shown in Figure 7–10B.

Consider point *c* which is the center of mass of a thin rod moving around axis 0.

The radial acceleration ($a_R = w^2 r$) is toward 0 as point *c* is forced to change direction. The tangential acceleration ($a_T = \alpha r$) is in the direction of motion in this situation as the velocity of *c* increases. Analysis of the direction of the tangential acceleration is essential for showing the correlation between these sets of acceleration components. If the rod had a negative acceleration (decreasing velocity) at this time, the tangential acceleration would be shown in the opposite direction.

To obtain a_X from a_R and a_T, we add the X components of both a_R and a_T. To obtain a_Y, we add the Y components of a_R and a_T (Fig. 7–10C and 7–10D). In this situation the equation would be

$$a_X = -a_R \cos \theta + a_T \sin \theta$$
$$a_Y = -a_R \sin \theta - a_T \cos \theta$$

Equations would be similar for obtaining rectangular components of acceleration for any moving point. Only the signs may change depending upon the direction of motion and the direction of tangential acceleration.

Similar equations may be used to convert rectangular components to radial and tangential components. In this example, the equations would be

$$a_R = -a_X \cos \theta - a_Y \sin \theta$$
$$a_T = a_X \sin \theta - a_Y \cos \theta$$

See if you can draw the diagram to illustrate these equations. Use Figure 7–10E as a guide.

A variety of recording and measuring devices have been developed to obtain kinematic parameters. Bernstein (1967) discussed the filming of synchronized lights placed on body parts; Nelson and associates (1969) described the utilization of stroboscopy; Karpovich and associates (1959, 1960) have developed electrogoniometers; and the process of cinematography was described by Sutherland and Hagy (1972) and reviewed by Miller and Nelson (1973).

Video analysis was described by Winter and associates (1972 and 1974). A report about an optoelectric system using pulsed light-emitting diode targets was presented by Woltring and Marsolais (1980). Morris (1973) summarized the technique of accelerometry used to measure acceleration directly. Smidt and co-workers (1971) used this technique to analyze several types of walking. These methods have been described by Dainty and Norman (1987). These techniques and others like them utilize the same basic procedure to obtain the desired kinematic values. This common procedure includes (1) obtaining the appropriate recordings of the movement by such means as photographs or videotapes, (2) making tracings or stick figures of the recordings, (3) taking accurate measurements, and (4) using the proper equations to calculate the needed parameters. Formerly, this procedure was quite tedious and time-consuming. With the development of computers, however, some of these steps have been combined, and the time for the reduction of data has been greatly decreased (Plagenhoef, 1966, 1968; Petak, 1971). Salek and Murdock (1985) discussed the importance of objective gait analysis. They compared visual observation with a quantitative measurement method (video) and found that the visual observation was not adequate. They stated that the modern gait laboratory depends upon (1) visual observation, (2) quantitative measurement, and (3) biomechanical analysis.

In the following problems we will apply the preceding steps to obtain some kinematic parameters of (1) elbow flexion and (2) lower limb motion during walking. Remember that any of the previously mentioned recording devices could supply the necessary recordings.

▶ **PROBLEM 7–9**

The kinematic parameters of elbow flexion vary as the conditions under which the limb functions are changed. Let's consider the differences in movement values of the unloaded limb to one with a weight held in the hand.

QUESTIONS:
Compare the kinematic parameters of elbow flexion for the conditions of an unloaded limb and one with 4.5 Kg mass held in the hand. Determine the values for the parameters listed in Table 7–1.

SOLUTION:
From the appropriate recording procedure, we may draw a figure representing the changes in position of the forearm in the two conditions (Fig. 7–12A and 7–

12B). A time interval between each successive line of 0.02 sec. was obtained from the recording method. From these drawings the kinematic parameters may be measured and calculated. The total angular displacement is obtained by measuring the change in position from the initial position θ_i to the final position θ_f. The angle may be measured directly or calculated using the formula $\Delta\theta = \theta_f - \theta_i$. Thus, the total displacement is

for unloaded limb: and for 4.5 Kg load:
$\Delta\theta = 125° - 0°$ $\Delta\theta = 125° - 0°$
$\quad = 125°$ $\quad = 125°$

By changing these values to radians, $\dfrac{125°}{57.3°} = 2.18$

rad., we obtain a total displacement of 125° or 2.18 rad. The time duration of the movement is obtained by counting the total number of time intervals on the stick diagrams and multiplying by the time of each interval, 0.02 sec. For the unloaded limb the duration of the movement was 8 times 0.02, or 0.16 sec.; for the loaded condition the duration was 16 times 0.02, or 0.32 sec.

Measurements of each individual line for the separate time intervals yield the values listed in Table 7–2 for the two conditions. The change in angle displacement ($\Delta\theta$) could either be measured directly or calculated from the formula $\Delta\theta = \theta_n - \theta_{n-1}$, where $n - 1$ is the beginning line of the interval and n is the end line of that interval. For the remaining solution, all values have been calculated for the unloaded limb. The student should determine the values for the loaded limb from the data given.

TABLE 7–1. KINEMATIC PARAMETERS FOR UNLOADED AND LOADED ELBOW FLEXION

	Unloaded	Loaded
1. Angular displacement (range of motion)		
2. Total duration of the movement		
3. Average angular velocity		
a. For the total ROM		
b. For the first quarter of motion		
c. For the second quarter of motion		
d. For the third quarter of motion		
e. For the fourth quarter of motion.		
4. Magnitude of maximum velocity		
5. Position of maximum velocity		
6. Magnitude of maximum acceleration		
7. Position of maximum acceleration		
8. Magnitude of maximum deceleration		
9. Position of maximum deceleration		

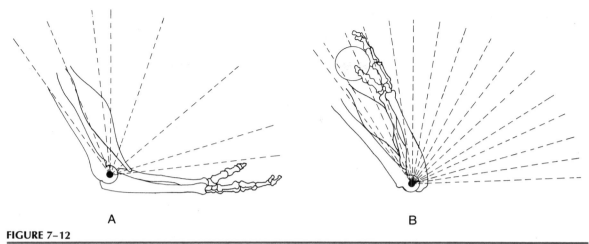

FIGURE 7-12

Tracings of forearm during elbow flexion from stroboscopic photographs: A, Unloaded. B, Loaded (time interval 0.02 seconds).

The average velocity for each interval and for the quarter intervals is calculated from the general equation

$$\bar{\omega} = \frac{\Delta\theta}{\Delta t}$$

The individual interval values are shown in Table 7-2 for the unloaded limb, while the quarter intervals are given in Table 7-1. The value of the maximum average angular velocity for an individual time interval can be found by looking in the $\bar{\omega}$ column in Table 7-2. Its position lies between the angular values of the two lines bordering the time interval with the largest change in displacement. The average value is assumed to occur at the midpoint between the two lines. In our problem for the unloaded limb, the maximum velocity occurs between 41.3° and 72° (0.720 and 1.256 rad.), or at 56.65° (0.989 rad.). From the stick drawing we can find the position of maximum velocity by finding the largest angle between successive time intervals.

For calculation of acceleration from objective measurements, three displacement data points are necessary for one acceleration of the limb. For successive time intervals, we must find the change in angular velocity, $\bar{\omega} = \omega_n - \omega_{n-1}$. Since the velocities were determined over separate time intervals, and the results are average values that are assumed to occur at the midpoint of the interval, the time interval (Δt) for calculating the acceleration is the midpoint of the initial interval to the midpoint of the final interval. For adjacent time intervals in one prob-

lem, this value is the same value as one interval (the last half of the initial interval and the first half of the final interval), or 0.02 sec. The average acceleration for each interval is found using the formula

$$\alpha = \frac{\omega_n - \omega_{n-1}}{\Delta t}$$

The values for each pair of time intervals are shown in the $\bar{\alpha}$ column in Table 7-2. The maximum acceleration of 545.5 rad./sec.^{2} is found at the midpoint angle of 18° (0.3141 rad.). The maximum deceleration of 366.64 rad./sec.^{2} is found at 96.2° (1.679 rad.).

The values of displacement, velocity, and acceleration may be "graphed" as shown in Figures 7-13A to 7-13C. Note that the acceleration is zero at the point of maximum velocity.

In the graphic approach, by measuring the slope (tangent) of the displacement time curve at each point on the graph, the average velocity may be established for that interval. From the velocity-time curve, the same procedure will yield the acceleration.

Theoretically, the curves will have a smooth curved line. In reality, however, the motion may be somewhat jerky. This movement will be reflected in the three graphs, especially in the acceleration curve.

Smoothing techniques have been developed to reduce data errors that occur from measurement and mathematical manipulation (Winter et al., 1974; Zernicke et al., 1976; Pezzack et al., 1977; Jackson,

TABLE 7–2. MEASURED AND CALCULATED KINEMATIC VALUES FOR THE UNLOADED AND LOADED FOREARM DURING ELBOW FLEXION

Line	Time	Unloaded					Loaded				
		θ^a	$\Delta\theta$	$\overline{\omega}^b$	$\Delta\overline{\omega}$	$\overline{\alpha}^c$	θ^a	$\Delta\theta$	$\overline{\omega}^b$	$\Delta\overline{\omega}$	$\overline{\alpha}^c$
1	0.00	0.0					0.0				
2	0.02	0.126	0.126	6.28	3.14	157.0	0.063				
3	0.04	0.314	0.188	9.42	10.91	545.5	0.162				
4	0.06	0.720	0.406	20.33	6.46	323.0	0.297				
5	0.08	1.256	0.536	26.79	−5.67	−283.65	0.443				
6	0.10	1.679	0.423	21.12	−7.33	−366.64	0.597				
7	0.12	1.955	0.276	13.79	−6.37	−318.6	0.768				
8	0.14	2.103	0.148	7.42	−3.52	−176.0	0.939				
9	0.16	2.182	0.079	3.9			1.092				
10	0.18						1.246				
11	0.20						1.400				
12	0.22						1.553				
13	0.24						1.705				
14	0.26						1.852				
15	0.28						1.988				
16	0.30						2.105				
17	0.32						2.182				

[a]In radians.
[b]In radians/second.
[c]In radians/second^2.

1979; Miller et al., 1980). The student should be able to graph the curves for elbow flexion in the loaded condition.

Similar calculations can be made from objective recordings of the gait—for example, for linear movement of the foot, and body center of mass, and for upper and lower limb movements. To obtain the kinematic characteristics of motion, the only necessary parameters to be recorded are displacement and time, since once displacement is measured over a given time interval, the average velocity and acceleration may be calculated. In Problem 7–9 all data would be more precise if smaller time intervals were used. This procedure, however, increases the number of measurements and calculations needed. A decision must be reached as to the level of precision necessary versus time and labor involved.

Kinetics

In the preceding action on kinematics, we studied and described motion. In this section we will study the forces that affect motion and their relationship to the resulting characteristics of motion. We may study force and motion by one of

three related approaches based on Newton's laws of motion. For analysis of force and instantaneous accelerations, the *acceleration approach* may be used. When force is acting over a period of time or a collision is involved, the *impulse-momentum approach* may be applied. The *work-energy approach* is used when a force acts over a distance. A full understanding of kinematic parameters is essential in order to use these approaches.

ACCELERATION APPROACH

Let's first look at the acceleration approach. When studying the principles of static equilibrium, we found that the resultant force acting on a body equaled zero. No acceleration was produced. What happens, however, when the forces are unbalanced and the resultant force is not zero?

Translatory Motion

In Chapter 2 we defined force as a push or pull, but we may also define force as the physical en-

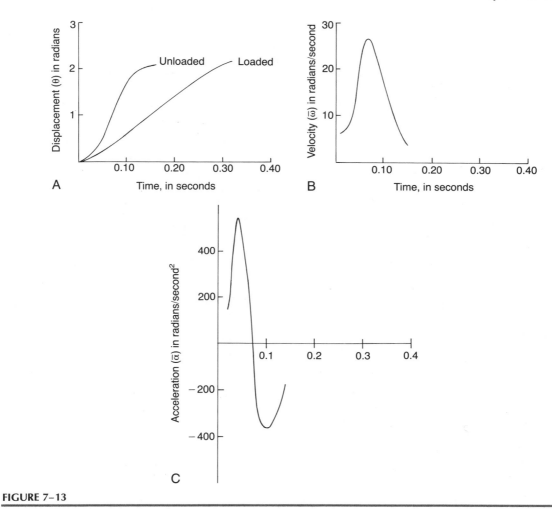

FIGURE 7–13

Graphs of forearm motion (unloaded): *A*, Angular displacement versus time. *B*, Angular velocity versus time. *C*, Angular acceleration versus time.

tity that tends to accelerate a body to which it is applied. Force is required to start or stop an object or to change its direction of motion. This results in a change in the object's velocity, which we have defined earlier as acceleration. Through experimentation, scientists have found that the acceleration produced is directly proportional to the resultant force acting on it and is in the direction of that force. Thus,

$$a \propto F$$

Statics treats those special cases in which the resultant force is zero. Hence, the acceleration is zero.

We stated in Chapter 2 that mass is the amount of substance in a body. However, mass, under normal circumstances, may be considered a property of the body that resists change in its velocity. This is directly related to Newton's first law of motion, the law of inertia. The mass of an object provides its tendency to remain at rest or in constant motion, or to follow a straight

F = 1000 N

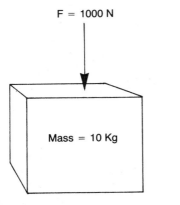

Mass = 10 Kg

FIGURE 7–14

Forces acting on a box.

path. Thus, mass represents the quantitative measure of the inertia of a body. An object with a large mass is more difficult to accelerate than one with a small mass. This indicates an inverse relationship of acceleration to mass, or a $\propto 1/m$. Newton, in this second law of motion, has combined the preceding two proportions relating force and mass to acceleration. Mathematically, the law may read $a = F/m$. Thus, to answer an earlier question, when the resultant force is not zero ($F \neq 0$), the body moves with an acceleration motion that is directly proportional to the resultant force and inversely proportional to the mass of the body.

▶ **PROBLEM 7–10**

QUESTION:

What is the acceleration of an object if a resultant force of 1000 N is applied to the object having a mass of 10 Kg?

SOLUTION:

We first draw a figure representing the object and the forces acting on it (Fig. 7–14). By using the formula $a = F/m$, we find that

$$a = 1000 \text{ N}/10 \text{ Kg} = 100 \text{ m/sec.}$$

By rearranging the preceding equation we find that

$$F/a = m$$

The ratio of F/a for a given body is always the same, but the ratio is different for different bodies. From this equation we see that mass is the constant proportionality between force and acceleration. Occasionally, the mass of a body can be determined by applying a known force to an object and measuring its resulting acceleration.

▶ **PROBLEM 7–11**

QUESTION:

What is the mass of an object that is accelerated at 2 m/sec.² by a 100 N force?

SOLUTION:

The accelerated object is shown in Figure 7–15. By using the equation $m = F/a$, we find that

$$m = \frac{F}{a} = \frac{100 \text{ N}}{2 \text{ m/sec.}^2}$$
$$m = 50 \text{ Kg}$$

▶ **PROBLEM 7–12**

QUESTION:

What is the mass of a body weighing 900 N?

SOLUTION:

When substituting into the formula $F/g = m$, we find that

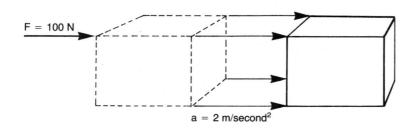

F = 100 N

a = 2 m/second²

FIGURE 7–15

Object accelerated at 2 m/sec.² by a 100 N force.

$$m = 900 \text{ N}/9.8 \text{ m/sec.}^2 = 91.8 \text{ Kg}$$

Often gravity is not the only force that acts on a body to affect its motion. If the magnitude of the force is unknown, we may calculate it by rearranging the formula to obtain $F = ma$. Thus, by knowing the weight of the body we may calculate its mass (m), and by observing its motion characteristic of acceleration, we may determine the unknown resultant force.

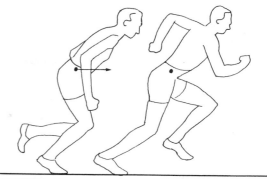

FIGURE 7–16

Acceleration of a runner.

▶ PROBLEM 7–13

QUESTION:

The maximum acceleration of a 700 N runner is 28 m/sec.^{2} What resultant force is necessary to obtain the maximum acceleration?

SOLUTION:

As in static problems, it is helpful to draw a diagram of the situation (Fig. 7–16). Next, the mass of the 700 N runner must be determined. Since $m = w/g$,

$$m = 700 \text{ N}/9.8 \text{ m/sec.}^2 = 71.4 \text{ Kg}$$

Thus, the mass is 71.4 Kg and the body is accelerated 28 m/sec.^{2} By substituting into the formula $F = ma$, the force to obtain this motion is

$$F = ma = 71.4 \text{ Kg} \times 28 \text{ m/sec.}^2$$
$$= 1999.2 \text{ N}$$

Remember that in this situation the force and acceleration, both vectors, act in the same direction.

Knowledge of any two terms of the equation allows for the third to be calculated. Thus, if the force and mass are known, the resulting acceleration can be found; if the acceleration and force are known, the mass can be determined; and if the mass and acceleration are known, the resultant force applied can be calculated.

By using the basic formula derived from Newton's second law of motion, $a = F/m$, we obtain the acceleration approach to solve problems in dynamics. This approach necessitates the use of instantaneous accelerations.

▶ PROBLEM 7–14

A patient is exercising his shoulder extensor muscles with wall pulleys (Fig. 7–17). Weights of 100 N, 50 N, and 25 N are loaded on the weight pan, which weighs 20 N. The patient is exerting an opposing force of 200 N.

QUESTION:

What is the resultant force of the entire system? What are the magnitude and direction of acceleration of the weights?

SOLUTION:

We must first draw a free body diagram, as shown in Figure 7–17. The weights acting downward will be negative in value and the force exerted through the rope will be positive. The next step is to find the resultant force. This is a linear system so that we may use $R_f = \Sigma F$. Then

$$R_f = (-100) + (-50) + (-25) + (-20) + 200$$
$$R_f = 5 \text{ N}$$

The resultant force is a positive one of 5 N, indicating an upward movement of the weights. Before we can solve for the acceleration, the mass of the weights must be found using the formula $m = w/g$. Thus,

$$m = \frac{195 \text{ N}}{9.8 \text{ m/sec.}^2}$$
$$m = 19.9 \text{ Kg}$$

Now the acceleration may be determined from the formula, $a = F/m$. Then

$$a = \frac{5 \text{ N}}{19.9 \text{ Kg}}$$
$$a = 0.25 \text{ m/sec.}^2$$

The instantaneous acceleration of the weights system at the time a 200 N force is applied is 0.25 m/sec.^{2} in an upward direction.

More often we would know the magnitude of weights and can measure the acceleration of the system. From this information we could determine the resultant force on the cord.

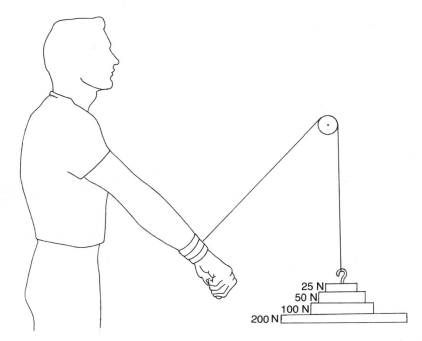

FIGURE 7–17

Patient exercising his shoulder extensor muscles with wall pulleys.

▶ **PROBLEM 7–15**

QUESTION:
In the weight system described in the previous problem, what would be the force in the cord if the acceleration at the beginning of movement was 0.5 m/sec.^{2} upward?
SOLUTION:
The free body diagram is the same as in the previous problem. The mass of the weight system was 19.9 Kg. The resultant force can be found using the formula F = ma.

$$F = ma$$
$$= 19.9 \text{ Kg} \times 0.5 \text{ m/sec.}^2$$
$$= 9.95 \text{ N}$$

The resultant force is 9.95 N and must be directed upward, since the acceleration is upward. The force transmitted through the cord is found using the formula R = ΣF.

$$9.95 \text{ N} = (-100 \text{ N}) + (-50 \text{ N})$$
$$+ (-25 \text{ N}) + (-20 \text{ N}) + T$$
$$9.95 \text{ N} = -195 \text{ N} + T$$
$$T = 195 \text{ N} + 9.95 \text{ N}$$
$$T = 204.95 \text{ N}$$

Thus, the force exerted through the cord is 204.95 N to obtain the acceleration of 0.5 m/sec.^{2} This can be compared with a force of 195 N to hold the system in static equilibrium with the acceleration equal to zero. Note that to increase the value of the acceleration, the force is increased in the cord. This in turn reflects an increased muscular force necessary to increase the tension in the cord. What does this tell you about speed of movement in an exercise program?

What would happen in the two previous problems if the pulley axis had a coefficient of friction of 0.05? Of 0.1? Can you calculate the resulting tension in the cord in these situations?

Rotatory Motion

The preceding portion of this chapter has been concerned with linear motion and has dealt with the body as a point. The motion of the limbs of the body, however, must be treated as lines moving about an axis. Just as in the section on kinematics, the equations relating force and motion are analogous to those of linear motion.

The acceleration approach to solving kinetic

problems may be used with rotational motion, as well. In this case, the cause of the angular acceleration is a torque (T) that is, the force (F) acting at a distance (d) from the axis of rotation. In statics, the clockwise moment, or torque, was balanced by counterclockwise moments resulting in an angular acceleration of zero. In the study of dynamics, these torques are not equal to zero. Hence, an acceleration is produced. The resultant torque has the same causal relation to angular acceleration that the resultant force does to linear acceleration.

The resistance to change in angular velocity depends upon the mass of the body and its distribution about the center of rotation. This resistance to change in angular velocity is called the *moment of inertia*. The moment of inertia (I) is analogous to mass in linear motion. If a body is divided into a large number of small particles, with each having a mass (m) and a perpendicular distance (r) from the axis of rotation, each particle has a contribution of mr^2 to the moment of inertia. The moment of inertia of the body will equal the sum of all such contributions. Thus, $I = \Sigma mr^2$. The moment of inertia is different if the body is rotated about a different axis since the distance (r) of each particle will change. The moment of inertia is also different for different shaped bodies. Unless a definite axis is specified, the moment of inertia has no meaning.

In the case of angular motion, the mass is not considered as concentrated at the center of mass for the purpose of computing its moment of inertia. A new term, called the *radius of gyration* (k) must be introduced (Fig. 7–18). This is the radial distance from the axis of rotation at which the mass of the body could be concentrated without altering the moment of inertia of the body about that axis. In the general formula, $I = \Sigma mr^2$, r^2 represents the average radii of many particles. We may substitute k for r, so that k represents the radius of gyration and Σm equals the sum of the mass of all the particles. To calculate the magnitude of the radius of gyration, we substitute in the formula. Thus, $I = mk^2$. Then

$$k = \sqrt{\frac{I}{m}}$$

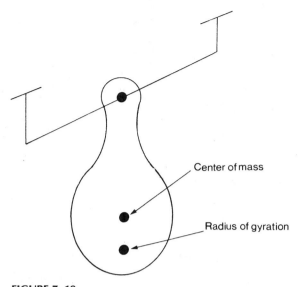

FIGURE 7–18

Radius of gyration.

The moment of inertia must be determined before the radius of gyration can be calculated. By using integral calculus, if the shape, composition, and axis of the rotation of a body are known, we can calculate the moment of inertia. Some (Fowler and Myer, 1958; Sears and Zymanski, 1949; McGill and King, 1989) texts give equations already derived for objects of certain shapes. Often one of these is selected if the body part resembles a specified shape. For example, the equation for the moment of inertia of a sphere may be used for the head, or the equation for the moment of inertia of a cylinder or truncated cone may be used for a limb segment. When applying these formulas, we may have to adjust the equation to apply to the specific axis of rotation. This is done by using the parallel axis theorem. The theorem states that the moment of inertia about an axis parallel to the axis for which the formula was derived equals the moment of inertia of the body at the original axis plus the product of the mass and square of the perpendicular distance between the parallel axes (Fig. 7–19).

For application, we must realize that the greater the mass or the greater the distance the

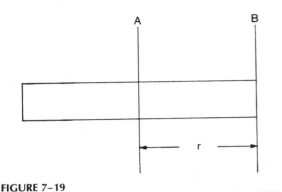

FIGURE 7–19

Parallel axis theorem.

mass is located from the axis of rotation, the greater will be the resistance to change in angular velocity. The radius of gyration in prosthetic and orthotic design is of great importance, as it provides control for the resistance of angular motion. The prosthesis must be designed so that it will swing properly, without too much resistance to motion. However, enough resistance must be provided to allow for movement coordination. In an above-knee (AK) prosthesis, if the leg portion moves either too slowly or too rapidly, the gait pattern will be disrupted. Proper mass and location of the mass will help the patient with a prosthesis control the limb more efficiently.

A heavy brace on the foot greatly affects the motion of the lower limb. A 2 N weight added to a shoe may have more effect on the limb swing than 10 N added to the thigh. From the equation $I = mk^2$, we see that increasing both the mass and the radius of gyration increases the moment of inertia. However, doubling the radius of gyration increases the moment of inertia by four. Thus, the distribution of the mass is of great importance.

Newton's second law of motion can now be shown to apply to angular as well as linear motion. The angular acceleration (α) depends directly upon the torque (T) producing it, and the moment of inertia (I) resisting it. Hence, $\alpha = T/I$. This equation may be rearranged in the following manner so that

$$T = I\alpha \text{ and } I = T/\alpha$$

As in linear motion, the acceleration approach for angular motion holds for instantaneous values.

▶ **PROBLEM 7–16**

Occasionally, the moment of inertia of a limb is determined by the angular acceleration method or quick release experimental method (Drillis, 1959; Drillis et al., 1964).

QUESTION:
What is the moment of inertia of the forearm?
SOLUTION:
We may set up the testing procedure as shown in Figure 7–20. The distance (d) from the cord connecting a force transducer to the wrist to the elbow joint axis is 25 cm. The force transducer directly measures 75 N of force (F) applied at the wrist. The acceleration (α) of the limb is measured immediately following the quick release of the cord connecting the wrist to the force transducer. Its magnitude is 290 rad./sec. From these data we may calculate the moment of inertia (I) of the limb segment.

$$T = I\alpha, \text{ or } I = T/\alpha$$
$$I = \frac{F \times d}{\alpha} = \frac{75 \text{ N} \times 0.25 \text{ m}}{290 \text{ rad./sec.}^2}$$
$$I = 0.065 \text{ Kgm}^2$$

Occasionally, we want to investigate the forces applied to a particle on a rotating body. We found earlier that the magnitude of acceleration of a particle revolving in a circle has an inward radial component of $\frac{v^2}{r}$. Since the direction of the acceleration is always changing (always points to the center of rotation), a force must be acting on the particle. If $a_R = \frac{v^2}{r}$, substituting into the acceleration formula (F = ma), the inward $F = m\frac{v^2}{r}$. This resultant force, which pulls the particle from its straight line path toward the center of rotation, is called *centripetal force*. For example, an object on a string whirling around in a circle has a force acting on it to keep it from continuing in a straight path (flying off at a tangent to the circular path). The string exerts the centripetal force to overcome the inertia of the object. According to Newton's third law, for every action there is an equal and opposite reaction. Thus, a force caused by the inertia of the object is said to act with equal magnitude and in an opposite direction to the centripetal force. This force is called *centrifugal force*. In the

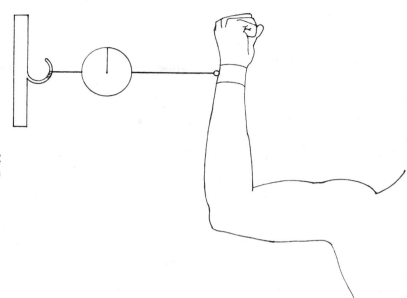

FIGURE 7–20

Quick release method to determine the moment of inertia of the forearm and hand.

case of the whirling object, the centrifugal force may become so great by increasing the velocity of the object that it will overcome the resisting force in the string, and the string will break.

In the human body, ligaments and muscles hold limbs together as they swing through their range of motion. Rapid motion of the limb will produce increased tension on these structures. The application of prostheses and orthotics must take this principle into account.

Equations of Motion

Now that you have an understanding of the principles of linear and angular acceleration, let's see how these concepts can be used to solve problems of motion.

The acceleration approach may be used to determine (1) the forces acting at the joints and (2) the moments around the joints caused by the muscles. The moments represent muscle groups rather than the force produced by each individual muscle. Some attempt, however, has been made to determine individual muscle force by using EMG and/or relating the muscle force to muscle cross section (Seireg and Arvikar, 1973; Pierrynowski and Morrison, 1985b; Cappozzo

et al., 1976; Hof et al., 1987; Davy and Audu, 1987).

The equations of motion were derived from Newton's second law and expanded by Euler (McGill and King, 1989). Hence, they are referred to as the Newton-Euler equations. Based upon these equations d'Alembert derived the principle that the resultant of the external forces and the kinetic reaction (inertial forces) acting on a body equal zero. This principle essentially brings dynamic solutions under the rule of statics similar to those in Chapter 4. You should remember that mass (m) may be considered the resistance to change in linear motion and that the moment of inertia (I) may be considered the resistance to change in angular motion. This resistance is the inertia, sometimes referred to as *reverse-effective forces,* and torques. The static equilibrium equations become dynamic equilibrium equations by including the inertial force of magnitude (mass × linear acceleration = ma) at the center of gravity in the equations for the first condition of equilibrium and the inertia moment of force (moment of inertia × angular acceleration = Iα) in the equation for the second condition of equilibrium. Since inertia resists the change in motion, the direction of these inertial forces are in the opposite direction of the accelerated motion.

The equations of motion in a two-dimensional system then become:

$$\Sigma F_X = ma_X, \text{ or}$$

$$\Sigma F_X + (-ma_X) = 0 \text{ if X is horizontal}$$

$$\Sigma F_Y + (-mg) = ma_Y, \text{ or}$$

$$\Sigma F_Y + (-mg) + (-ma_Y) = 0 \text{ if Y is vertical}$$

$$\Sigma M = I\alpha, \text{ or}$$

$$\Sigma M + (I\alpha) = 0$$

If $\alpha = 0$, the motion is linear. If a_x and $a_y = 0$, then the motion is rotatory. If $a_x = 0$, $a_y = 0$ and $\alpha = 0$, then these equations are the same as the static equilibrium equations.

Since the forces acting on a body cause the resulting motion of the body, the direct way to study motion would be as shown in the following diagram (Fig. 7–21).

The magnitude of the internal forces acting on the body, however, are not accessible by direct measurement (Groh and Baumann, 1976). We may determine these forces and external force and kinematic data by using the equations of motion. Displacement values may be determined by photographic or electrogoniometric measurements. The velocities and accelerations of the body may then be calculated from this displacement information. The accelerations, however, may also be determined directly by accelerometers. Since the forces that cause the motion are determined by evaluating the resulting motion, the process often is called *inverse dynamics.*

Inverse Dynamics

The first step in the inverse dynamic procedure is to define the system under consideration. It is the whole body, the foot, one limb, the trunk, an implement, or a series of segments. Should the system be treated as a particle (point), a rigid body (lever), or a link system (series of levers)?

Next, all external forces acting upon the system must be identified. In the acceleration approach, a particular instant of motion is assessed. We may consider the system as though we have taken a snapshot. Therefore, a two-dimensional free body diagram for each segment of the system must be drawn. As you remember from statics, the free body diagram is a sketch in which all the forces acting upon the body are carefully drawn with respect to their location, direction, and magnitude. The free body diagram identifies the body whose motion is being analyzed and defines the system under consideration. It shows all the forces acting on the

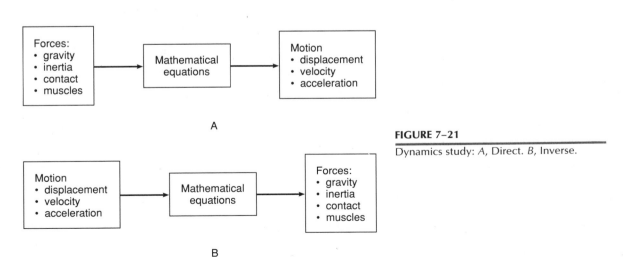

A

B

FIGURE 7–21

Dynamics study: *A,* Direct. *B,* Inverse.

body, the lines of action of the known and unknown forces, and the predominant moments acting on each segment.

Certain assumptions must be made when using this approach. For the purposes of this text and often for many motions, the motion will be examined in one plane. The body is considered as a rigid-body linked system with frictionless pin joints. Each segment has a fixed mass with the center of mass at a fixed point. The moment of inertia of each segment for a given axis remains constant.

Certain assessments must be made as accurately as possible. These include the assessment of the segment masses, the location of the centers of mass, the moments of inertia, and the location of the joint centers.

The forces acting on the body may be muscular, gravitational, contact, or inertial. Gravitational forces reflect the weight of each segment, or the mass times the gravitational acceleration (mg). The contact forces may be with the ground, an adjacent segment, or other object exerting force on the segment. Ground reaction forces may be determined from force platform records that provide the vertical and horizontal components of the force applied by the body to the ground. As discussed earlier, the inertial forces are ma_x and ma_y for linear motion and $I\alpha$ for angular motion. The muscle moment of force and joint reaction forces are to be calculated. The direction of the forces and moments are important. The forces acting upward or to the right are given a positive (+) sign, while those acting downward or to the left are given a negative (−) sign. Conventions for moments of force or torque are less straightforward. The following are some of the conventions used by researchers.

The right-hand screw rule is based on the right thumb pointing upward with the fingers curving in a counterclockwise manner. Thus, counterclockwise (CCW) is considered positive and clockwise (CW) is considered negative. Some researchers use the right-hand rule for studying the right side of the body and a similar left-hand rule for studying the left side of the body (Bresler and Frankel, 1950). Other researchers consider the movement toward extension as positive and the movement toward flexion as negative (Winter, 1979; Winter et al., 1974). Setting the convention you will use before you begin and being consistent with that system as you attack the problem is essential.

All possible motion of a rigid segment can be described in terms of the linear motion of the center of mass of the segment and rotational motion around the center of mass. Therefore, the accelerations obtained should be the linear acceleration components of the segment's center of mass (a_x and a_y) and the rotational acceleration of the segment. Depending on the specific problem being studied, adjustments may be used to compute the moments around a joint center by using appropriate distances and the parallel axis theorem for the moment of inertia. The equations of motion based upon the acceleration approach may be used to calculate forces on swinging and supported moving objects.

▶ PROBLEM 7–17

We may consider a simple example of a thin rod of 1 Kg mass 0.3 m long with a frictionless axis fixed to a surface at one end (0) and free to move at the other (Fig. 7–22). The rod may be allowed to fall around the axis. We would like to determine the reaction force at the axis and evaluate the moments acting on the rod. To do this, we use the equations of motion. Figure 7–22 may be used as the free body diagram. The following values have been obtained from appropriate measuring procedures when the rod is at 30° with the horizontal.

position $\theta = 30°$
angular velocity (ω) = 7 rad./sec.²
angular acceleration (α) = 42.43 rad./sec.²
gravitational acceleration (g) = 9.8 m/sec.²
horizontal acceleration of the center of mass a_x = 3.18 m/sec.²
vertical acceleration of the center of mass (a_y) = 9.18 m/sec.²

The moment of inertia for a thin rod around the center of mass (I_c) is calculated as $ml^2/12 = 0.0075$ Kgm². For a rod around the axis (I_o), it is calculated as $ml^2/12 + m(1/2)^2 = ml^2/3 = 0.03$ Kgm².

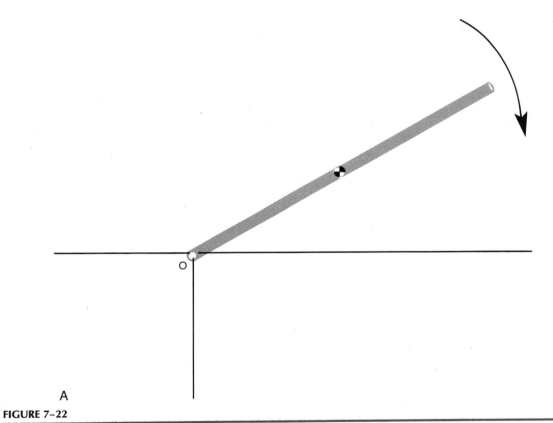

A

FIGURE 7–22

A, Thin rod rotating around fixed axis O, free fall.

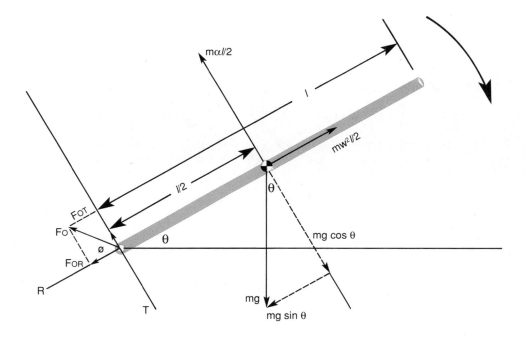

B

FIGURE 7–22

Continued B, Radial and tangential force components.

Illustration continued on following page

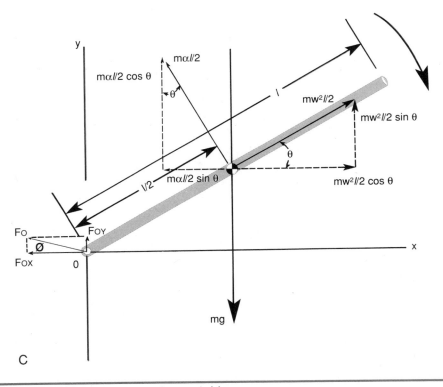

FIGURE 7–22

Continued C, X and Y components of radial and tangential forces.

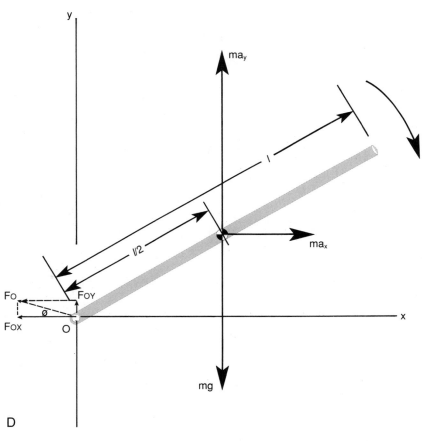

FIGURE 7–22

Continued D, X and Y force components.

Three similar approaches to this problem may be used. We may find the forces and moment by using:

1. The rod and a line perpendicular to it as the coordinate axes, and the radial (a_R) and tangential (a_T) acceleration components (Fig. 7–22B),
2. The X and Y axes and the radial (a_R) and tangential (a_T) acceleration components (Fig. 7–22C), or
3. The X and Y axes and the rectangular acceleration components (a_X and a_Y) (Fig. 7–22D).

Note that the force of inertia may be in the opposite direction of acceleration since it resists change in motion. For this example we may see how all three approaches may be used. Since the motion of the rod is rotatory around a fixed axis with no linear motion, it is convenient to use the radial (R) and tangential (T) components with the rod and perpendicular line as the coordinate axes. We will begin with this approach.

APPROACH NO. 1

F_{oR} represents the radial force component at 0.
F_{oT} represents the tangential force component at 0.
F_o represents the magnitude of reaction force at 0.

Remember that $w^2 l/2 = a_R$ and $\alpha l/2 = a_T$

$$F_{oR} + (mw^2 l/2) + (-mg \sin \Theta) = 0$$
$$F_{oR} + (1 \text{ Kg}) (7 \text{ rad./sec.})^2 (0.03/2 \text{ m})$$
$$- (1 \text{ Kg}) (9.8 \text{ m/sec.}^2) (0.05) = 0$$
$$F_{oR} + (7.35 \text{ N}) - (4.9 \text{ N}) = 0$$
$$F_{oR} + 2.45 \text{ N} = 0$$
$$F_{oR} = -2.45 \text{ N}$$

$$F_{oT} + (m\alpha l/2) + (-mg \cos \Theta) = 0$$
$$F_{oT} + (1 \text{ Kg}) (42.43 \text{ rad./sec.}^2) (0.3/2 \text{ m})$$
$$- (1 \text{ Kg}) (9.8 \text{ m/sec.}^2) (0.866) = 0$$
$$F_{oT} + (6.36 \text{ N}) - (8.49 \text{ N}) = 0$$
$$F_{oT} - 2.13 \text{ N} = 0$$
$$F_{oT} = 2.13 \text{ N}$$

$$F_o = \sqrt{(F_{oR})^2 + (F_{oT})^2}$$
$$F_o = \sqrt{(-2.45)^2 + (2.13)^2}$$
$$F_o = \sqrt{(6.0) + (4.54)}$$
$$F_o = \sqrt{10.54}$$
$$F_o = 3.25 \text{ N}$$

$$\tan \phi = F_{oR}/F_{ox}$$
$$\tan \phi = 2.13/-2.45$$
$$\tan \phi = -0.869$$
$$\phi = 41° \text{ with the rod.}$$

APPROACH NO. 2

F_{TX} represents the total forces acting in the X direction.
F_{TY} represents the total forces acting in the Y direction.
F_{ox} represents the X force component $a_T = 0$.
F_{oY} represents the Y force component $a_T = 0$.

$$F_{ox} + (mw^2 l/2 \cos \Theta) +$$
$$(-m\alpha l/2 \sin \Theta) = 0$$
$$F_{ox} + (1 \text{ Kg}) (7 \text{ rad./sec.})^2$$
$$(0.3/2 \text{ m}) (0.866) - (1 \text{ Kg})$$
$$(42.43 \text{ rad./sec.}^2) (0.3/2 \text{ m}) (0.05) = 0$$
$$F_{ox} + (6.36 \text{ N}) - (3.18 \text{ N}) = 0$$
$$F_{ox} + 3.18 \text{ N} = 0$$
$$F_{ox} = -3.18 \text{ N}$$

$$F_{oY} + (mw^2 l/2 \sin \phi) + (m\alpha l/2 \cos \Theta)$$
$$+ (-mg) = 0$$
$$F_{oY} + (1 \text{ Kg}) (7 \text{ rad./sec.})^2 (0.3/2 \text{ m}) (0.5)$$
$$+ (1 \text{ Kg}) (42.43 \text{ rad./sec.}^2) (0.3/2 \text{ m}) (0.866)$$
$$- (1 \text{ Kg}) (9.8 \text{ m/sec.}^2) = 0$$
$$F_{oY} + (3.68 \text{ N}) + (5.51 \text{ N}) - (9.8 \text{ N}) = 0$$
$$F_{oY} - 0.63 \text{ N} = 0$$
$$F_{oY} = 0.63 \text{ N}$$

$$F_o = \sqrt{(-3.18)^2 + (0.62)^2}$$
$$F_o = \sqrt{(10.1) + (0.40)}$$
$$F_o = \sqrt{10.51}$$
$$F_o = 3.24 \text{ N}$$
$$\tan \Theta = F_{oY}/F_{ox}$$
$$\tan \Theta = 0.63/-3.18$$
$$\tan \Theta = -0.198$$
$$\Theta = 11.2° \text{ with the X axis or } 41.2° \text{ with the rod}$$

APPROACH NO. 3

$$F_{ox} + (ma_x) = 0$$
$$F_{ox} + (1 \text{ Kg}) (3.18 \text{ m/sec.}^2) = 0$$
$$F_{ox} + 3.18 \text{ N} = 0$$
$$F_{oX} = 3.18 \text{ N}$$

$$F_{oY} + (ma_Y) + (-mg) = 0$$
$$F_{oY} + (1 \text{ Kg}) (9.18 \text{ m/sec.}^2) =$$
$$(1 \text{ Kg}) (9.8 \text{ m/sec.}^2) = 0$$
$$F_{oY} + (9.18 \text{ N}) - (9.8 \text{ N}) = 0$$
$$F_{oY} - 0.63 \text{ N} = 0$$
$$F_{oY} = 0.63 \text{ N}$$

These components would provide the same magnitude and direction as in approach no. 2.

There are also different ways by which we may solve for the moments. We can calculate the moments (1) around the axis O and (2) around the center of mass.

SOLUTION NUMBER ONE

M_o represents the amount of force other than gravity and inertia.

$$M_o + (-mgl/2 \cos \theta) + (I_o\alpha) = 0$$
$$M_o - (1 \text{ Kg})(9.8 \text{ m/sec.}^2)(0.03/2 \text{ m})(0.866)$$
$$+ (0.03 \text{ Kgm}^2)(42.43 \text{ rad./sec.}^2) = 0$$
$$M_o - 1.273 \text{ Nm} + 1.273 \text{ Nm} = 0$$
$$M_o = 0$$

SOLUTION NO. 2A

M_C represents the moment of force other than gravity and inertia.

$$M_C + (F_{oT}\tfrac{1}{2}) + (I_c\alpha) = 0$$
$$M_C + (-)(2.13 \text{ N})(0.3/2 \text{ m})$$
$$+ (0.0075 \text{ Kgm}^2)(42.43 \text{ rad./sec.}^2) = 0$$
$$M_C - 0.32 \text{ Nm} + 0.32 \text{ Nm} = 0$$
$$M_C = 0$$

SOLUTION NO. 2B

$$M_C (-F_{ox}l/2 \sin \theta) + (-F_{oy}l/2 \cos \theta) + I_c\alpha) = 0$$
$$M_C - (3.18 \text{ N})(0.3/2 \text{ m})(0.5)$$
$$- (0.63 \text{ N})(0.3/2 \text{ m})(0.866)$$
$$+ (0.0075 \text{ Kgm}^2)(42.43 \text{ rad./sec.}^2) = 0$$
$$M_C - (0.238 \text{ Nm}) - (0.082 \text{ Nm}) + (0.32 \text{ Nm}) = 0$$
$$M_C = 0$$

The moment equations show that the only moments acting on the rod around the fixed axis are the pull of gravity and the resistance of inertia.

This problem is a simple case in which no kinematic measurements need to be taken in order to determine the values for motion. In this situation only gravity and inertia should be creating moments of force around the fixed axis. Thus, from the moment equation:

$$mgl/2 \cos \theta - I_o\alpha = 0$$

Specifically for a thin rod $I_o = ml^2/3$

$$mgl/2 \cos \theta - (ml^2/3)\alpha = 0$$

Therefore,

$$mgl/2 \cos \theta = ml^2/3\alpha$$

and

$$\alpha = 3g/21 \cos \theta$$

From this equation and integral calculus (McGill and King, 1989)

$$\omega^2 = 3g/1 \sin \theta$$
$$\omega = \sqrt{3g/1 \sin \theta}$$

Note that the moment of inertia for the specific object must be substituted into the original equation for I_o to obtain the equations for the object moving freely around a fixed axis.

▶ PROBLEM 7–18

Let's consider the thin rod of 1 Kg mass being moved around a fixed axis (O) with velocity of 5.6 rad./sec. and an instantaneous acceleration of 34.9 rad./sec.^{2} at an angle of 30° with the horizontal (Fig. 7–23). Do not be concerned with what is causing the acceleration at this time. We will be determining (1) the reaction force components at O caused by gravity and inertia and (2) the moment of force needed to cause such motion. The reaction force components at O developed by the force causing the acceleration of the rod cannot be determined until the magnitude of the moment of this force, its point of application, its line of application, and its magnitude are known.

The following values have been obtained from physical measurements of the rod and from appropriate measuring procedures at the specific instant the counterclockwise rotating rod is at 10°.

m = 1 Kg	θ = 30°
l = 0.3 m	ω = 5.6 rad./sec.
l/2 = 0.15 m	α = 34.9 rad./sec.^{2}
$I_C = ml^2/12 = 0.0075$ Kgm^2	a_X = −6.67 m/sec.^{2}
$I_o = ml^2/3 = 0.03$ Kgm^2	a_Y = 2.15 m/sec.^{2}

Since this is rotatory motion, the radial (a_R) and tangential (a_T) acceleration components may be more convenient to use. However, any of the ap-

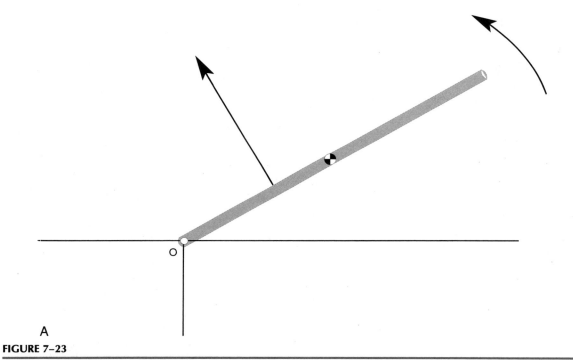

A

FIGURE 7–23

A, Thin rod rotating around fixed axis O, added moment.

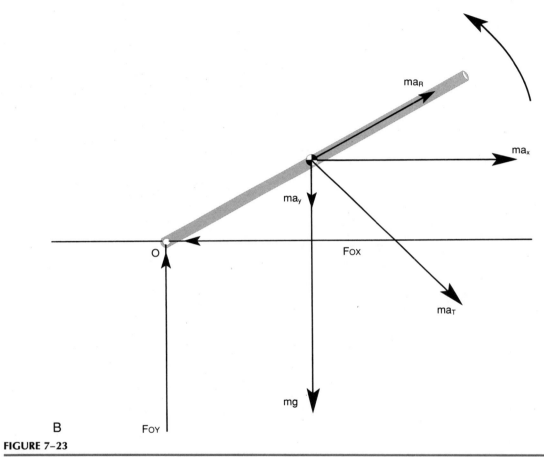

B

FIGURE 7–23

Continued B, Inertial components, weight, and force components at axis.

Illustration continued on following page

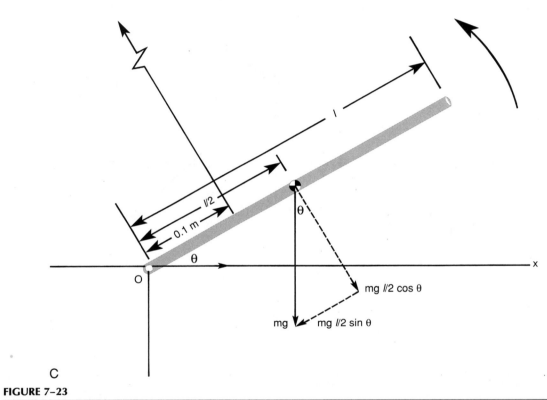

C

FIGURE 7–23

Continued C, Weight components, lever arm lengths, and position (Θ).

proaches presented in Problem 7–17 may be used. This problem only differs from Problem 7–17 in that an additional external force is causing the rod to rotate counterclockwise around the fixed axis. This additional force is being resisted by gravity and inertia.

Always remember that inertia resists the change of a body being at rest or having a constant velocity.

We will solve for the force values for this problem by using the rectangular acceleration components, a_x and a_y.

$$F_{ox} + (-ma_x) = 0$$
$$F_{ox} + (1 \text{ Kg})(6.67 \text{ m/sec.}^2) = 0$$
$$F_{ox} + 6.67 \text{ N} = 0$$
$$F_{ox} = -6.67 \text{ N}$$

$$F_{ox} + (-ma_Y) + (-mg) = 0$$
$$F_{oY} - (1 \text{ Kg})(2.15 \text{ m/sec.}^2)$$
$$- (1 \text{ Kg})(9.8 \text{ m/sec.}^2) = 0$$
$$F_{oY} - (2.15 \text{ N}) - (9.8 \text{ N}) = 0$$
$$F_{oY} - 11.98 = 0$$
$$F_{oY} = 11.98$$

The magnitude of the reaction force without the additional motor force components can be calculated using the Pythagorean theorem.

$$F_o = \sqrt{-(6.67)^2 + (11.98)^2}$$
$$F_o = \sqrt{(44.49) + (143.5)}$$
$$F_o = \sqrt{188.0}$$
$$F_o = 13.71 \text{ N}$$

The direction can be determined by using the tangent, sine, or cosine functions.

$$\text{Tan } \phi = 11.98/6.67$$
$$\text{Tan } \phi = 1.79$$
$$\phi = 60.9° \text{ with the X axis}$$

The moments acting around the axis (O) are gravity ($mg \, l/2 \cos \Theta$), inertia ($I_o\alpha$), and the additional external moment (M_o).

$$M_o + (-mg \, \tfrac{1}{2} \cos \Theta) + (-I_o\alpha) = 0$$
$$M_o - (1 \text{ Kg})(9.8 \text{ m/sec.}^2)(0.3/2 \text{ m})(0.866)$$
$$- (0.03 \text{ Kgm}^2)(34.9 \text{ rad./sec.}^2) = 0$$
$$M_o - 1.27 \text{ Nm} - 1.05 \text{ Nm} = 0$$
$$M_o - 2.32 \text{ Nm} = 0$$
$$M_o = 2.32 \text{ Nm}$$

The additional external moment causing the counterclockwise motion is 2.32 Nm.

Suppose that this additional moment is caused by a force applied at 90° to the rod a distance of 0.1 m from the axis, O (Fig. 7–23C). Knowing the magnitude of the moment, the point of application of the force, and the line of application of the force, we may calculate the magnitude of the force (B).

$$M_o = 2.32 \text{ Nm}$$
$$(B)(0.1 \text{ m}) = M_o$$
$$(B)(0.1 \text{ m}) = 2.32 \text{ Nm}$$
$$B = 2.32 \text{ Nm}/0.1 \text{ m}$$
$$B = 23.2 \text{ N}$$

We now have sufficient information to calculate the total force acting at the axis (O).

Since we know that the force (B) is perpendicular to the rod which is at Θ degrees with the X axis, we can determine that B_x equals $B \sin \Theta$, and B_Y equals $B \cos \Theta$.

Therefore the additional force components acting at O are

$$B_{ox} = B \sin \Theta$$
$$B_{ox} = (23.2 \text{ N})(0.5)$$
$$B_{ox} = 11.6 \text{ N}$$
$$B_{oY} = B \cos \Theta$$
$$B_{oY} = (23.2 \text{ N})(0.866)$$
$$B_{oY} = 20.1 \text{ N}$$

The total force components (T_{ox} and T_{oy}) acting at O are

$$T_{ox} = F_{ox} + B_{ox}$$
$$T_{ox} = 6.67 \text{ N} + 11.6 \text{ N}$$
$$T_{ox} = 18.27 \text{ N}$$

$$T_{oY} = F_{oY} + B_{oY}$$
$$T_{oY} = 11.98 + 20.1 \text{ N}$$
$$T_{oY} = 32.1 \text{ N}$$

$$T_o = \sqrt{(18.27)^2 + (32.1)^2}$$
$$T_o = \sqrt{(333.8) + (1030.4)}$$
$$T_o = \sqrt{1364.2}$$
$$T_o = 36.9 \text{ N}$$

The total force at the axis (O) is 36.9 N (8.3 lb.) with a horizontal component of 18.27 N and a vertical component of 32.1 N.

The problem was solved using the rectangular ac-

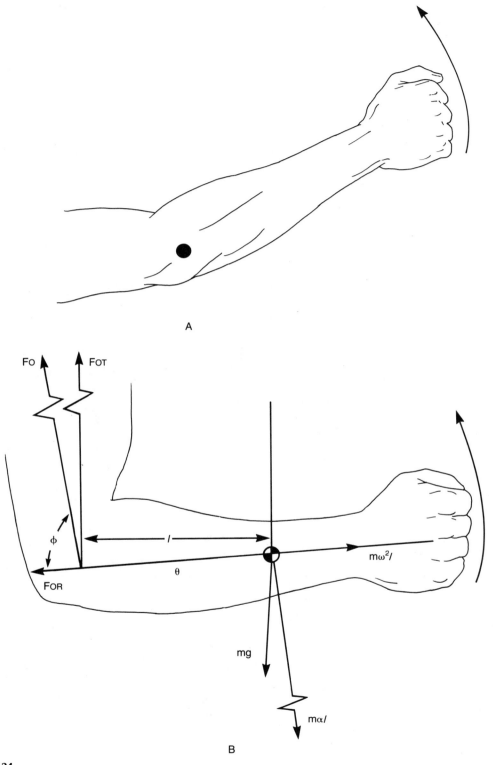

A

B

FIGURE 7–24

See legend on opposite page

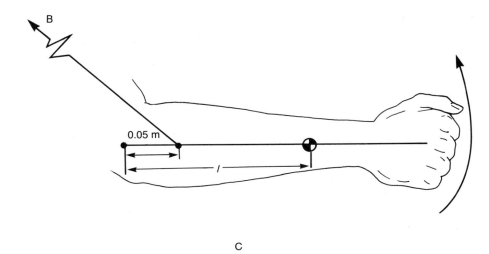

FIGURE 7–24

Elbow flexion forces.

celeration component. Try solving the problem using the radial and tangential components. The moment and total force at the axis (O) should be the same values. The force components in the radial and tangential directions, however, would be different from the X and Y components.

What would happen to the force at the axis in this problem if the point of application was at 0.05 m from O? What would happen if the line of force (B) were horizontal? Vertical?

▶ PROBLEM 7–19

We may extend the preceding problem by replacing the thin rod by a forearm and hand. The fixed axis will be the elbow joint. The unloaded limb resting on a table is moved from extension to flexion (Fig. 7–24). At the instant the forearm reaches the position of 10° with the horizontal, it is traveling with an angular velocity of 5.2 rad./sec. and with an instantaneous acceleration of 220 rad./sec.² The combined mass of the forearm and hand is 1.5 Kg, and the center of mass is located 0.18 m from the axis of the elbow. The combined moment of inertia of the forearm and hand from Table A-7 in Appendix A is 0.0589 Kgm². The kinematic values are given:

$$m = 1.5 \text{ Kg}$$
$$l = 0.18 \text{ m}$$
$$I_o = 0.0589 \text{ Kgm}^2$$
$$I_c = 0.0190 \text{ Kgm}^2$$

$$\theta = 10°$$
$$\omega = 5.2 \text{ rad./sec.}$$
$$\alpha = 220 \text{ rad./sec}^2$$
$$a_X = 11.68 \text{ m/sec.}^2$$
$$a_Y = 38.1 \text{ m/sec.}^2$$

We again may solve for the forces by using radial and tangential acceleration components or their vertical and horizontal components. For the first equation, the reaction forces at the elbow joint are only the result of gravity and inertia and do not include the reaction to muscle force.

Joint component + weight component + radial inertia = 0

$$F_{oR} + (-mg \sin \theta) + (m\omega^2 l) = 0$$

$$F_{oR} - (1.5 \text{ Kg})(9.8 \text{ m/sec.}^2)(0.1736)$$
$$+ (1.5 \text{ Kg})(5.2 \text{ rad./sec.})^2(0.18 \text{ m}) = 0$$

$$F_{oR} - 2.55 \text{ N} + 7.3 \text{ N} = 0$$

$$F_{oR} + 4.76 \text{ N} = 0$$

$$F_{oR} = -4.75 \text{ N}$$

The sum of the total tangential forces (F_{TT}) equals zero.

$$\Sigma F_{TT} = 0$$

Joint component + weight component + tangential inertia = 0

$$F_{oR} + (-mg \cos \Theta)$$
$$+ (ma1) = 0$$
$$F_{oT} - (1.5 \text{ Kg})(9.8 \text{ m/sec.}^2)(0.9848) - (1.5 \text{ Kg})$$
$$(220 \text{ rad./sec.}^2)(0.18 \text{ m}) = 0$$
$$F_{oT} - 14.48 \text{ N} - 59.4 \text{ N} = 0$$
$$F_{oT} - 73.88 \text{ N} = 0$$
$$F_{oT} = 73.88 \text{ N}$$
$$F_o = \sqrt{(F_{oR})^2 + (F_{oT})^2}$$
$$F_o = \sqrt{(-4.75)^2 + (73.88)^2}$$
$$F_o = \sqrt{(22.56) + (5458.25)}$$
$$F_o = \sqrt{5480.82}$$
$$F_o = 74.03 \text{ N}$$
$$\tan \phi = 73.88 \text{ N}/4.75 \text{ N}$$
$$\tan \phi = 15.55$$
$$\phi = 86°$$

The sum of the total moments (M_{oT}) acting around the elbow joint at this instant can be solved as follows:

External moments + gravity + inertia = 0

$$M_o + (-mgl \cos \Theta) + (-I_o \alpha) = 0$$
$$M_o - (1.5 \text{ Kg})(9.8 \text{ m/sec.}^2)(0.18 \text{ m})(0.9848)$$
$$- (0.0589 \text{ Kgm}^2)(220 \text{ rad./sec.}^2) = 0$$
$$M_o - 2.61 \text{ Nm} - 12.96 \text{ Nm} = 0$$
$$M_o - 15.57 \text{ Nm} = 0$$
$$M_o = 15.57 \text{ Nm}$$

The moment of 15.57 Nm is the result of all the muscles and other tissue at the elbow joint. If the moment is calculated using I_c, the value is approximately 17.48 N, a difference possibly caused by the estimation of body values. We cannot tell exactly how much each flexor muscle contributes to the moment. In fact, the contribution of each muscle may change throughout the motion. We cannot tell whether antagonistic muscles, joint tissues, and/or joint damage are creating countermoments that must be overcome by the elbow flexors to obtain this resulting moment.

To determine a rough estimate of what might be the minimum elbow flexor muscle force needed to produce a moment of 15.57 Nm, we may make some assumptions.

We may assume that (1) the friction in the joint is negligible, (2) the joint tissues are not resisting the motion, and (3) the antagonistic muscles are not contracting at this instant. Electromyography may as-sist in estimating the activity of the antagonistic muscles.

If we can accept these assumptions and can place the point of application of the combined elbow flexors at 0.05 m and the combined line of application at 40°, we may roughly determine the combined force of the elbow flexors.

Some authors (Seireg and Arvikar, 1973; Hof et al., 1987; Davy and Audu, 1987) have extended these assumptions to determine the force developed by each major individual elbow flexor muscle by using electromyography and more assumptions related to muscle cross-section measurements, each muscle's length, and each muscle's angle of pull.

Let's roughly determine the elbow flexor muscle force (B). Let B_T equal the muscle force component perpendicular to the forearm, and B_R equal to the muscle force component parallel to the forearm.

$$M_o = (B_T)(0.05 \text{ m})$$
$$M_o = 15.57 \text{ Nm}$$
$$(B_T)(0.05 \text{ m}) = 15.57 \text{ Nm}$$
$$B_T = 15.57 \text{ Nm}/0.05 \text{ m}$$
$$B_T = 311.4 \text{ N}$$

Since B is at 40° with the forearm, B_T equals B sin 40.

$$B_T = B \sin 40$$
$$B = B_T/\sin 40$$
$$B = 311.4 \text{ N}/0.643$$
$$B = 484.3 \text{ N}$$

B_R may be determined by using

$$B_R/B = \cos 40°$$
$$B_R = B \cos 40°$$
$$B_R = (484.3 \text{ N})(0.766)$$
$$B_R = 371 \text{ N}$$

Since B_R is directed to the left in our figure, B_R would be −371 N.

We may now add the muscle force components B_T and B_R to the already determined reaction force components to obtain rough estimates of the total force (T_o) at the joint.

To find the total radial force component at this joint:

$$T_{oR} = B_R + F_{oR}$$
$$T_{oR} = (-371 \text{ N}) + (-4.75 \text{ N})$$
$$T_{oR} = -375.75 \text{ N}$$

To find the total tangential force component at this joint:

$$T_{oT} = B_T + F_{oT}$$
$$T_{oT} = (311.4 \text{ N}) + (73.88 \text{ N})$$
$$T_{oT} = 385.28 \text{ N}$$

To find the total force at the joint:

$$T_o = \sqrt{(-375.75)^2 + (385.28)^2}$$
$$T_o = \sqrt{(141188.0) + (148440.7)}$$
$$T_o = \sqrt{289628.7}$$
$$T_o = 538.17 \text{ N}$$

To find the line of application of this force:

$$\tan \Theta = T_{oT}/T_{oR}$$
$$\tan \Theta = 385.28/375.75$$
$$\tan \Theta = 1.025$$
$$\Theta = 45.7° \text{ with the axis of the forearm.}$$

Thus, an individual flexing the elbow at the given kinematic characteristics would need a minimum of 484.3 N (108.9 lb.) of muscle force and would have a minimum force of 538.17 N (121 lb.) at the joint.

We may use the equations of motion to determine (1) the elbow extensor force required to stop elbow flexion or (2) determine the minimum elbow flexor muscle force and force at the joint if a weight is held in the hand during elbow flexion.

▶ **PROBLEM 7–20**

Often the lower limb is likened to a pendulum during the swing phase of gait. The following example is the basic situation of a thin rod swinging around a fixed point (Fig. 7–25). This example will later be expanded to relate to a swinging limb.

$$m = 1 \text{ Kg}$$
$$l = 0.3 \text{ m}$$
$$l/2 = 0.15 \text{ m}$$
$$I_o = ml^2/3 = 0.03 \text{ Kgm}^2$$
$$I_c = ml^2/12 = 0.0075 \text{ Kgm}^2$$

At the instant the rod moving counterclockwise is at 60° with the horizontal, it has an angular velocity of 9.21 rad./sec. and an instantaneous acceleration of 24.5 rad./sec.[2] The rectangular acceleration components are $a_x = 9.54$ m/sec.[2] and $a_Y = -9.16$ m/sec.[2].

The forces acting in this situation are gravity, inertia around the axis, and the contact at the fixed axis. The forces at the fixed axis may be resolved into rectangular components F_R and F_T, or F_X and F_y.

Let's solve for the radial and tangential components:

Contact force component + weight component + radial inertia = 0

$$F_{oR} + (-mg \sin \Theta) + (ml/2\omega^2) = 0$$
$$F_{oR} = (1.0 \text{ Kg})(9.8 \text{ m/sec.}^2)(0.866)$$
$$- (1.0 \text{ Kg})(0.15 \text{ m})(9.21 \text{ rad./sec.})^2 = 0$$
$$F_{oR} - 8.49 \text{ N} - 12.71 \text{ N} = 0$$
$$F_{oR} - 21.21 \text{ N} = 0$$
$$F_{oR} = 21.21 \text{ N}$$

Contact for component + weight component + tangential inertia = 0

$$F_{oT} + (mg \cos \Theta) + (-m \tfrac{1}{2}\alpha) = 0$$
$$F_{oT} + (1.0 \text{ Kg})(9.8 \text{ m/sec.}^2)(0.5)$$
$$- (1.0 \text{ Kg})(0.15 \text{ m})(24.5 \text{ rad./sec.}^2) = 0$$
$$F_{oT} + 4.9 \text{ N} - 3.68 \text{ N} = 0$$
$$F_{oT} + 1.22 \text{ N} = 0$$
$$F_{oT} = 1.22 \text{ N}$$

Now let's solve for the moments:
External moment + gravity moment + inertial moment = 0

$$M_o + (mg \tfrac{1}{2} \cos \Theta) + (-I_o\alpha) = 0$$
$$M_o + (1.0 \text{ Kg})(9.8 \text{ m/sec.}^2)(0.15 \text{ m})(0.05)$$
$$- (0.03 \text{ Kgm}^2)(24.5 \text{ rad./sec.}^2) = 0$$
$$M_o + 0.735 \text{ Nm} - 0.735 \text{ Nm} = 0$$
$$M_o = 0$$

No forces other than gravity and inertia are acting to cause moments around the fixed axis.

To find the force at the axis we use the Pythagorean theorem:

$$F_o = \sqrt{(F_{oR})^2 + (f_{oT})^2}$$
$$F_o = \sqrt{(21.21)^2 + (-1.22)^2}$$
$$F_o = \sqrt{(449.86) + (1.49)}$$
$$F_o = \sqrt{(451.35)}$$
$$F_o = 21.24 \text{ N}$$

The direction of F_o can be found by using the tangent function:

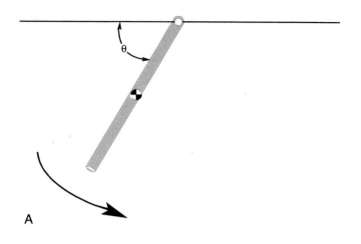

A

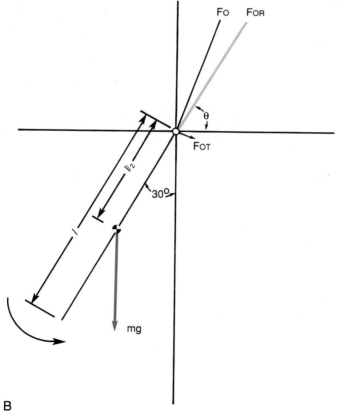

B

FIGURE 7–25

A, Swinging rod. *B,* Forces acting on rod.

$\tan \phi = 1.22/21.21$

$\tan \phi = 0.0575$

$\phi = 3.29°$ with the radial axis or 63.29 with the X axis

A force of 21.24 N (4.8 lb.) is needed to support the swinging 1 Kg rod.

If the knee acted as a fixed stationary axis, we could solve for the forces and moments acting on and around the joint in the same manner as the previous thin rod problem. The values for lengths, mass, and moment of inertia around the axis can be found in Tables A–5 to A–7 in Appendix A. The angular positions for each instant in time may be obtained from photographic or goniometric recordings. The angular velocity and acceleration may be calculated from the position-time data. Such a situation could occur as an indivdiual sits at the edge of a treatment table or exercise chair with the leg free to swing (Fig. 7–26). The "ideal" mechanical situation might be that the leg and foot could swing as freely as the thin rod. However, such is not the case. Active and passive tissues provide forces and moments that either enhance or restrict the motion of the leg and foot. The forces and moments during a resistance exercise with weight at the ankle can be calculated. A better estimate of muscle force during motion may be made using the preceding methods. Can you give examples of similar situations?

Plane Motion

The preceding examples were related to motion around a fixed axis. We may consider the situation in which plane motion occurs. Plane motion is defined as the combined linear and rotatory motion in a single plane. The swinging leg during gait may be an example. The hip, knee, and ankle axes are not fixed as the segments rotate around the joints. Thus, the joint axes and segments have combined motion primarily in a single plane.

In this situation the components of linear acceleration are added to the equations of motion as appropriate (Younger, 1958).

The equations for force would then be as follows where a_{jx} and a_{jy} represent the rectangular acceleration of the joint center. The distance to the center of the mass is l_c.

Joint component + joint acceleration component + radial acceleration component + tangential acceleration component = 0

$$F_{ox} + ma_{jx} + m\, l_c\, \omega^2 \cos\theta + m\, l_c\, \alpha \sin\theta = 0$$

Joint component + joint acceleration component + radial acceleration component + tangential acceleration component = 0

$$F_{oY} + ma_{jy} + m\, l_c\, \omega^2 \sin\theta + m\, l_c\, \alpha \cos\theta = 0$$

If the limb is acting as a linearly moving rigid body, these rectangular acceleration components should be the same for the segment's center of mass. Any angular motion of the segment around the joint center will also be reflected at the center of mass of the segment. Therefore, the rectangular components of the segment's center of mass (a_{cx} and a_{cy}) would represent the combined acceleration of the linear and angular movement with respect to the joint center.

The force equations then may be

$$F_{ox} = ma_{cx}, \text{ or}$$

$$F_{ox} + ma_{cx} = 0, \text{ and}$$

$$F_{oY} + (-mg) = ma_{cy}, \text{ or}$$

$$F_{oY} + (-mg) + ma_{cy} = 0$$

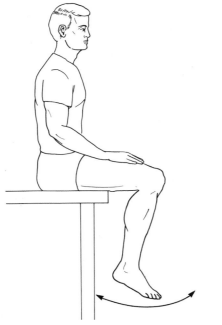

FIGURE 7–26

Swinging leg.

▶ PROBLEM 7–21

Assume that the ankle is fixed with the foot and leg acting as a single unit. Tables A–5 to A–7 in Appendix A allow for the determination of this segment mass, location of center of mass, and movement of inertia. Kinematic analysis may provide the movement characteristics for the swinging segment. Let's evaluate the knee joint forces and moments when the foot and leg is swinging forward at the position of 75° with the horizontal just prior to heel strike (Fig. 7–27). The subject weighs 667 N (150 lbs.).

$M = 4$ Kg	$\theta = 75°$ with horizontal
$l = 0.50$ m	$\omega = 3.2$ rad./sec.^{2}
$l_c = 0.24$ M	$\alpha = -38.4$ rad./sec.^{2}
$l_o = 0.3332$ Kgm^2	$a_{KX} = 2.05$ m/sec.^{2}
$l_c = 0.1077$ Kgm^2	$a_{KY} = -0.5$ m/sec.^{2}
	$a_{CX} = -11.6$ m/sec.^{2}
	$a_{CY} = 0.6$ m/sec.^{2}

Let's first solve for the joint force:

$$F_{ox} + (ma_{Kx})$$
$$+ (ml_c\ \omega^2 \cos\theta)\ ml_c\ \alpha \sin\theta = 0$$
$$F_{ox} + (4\ \text{Kg})(2.05\ \text{m/sec.})$$
$$+ (4\ \text{Kg})(0.24\ \text{m})(3.2\ \text{rad./sec.})^2(0.2588) + (4\ \text{Kg})$$
$$(0.24\ \text{m})(38.4\ \text{rad./sec.}^2)(0.966) = 0$$
$$F_{ox} + 46.33\ \text{N} = 0$$
$$F_{ox} = -46.33\ \text{N}$$

$$F_{oY}(ma_{KY}) + (-ml_c\omega^2 \sin\theta)$$
$$+ (ml_c\ \alpha \sin\theta) + (-mg) = 0$$
$$F_{oY} + (4\ \text{Kg})(0.5\ \text{m/sec.}^2)$$
$$- (4\ \text{Kg})(0.24\ \text{m})(3.2\ \text{rad./sec.})^2(0.966)$$
$$+ (4\ \text{Kg})(0.24\ \text{m})(38.4\ \text{rad./sec.}^2)$$
$$- (4\ \text{Kg})(9.8\ \text{m/sec.}^2) = 0$$
$$F_{oY} + 2\ \text{N} - 9.49\ \text{N}$$
$$+ 9.5\ \text{N} - 39.2\ \text{N} = 0$$
$$F_{oY} - 37.19\ \text{N} = 0$$
$$F_{oY} = 37.19\ \text{N}$$

We may find the force at the joint by using the Pythagorean theorem:

$$F_o = \sqrt{(F_{ox})^2 + (F_{oy})^2}$$
$$F_o = \sqrt{(-46.33)^2 + (37.19)^2}$$
$$F_o = \sqrt{(2146.5) + (1381.1)}$$
$$F_o = \sqrt{3529.6}$$
$$F_o = 59.4\ \text{N}$$

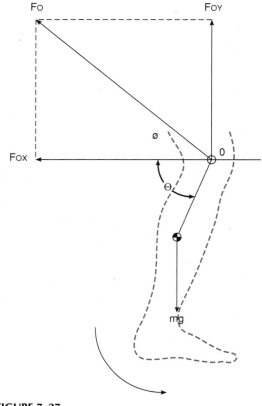

FIGURE 7–27

Swing phase of gait.

The line of application of the force may be determined by using the tangent function:

$$\tan\phi = F_{oY}/F_{ox}$$
$$\tan\phi = 37.19\ \text{N}/-46.33\ \text{N}$$
$$\tan\phi = 0.803$$
$$\phi = 38.8°\ \text{with the X axis}$$

The force components may also be determined using the rectangular acceleration components for the center of mass (a_{CX} and a_{CY}.)

$$F_{ox} + (-ma_{CX}) = 0$$
$$F_{ox} + (4\ \text{Kg})(11.6\ \text{m/sec.}^2) = 0$$
$$F_{ox} + 46.4\ \text{N} = 0$$
$$F_{ox} = -46.4\ \text{N}$$

$$F_{oY} + (ma_{CY}) + (-mg) = 0$$

$$F_{oY} + (4 \text{ Kg})(0.6 \text{ m/sec.}^2)$$

$$- (4 \text{ Kg})(9.8 \text{ m/sec.}^2) = 0$$

$$F_{oY} + 2.4 \text{ N} - 39.2 \text{ N} = 0$$

$$F_{oY} - 36.8 \text{ N} = 0$$

$$F_{oY} = 36.8 \text{ N}$$

To analyze the moments we may use the knee axis or the center of mass as the center of rotation.

For the moments around the knee axis (O), we use the moment of inertia (I_o) which is determined for that axis (Table A–7). The forces at the knee joint in this situation do not create moments around the joint. Their force arm would be zero.

External moment + gravity + angular inertia + linear inertia = 0

$$M_o + (-mg \, l_C \cos \Theta) + (I_o\alpha) +$$

$$(ma_{CX} \, l_C \sin \Theta) + (ma_{CY} \, l_C \cos \Theta) = 0$$

$$M_o - (4 \text{ Kg})(9.8 \text{ m/sec.}^2)$$

$$(0.24 \text{ m})(0.2588)$$

$$+ (0.3332 \text{ Kgm}^2)(38.4 \text{ rad./sec.}^2)$$

$$+ (4 \text{ Kg})(11.6 \text{ m/sec.})(0.24 \text{ m})(0.966)$$

$$+ (4 \text{ Kg})(0.6 \text{ m/sec.})$$

$$(0.24 \text{ m})(0.2588) = 0$$

$$M_o - 2.43 \text{ Nm} + 12.8 \text{ Nm}$$

$$+ 10.76 \text{ Nm} + 0.15 \text{ Nm} = 0$$

$$M_o + 21.28 \text{ Nm} = 0$$

$$M_o = -21.28 \text{ Nm}$$

These calculations show that a moment of 10.34 Nm (7.6 ft-lb.) is being used at this instant to decelerate the foot and leg before heel strike. Do not consider this value to be the maximum torque needed to decelerate the segment during gait. The angular acceleration value is not the maximum deceleration value. This point occurs slightly later in the swing phase.

Using the same assumptions mentioned earlier in the chapter, we may roughly determine the hamstring muscle force needed to decelerate the swinging limb at this instant. In this situation the hamstring muscles attach 0.06 m from the knee axis at a 10° angle with the leg; the quadriceps are not active; and the other tissues around the knee joint are producing only negligible moment effects.

The moment equals the hamstring muscle force component perpendicular to the limb (H sin 10°) times the lever arm distance (0.06 m).

$$M_o = (H \sin 10°)(0.06 \text{ m}) = 21.28 \text{ Nm}$$

$$H = 21.28 \text{ Nm}/(0.06 \text{ m})(0.174)$$

$$H = 2038.3 \text{ N}$$

The estimated hamstring muscle force needed at this instant of the swing phase during normal gait is 2038.3 N (458 lb.).

What would happen to this muscle force if the subject were jogging, running, or sprinting?

In the previous examples, we determined the forces and moments acting on a body allowed to swing freely around a point. Let us now consider a situation in which the swinging body makes contact with a surface. In this situation a contact force (R) is added to the system. This force may be resolved into one force component perpendicular to the surface (normal component) and one parallel to the surface (tangential component).

A common example of such a situation is the stance phase of gait. During stance, the floor reaction force is applied to the foot. This force sets up a moment around the foot's center of mass. A joint force at the ankle joint also contributes to the moment around the center of mass. By use of a force platform the floor reaction force components can be determined. The length, mass, and moment of inertia of the foot can be obtained from Tables A–5 to A–7 in Appendix A. The force components at the ankle joint and the moment around the joint or center of the mass can then be calculated from the equations of motion.

▶ **PROBLEM 7–22**

Immediately following heel strike we may calculate the reaction forces at the ankle joint and the moments around the ankle joint (Fig. 7–28). The reaction force components in this situation are the sum of the ground reaction components, gravitational components, and inertial components. The muscle force components are not yet included.

The estimates of the physical characteristics of the foot are varied. Difficulty seems to exist in accurately determining these characteristics. For this problem we will use the following physical and kinematic values.

BW = 667 N	Θ = 20°
m = 1.2 Kg	ω = 2.0 rad./sec.
I_o = 0.0646 Kgm^2	α = −35.0 rad./sec.
l_1 = 0.023 m	a_{XC} = 2.03 m/sec.^{2}
l_2 = 0.06 m	a_{CY} = 2.85 m/sec.^{2}d
l_3 = 0.013 m	R_X = −36 N
l_4 = 0.07 m	R_Y = 182 N

Ankle joint force + ground reaction force + inertia

$$F_{ox} + (-R_x) + (-ma_{cx}) = 0$$

$$F_{ox} - 36 \text{ N} - (1.2 \text{ Kg})(2.03 \text{ m/sec.}) = 0$$

$$F_{ox} - 36 \text{ N} - 2.44 \text{ N} = 0$$

$$F_{ox} - 38.44 \text{ N} = 0$$

$$F_{ox} = 38.44 \text{ N}$$

Ankle joint force + ground reaction force + gravity + inertia

$$F_{oY} + (R_Y) + (-mg) + (-ma_{cY}) = 0$$

$$F_{oY} + (182 \text{ N}) - (1.2 \text{ Kg})(9.8 \text{ m/sec.}^2)$$
$$- (1.2 \text{ Kg})(2.85 \text{ m/sec.}^2) = 0$$

$$F_{oY} + 182 \text{ N} - 11.76 \text{ N}$$
$$- 3.42 \text{ N} = 0$$

$$F_{oY} + 166.82 \text{ N} = 0$$

$$F_{oY} = -166.82 \text{ N}$$

The ankle reaction force components are 38.44 N forward horizontally and 166.82 N downward.

Now let's solve for the moments:

External moments + reaction moments + gravity + angular inertia + linear inertia = 0

$$M_o + (-R_x)(l_1 + l_2) + (-R_Y)(l_3) + (-mg)(l_4)$$
$$+ (l_o\alpha) + (ma_{cx}l_1) + (Ma_{cY}l_4) = 0$$

$$M_o - (36 \text{ N})(0.083 \text{ m}) - (182 \text{ N})(0.013 \text{ m})$$
$$- (1.2 \text{ Kg})(9.8 \text{ m/sec.}^2)(0.07 \text{ m})$$
$$+ (0.0646 \text{ Kgm}^2)(35 \text{ rad./sec.}^2)$$
$$+ (1.2 \text{ Kg})(2.03 \text{ m/sec.}^2)(0.023 \text{ m})$$
$$+ (1.2 \text{ Kg})(2.85 \text{ m/sec.}^2)(0.07 \text{ m}) = 0$$

$$M_o - 3.0 \text{ Nm} - 2.37 \text{ Nm} - 0.82 \text{ Nm}$$
$$+ 2.26 \text{ N} + 0.056 \text{ Nm} + 0.24 \text{ Nm} = 0$$

$$M_o - 3.62 \text{ Nm} = 0$$

$$M_o = 3.62 \text{ Nm}$$

At this instant following heel strike an external moment of 3.62 Nm is needed to control the movement of the foot.

If the combined ankle dorsiflexors act upward 0.03 m from the ankle joint the muscle force may be calculated as follows:

$$M_o = (A)(0.03 \text{ m}) = 3.62 \text{ Nm}$$

$$A = 3.62 \text{ Nm}/0.03 \text{ m}$$

$$A = 120.7 \text{ N}$$

The muscle force is determined to be 120.7 N (27.1 lb.) to control the ankle movement at this instant. This also provides an additional vertical force into the ankle joint. It does not add further force to the horizontal components of force in the joint at this time.

The total ankle joint force (F_T) would be the sum of the ground reaction force, gravity, inertia, and the muscle force.

$$F_T = 182 \text{ N} - 11.76 \text{ N} - 3.42 \text{ N} + 120.7 \text{ N}$$

$$F_T = 287.52 \text{ N} \ (64.6 \text{ lb.})$$

So far we have only been applying the equations of motion to the distal segment of a limb either free to swing or in contact with a surface. Since the limbs are a series of jointed segments, we may need to calculate the forces and moments acting on each segment of the entire limb. The equations of motion used for a proximal segment are similar to those used for a distal segment.

If you remember, we first studied the freely swinging limb segment that had inertia, gravity, and muscle forces causing moments of force around its proximal joint. Next we studied a distal limb segment that had a contact (reaction) force at its distal end. This contact provided two additional force components that produced moments of force around the proximal joint (or center of mass).

In accordance with Newton's third law, the joint reaction forces at the proximal end of the distal segment produce reaction forces equal in magnitude and opposite in direction on the distal end of the next proximal segment. Also, the resultant muscle force and muscle moments of force are applied to the next proximal segment with equal magnitude but in the opposite direction. The free body diagram for a segment with contact forces at each end is shown in Figure 7–29.

To evaluate the force and moments on a proximal segment, the approach is similar to the process used when the distal segment with contact at the distal end was studied. In this case the distal joint reaction forces are treated like the ground reaction forces. Assuming that the muscles are single-joint muscles, the resultant moment on the distal segment is added to moment equations for the proximal segment. Thus, the previous moment equation of motion around the proximal joint becomes:

Proximal moment + distal moment + distal reaction + gravity + angular inertia + linear inertia = 0

$$M_{o2} + M_{o1} + R_x l_1 \sin \theta + R_y l_2 \cos \theta + mgl_3 \cos \theta$$
$$+ (-l_o\alpha) + (-ma_x l_4) + (-ma_y l_5) = 0$$

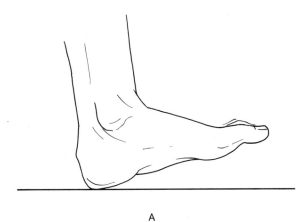

A

FIGURE 7–28

A, Heel strike of gait. *B,* Forces
acting on foot.

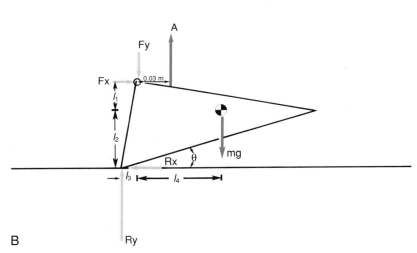

B

A similar equation may be written if the moments
are calculated around the center of mass. In this approach the moments developed by the proximal
joint reaction force components are added to the
equation, and the moments produced by the linear
inertia components acting at the center of mass and
the moment caused by gravity are eliminated. The
moment equation then becomes proximal moment
+ distal moment + distal reaction + proximal reaction + angular inertia:

$$M_{o2} + M_{o1} + (R_x l_1) + (R_y l_2)$$
$$- (F_x l_4) + (F_y l_5) + (-I_c \alpha) = 0$$

An important dynamic variable for studying
human movement is the determination of the moments of force at each joint during the course of

movement. You have been shown how to obtain
these values. Winter (1980) presented a principle
that algebraically sums the moments of force of the
ankle, knee, and hip to provide a "support moment." The support moment appears to be consistent across a variety of subjects and patients, although the individual joints may vary. This principle
shows how one joint can compensate for a reduced
moment of force at another joint.

Impulse-Momentum Approach

A second method used to solve kinetic problems
is the *impulse-momentum approach.* This ap-

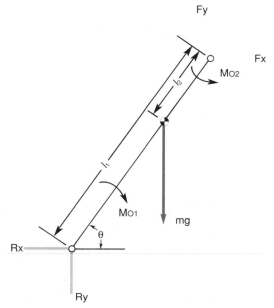

FIGURE 7–29

Forces and moments on segment. Inertia not included.

proach is particularly helpful when the force acts over a period of time. It is essential when a collision is involved.

We learned earlier that acceleration is the change in velocity per unit time. Thus, if we substitute the term $\dfrac{\Delta v}{\Delta t}$ for a in the acceleration equation, we obtain the momentum equation, F $= \dfrac{m\Delta v}{t}$, where mΔv represents the change in momentum of the body. This equation may be further manipulated so that

$$Ft = m\Delta v, \text{ or } Ft = mv_2 - mv_1$$

A more sophisticated mathematical derivation leads to an identical final equation.

The product of force and time is called the *impulsive force,* or impulse. A greater force, a force applied over a longer time, or a combination of both will increase the value of the momentum. The velocity vector will point in the same direction as the resultant force. Thus, depending upon the direction of force, the motion characteristic of velocity may be increased or retarded.

In many instances, to produce an increased change in momentum, one attempts to apply a force for a longer period of time. This is especially true in athletics. The preparatory movement and the follow-through increase the duration during which the force is applied. In activities such as baseball, tennis, and golf, a large amount of force is directly related to the shortness of the collision time of the implement on the ball. The impulse involved to stop a moving object corresponds directly to the change of momentum of the object. The force and time of the impulse are inversely related. A longer time taken to stop a moving object will require less force by allowing an increased time for the momentum to change. On the other hand, an increased force will reduce the duration necessary to stop the object.

▶ **PROBLEM 7–23**

Suppose a 0.2 Kg baseball is thrown at a velocity of 35 m/sec.

QUESTIONS:
What impulse is necessary to stop the baseball? If the force were constant, what would be the force applied to stop the ball in 0.001 sec.? What would be the force if the time to stop the ball took 0.05 sec.?

SOLUTION:
The two positions of the ball are shown in Figure 7–30. We may establish the change of momentum and the impulse needed to cause this change.

$$Ft = m\Delta v$$
$$Ft = m(v_2 - v_1)$$
$$Ft = 0.2 \text{ Kg}(0.0 \text{ m/sec.} - 35 \text{ m/sec.})$$
$$Ft = -7 \text{ Kgm/sec.} = -7 \text{ N sec.}$$

The negative impulse indicates a force tending to retard the velocity. With the force constant we may determine its magnitude as the momentum changes in 0.001 sec.

$$F = \frac{-7 \text{ N sec.}}{0.001 \text{ sec.}} = -7000 \text{ N}$$

A force of 7000 N (1574 lb.) is needed to stop within 0.001 sec. a baseball moving at an original velocity of 35 m/sec.

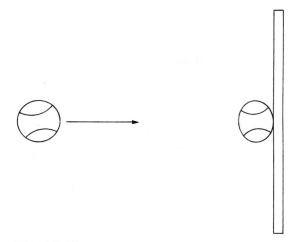

FIGURE 7–30

Impulsive force to stop a ball.

If the ball is stopped over a time period of 0.05 sec., we may begin with the impulse value of the previous part of the problem. If Ft = −7 N sec., then

$$F = \frac{-7 \text{ N sec.}}{0.05 \text{ sec.}} = -140 \text{ N}$$

Thus, with the time period over which to change the momentum increased, less force is required to stop the ball. If the ball happens to strike a bony body part, such as the tibia, hip, or head, less time is taken to change the momentum of the ball than if it hits a soft tissue area. Thus, less force is imparted by the ball to the body if it strikes a soft body area. Commonly, while attempting to catch a ball, the beginner will hold the hands and arms rigid. By not allowing a give in the joints, the time factor in catching is decreased and the force of impact is increased. Hence, the chance of being injured or dropping the ball is increased. This same principle illustrates that a fall from a small height may have disastrous results if one lands on a body part that does not provide much shock absorption.

▶ **PROBLEM 7–24**

Let's consider the force resulting from a fall on the hip. Suppose a 100 Kg man with a center of mass 1 m above the ground falls on his hip after tripping on a rug.

QUESTION:
What is the force of the floor on the hip if it acts for 0.1 sec. to stop the fall?
SOLUTION:
Figure 7–31 shows the extreme positions of the movement. The center of mass of the body falls freely for 0.9 m. The velocity at the instant the hip strikes the floor may be calculated from kinematic problems. Since the acceleration is caused by gravity, to solve for the time (t) we may write

$$s = \tfrac{1}{2}gt^2 \text{ or } t^2 = \frac{2s}{g}$$

$$t^2 = \frac{2 \times 0.9 \text{ m}}{9.8 \text{ m/sec.}^2}$$

$$t^2 = \frac{1.8 \text{ m}}{9.8/\text{sec.}^2}$$

$$t^2 = 0.184 \text{ sec.}^2$$

$$t = 0.43 \text{ sec.}$$

The duration of the 0.9 m fall was 0.43 sec. The average velocity ($\bar{v}$) can be found by

$$\bar{v} = \frac{s}{t}$$

$$\overline{N} = \frac{0.9 \text{ m}}{0.43 \text{ sec.}}$$

$$\bar{v} = 2.09 \text{ m/sec.}$$

To obtain the impact velocity, we use the formula

$$\bar{v} = \frac{v_f - v_o}{2}$$

Since $v_o = 0$, then

$$2.09 \text{ m/sec.} = \frac{v_f - 0}{2}$$

$$v_f = 4.18 \text{ m/sec.}$$

With the original velocity of zero, the final velocity of 4.18/sec., and the mass of 100 Kg, we may now use the impulse-momentum formula to find the impulse and force.

$$Ft = m(v_f - v_o)$$

$$= 100 \text{ Kg} \times (4.19 \text{ m/sec.} - 0)$$

$$Ft = 418 \text{ Ns}$$

The impulse is 418 Ns. Since the unknown force acts for 0.1 sec., this force is found by

$$F = \frac{418 \text{ Ns}}{0.1 \text{ sec.}}$$

$$F = 4180 \text{ N}$$

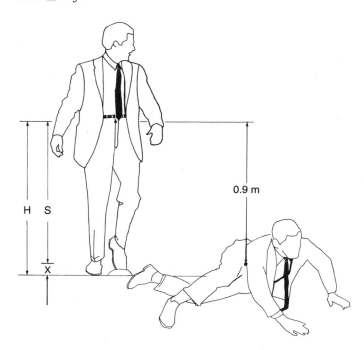

0.9 m

H   S

X

FIGURE 7–31

Forces involved during a fall on the hip.

Hence, a fall on the hip may impart a force of 4180 N (940 lb.) on the bony area. A force of this magnitude may be sufficient to cause a fracture of the hip.

If a person jumps or falls, he or she may lengthen the time of impact and decrease the force involved in changing the momentum by bending the knees and hips, or rolling with the fall. The ankle bones or leg bones may be broken, according to Benedek and Villars (1973), even with jumps from heights of 2 m, if the person lands stiffly with no "give" in the limb joints. Landing surfaces and protective equipment such as are used in athletics and the helmet for a child with cerebral palsy are designed to provide increased time for the duration of the force in an attempt to reduce injuries.

The equation may be rearranged to show that the velocity varies directly with the resultant force and time and indirectly with the mass.

$$v = \frac{Ft}{m}$$

This equation indicates that a large mass must have a greater impulse to obtain the same velocity as a small mass. Without the use of calculus, this equation should be used only if the force is constant during the time period involved.

The previous examples were concerned with the momentum and impulse applied to a single body. The momentum approach may also be applied when there is an interaction between two or more bodies, as in a collision. If the equation

$$mv_f - mv_i = Ft$$

is applied to a system of bodies in which the sum of all forces acting on the system is zero, the right side of the equation (Ft) is zero. The equation then becomes

$$(mv)_f = (mv)_i = 0, \text{ or } (mv)_f = (mv)_i$$

This final equation is known as the principle of *conservation of momentum.* That is, in a system in which the sum of forces equals zero, the momentum of the system remains constant. The final momentum equals the initial momentum. Note that no values for the application of force are necessary in this equation. If we consider the collision of two bodies in a system, we must take into account their individual masses and velocities for both the initial and final momentum. The equation then becomes expanded to

$$m_1v_{1f} + m_2v_{2f} = m_1v_{1i} + m_2v_{2i}$$

where m_1 and m_2 are the masses of the separate bodies, v_{1i} and v_{2i} are their initial velocities, and v_{1f} and v_{2f} are their final velocities.

For angular motion, if we substitute $\Delta\omega/t$ for α, we obtain the angular momentum equation:

$$T = \frac{I\Delta\omega}{t}$$

Here, $I\Delta\omega$ represents the angular momentum of the rotating body. The torque applied to a rotating body is directly proportional to the product of its moment of inertia and angular velocity and inversely proportional to its duration. The angular impulse is the torque times the duration of torque application, which equals the angular momentum:

$$Tt = I\Delta\omega, \text{ or}$$

from the formula $T = I\alpha$ we have

$$T = I\,d\omega/dt$$

If both sides of the equation are multiplied by dt, then

$$T\,dt = d\,(I\omega)$$

if the momentum changes as the torque is applied

$$\int_{t_1}^{t_2} T\,dt = (I\omega_2) - (I\omega_1)$$

If the force is constant for a long period of time then

$$Tt = I\omega_2 - I\omega_1$$

The change in angular momentum of a rotating body depends upon the magnitude and direction of the torque, and the duration of the torque applied.

A common example of angular impulse occurs during the gait cycle. Electromyographers have studied the coordinated action of the lower limb muscles. The muscles exert a force over a period of time. The force in this case produces a torque that changes the angular momentum of the limb.

▶ **PROBLEM 7–25**

Let's consider the recovery leg of a runner. The moment of inertia of the leg and foot is $0.3332\ \text{Kgm}^2$ (from Table A–7 in Appendix A). As the leg swings through, it must change from a rapid angular velocity to approximately zero velocity at foot strike. An angular impulse created by hamstring muscle force produces the change in momentum of the leg.

QUESTIONS:
What is the impulse necessary to change the velocity of the leg from 10.5 rad./sec. to 0 rad./sec.? What torque is exerted? What is the force exerted by the hamstring muscles to stop the leg swing if they attach 0.05 m from the knee axis?

SOLUTION:
The free body diagram is shown in Figure 7–32. The impulse-momentum equation can be used to determine the impulse.

$$Tt = I(\omega_f - \omega_0)$$
$$= 0.3332\ \text{Kgm}^2\ (0 - 10.5\ \text{rad./sec.})$$
$$= -3.5\ \text{Kgm}^2/\text{sec.}$$

If the time to stop the movement is 0.13 sec., the torque is then

FIGURE 7–32

Deceleration of a swinging leg during running.

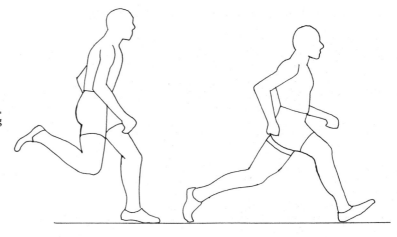

$$T = \frac{-3.5 \text{ Km}^2/\text{sec.}}{0.13 \text{ sec.}}$$

$$= -26.9 \text{ Kgm}^2/\text{sec.}^2 = -26.9 \text{ Nm}$$

The minus sign indicates deceleration of the limb. With the muscle attachment 0.05 m from the joint axis, the muscle force can be calculated by the formula

$$Fd = T, \text{ or } F = T/d$$

Then $$\qquad F = \frac{26.9 \text{ Nm}}{0.05 \text{ m}}$$

$$F = 538 \text{ N}$$

The muscle force needed to stop the leg swing is 538 N (121 lb.). What would happen if this were a faster runner with an initial angular velocity of 12.2 rad./sec.?

The impulse-momentum approach may be used to understand rotator cuff lesions in throwing. The velocity involved in the angular momentum of the arm and ball is directed backward, to counterclockwise (Fig. 7–33A), during the cocking phase of the motion. Suddenly the direction of the angular velocity is changed by the internal rotator muscles as the throwing phase begins (Fig. 7–33B). The rapid change in angular momentum may produce immediate muscle or joint damage (Slocum, 1959; Tullos and King, 1972), or fracture of the humerus (Tullos and King, 1973).

Careful observation of exercise programs reveals that angular momentum may play an important role in performance of the exercise. A brief but forceful muscular contraction at the beginning of the movement may produce sufficient impulse to allow the body part and exercise weight to move through the range of motion without further muscular contraction. Usually, this practice is not a recommended method of strength training. Momentum of a body part is often used in stretching exercises. In this instance, an increased force is necessary to stop the body part. If the momentum caused by a large mass or velocity is too great, the tissues may not be capable of supplying sufficient force to stop the movement. The force needed may be greater than the rupture strength of the tissues, and the tissues may tear. Prolonged stretching of low velocity will offer less chance of injury.

Similar to linear momentum, the angular mo-

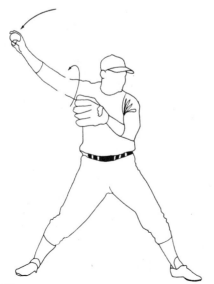
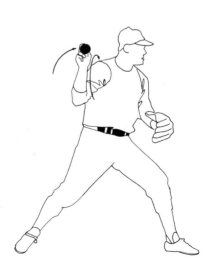

FIGURE 7–33

Forces across the shoulder while throwing a ball.

mentum is conserved if outside forces are not applied. Thus, $(I\omega)_f = (I\omega)_i$. An important aspect of this conservation appears if the radius of a rotating system is changed, hence changing the moment of inertia. For example, if no angular impulse is applied, and the radius is decreased, in order to conserve angular momentum the angular velocity must increase.

Common examples of this occur in athletic events such as gymnastics, diving, and skating. Suppose the athlete is spinning slowly with the limbs extended. When he or she pulls the limbs into the body, the moment of inertia (I) of the body decreases. Since $I\omega$ must remain constant as the moment of inertia decreases, the angular velocity must increase. The athlete will spin much faster. To slow the angular velocity, the limbs are again extended. This principle also occurs in human locomotion, as will be mentioned later. The momentum approach may be used if the torque applied is constant over the time period or if we are concerned with the conservation of momentum. It is particularly useful if there is no net external force acting on the system.

Work-Energy Approach

Reformulation of Newton's second law provides a third approach to solving problems in dynamics. This is called the *work-energy approach*. Its formulation arises when the forces acting on the system are known as a function of the position of the body. In many instances, the force on a body is known in terms of the location of the body. Hence, the work-energy approach is more convenient to solve for motion.

Before we develop the formula, we must define some related terms. Few terms are used with more confusion and variety of meanings than work, energy, and the related concept of power.

WORK

In mechanics the term *work* does not refer to muscular or mental effort as it is applied in everyday language but has a very specific mean-ing. Basically, work is a force overcoming a resistance and moving an object through a distance. The unit of measure for work in SI is the joule (see Table 1–1). Its value is determined by multiplying the force (F) by the displacement (s) of the object (Fig. 7–34A). Thus, we may write

$$\text{Work} = \text{Force} \times \text{Distance}$$
$$W = Fs$$

If the force is not in the same direction as the displacement, the component of force, $F \cos \theta$, in the direction of the displacement must be

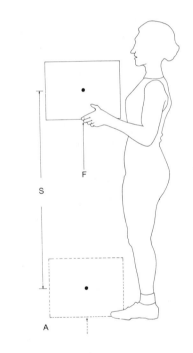

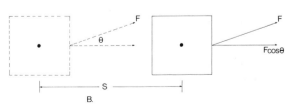

FIGURE 7–34

Examples of linear work: *A*, $W = F_s$. *B*, $W = F \cos \theta \times S$.

used to determine the work done (Fig. 7–34B). Then,

$$W = F \cos \Theta \times s$$

In situations where the force is not constant during displacement, infinitesimal portions must be considered to determine the work. Therefore,

$$dW = (F \cos \Theta) \, dx$$

the total work done in a finite displacement would be

$$W = \int dW = \int_{X_1}^{X_2} F \cos \Theta \, dx$$

Work done on a spring as in Figure 7–37B would be as follows. The angle of application of force would be zero. Thus, the cos Θ would equal 1:

$$W = \int_o^x F dx$$

Since F depends upon the amount of stretch on the spring, then

$$F = Kdx, \text{ then}$$

$$W = \int_o^x Kxdx = \tfrac{1}{2}Kx^2$$

The displacement must be along the same line and opposite in direction to the resisting force of the object. For example, movement perpendicular to the force of gravity will produce no work against gravity. A component of applied force must be parallel to elastic resistance such as spring or friction for work to be done.

When work is done, its unit of measure in the English system is the foot-pound. We must not, however, confuse work with torque, which also has been defined as a force times distance and has similar units. The resultant force producing work is concerned with a displacement, s (Fig. 7–35A), and lies along the same line as the distance the object is moved. The resultant force producing torque, on the other hand, is perpendicular to a lever arm distance, as shown in Figure 7–35B. Thus, the distances referred to in the two equations are different.

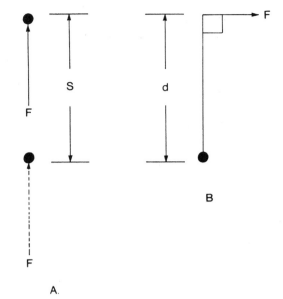

A.

FIGURE 7–35

Differences between work and torque: *A*, Work (F × S). *B*, Torque (F × d).

A force producing torque may also do work, but as shown in Figure 7–36, the correct distance must be used. The distance (r) is used to determine the torque, and the displacement (s) is used to calculate the work done. By using the conversion equations of angular to linear motion, the work done during angular motion can be calculated by multiplying the torque times the angular displacement.

Since W = Fs; s = Θr; and T = Fr, then W = FrΘ = TΘ.

If the torque is not constant through the angular displacement, then

$$dW = Fds = (Fr) \frac{ds}{r} = Td\Theta$$

$$dW = Fds = (Fr) \frac{ds}{r} = Td\Theta$$

$$dW = Td\Theta$$

$$W = \int_o^\Theta Td\Theta$$

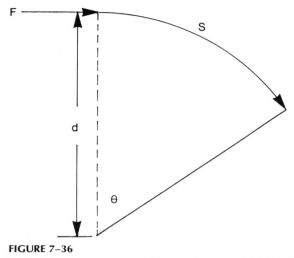

FIGURE 7–36

Work during angular motion.

Usually, we consider work as using a force to lift an object against gravity (Fig. 7–37A). However, this is not the only way to do work. By definition, if a resultant force moves a resistance through a distance parallel to the line of action of the force, work is done. Thus, for example, a spring (Fig. 7–37B), friction (Fig. 7–37C), and a balloon all offer resistance (Fig. 7–37D). Work is done as the resistance is overcome and movement occurs. Work is also done as an object is accelerated.

By referring to Newton's second law we see that force causes acceleration of an object and the accelerated motion is parallel to the force. The resistance in this case is the mass, or property of inertia

$$W = Fs = mas$$

This action meets the definition of work. The same holds true for angular acceleration, where

$$W = T\theta = I\alpha\theta.$$

Therefore, there are many ways to produce work, not only the case of lifting an object against the force of gravity.

The term *negative work* is used when a force acts parallel to the movement but in the opposite direction to the movement. Examples of this

concept are a weight being lowered from a height with the force controlling the descent (Fig. 7–38A), a spring gradually being released (Fig. 7–38B), and deceleration of a moving object (Fig. 7–38C).

ENERGY

Any object that has the ability to do work possesses *energy*. In fact, the common definition of energy is the capacity to do work. This means that if an object has the ability to produce a force through a distance, it possesses energy of some form. Examples are heat, light, nuclear, electrical, and mechanical energy. In this book we will consider only mechanical energy.

The ability to do work because of position or form is called *potential energy* (PE). A body contains stored-up energy because of its height or because of deformation. A 50 Kg barbell held above your head possesses a certain potential energy in relation to the floor. To lift the 50 Kg barbell 2 m above the floor, 1000 J of work is done. The potential energy (PE) of the barbell at this height equals the force needed to overcome gravity (F) times the height (h) above the floor, or

$$PE = F \times h = mgh$$

Thus, the barbell at this position has 1000 J of potential energy. As you can see, the units to measure energy are the same as those used to measure work, and the work done equals the potential energy of the object (W = PE). When work is done on a body to overcome gravity, its potential energy is increased.

To determine the potential of a deformed body such as a spring or balloon, the same basic computation is used as for gravity, with only slight modification. When determining the potential energy caused by gravity, the force is constant, except when at miles distant from the earth. However, for a deformed body, such as a spring or balloon, the resistance to deformation increases as the elastic body is stretched, and the magnitude of the force necessary to overcome the resistance increases as the distortion increases. For these cases, the average force

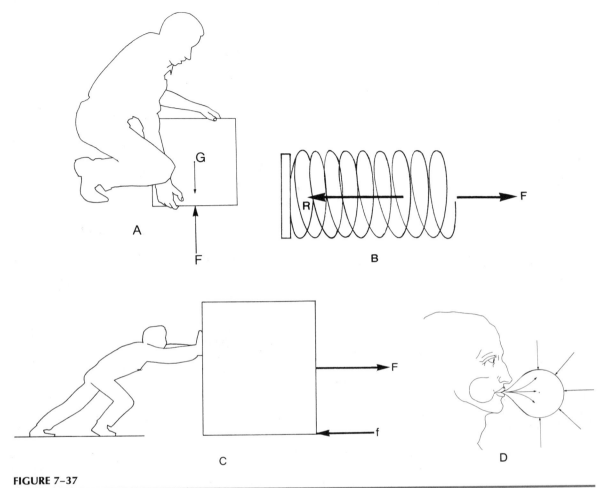

FIGURE 7–37

Examples of work: *A,* Lifting against gravity. *B,* Overcoming force of spring. *C,* Pushing against gravity. *D,* Stretching elastic balloon.

through the distance of distortion gives the potential energy of the deformed body. Then

$$W = \tfrac{1}{2}Ks$$

where K is a proportionality constant called a force constant, which is different for different elastic materials.

We have shown that work is related to potential energy. We have also seen that work is done by accelerating an object. For simplicity, suppose this acceleration is constant. Newton's second law may not be used to relate work to motion.

$$W = Fs = mas$$

and, for uniform acceleration,

$$s = \frac{v_f^2 - v_i^2}{2a}$$

$$W = \frac{m(v_f^2 - f_i^2)}{2} = \tfrac{1}{2}mv_f^2 - \tfrac{1}{2}mv_i^2$$

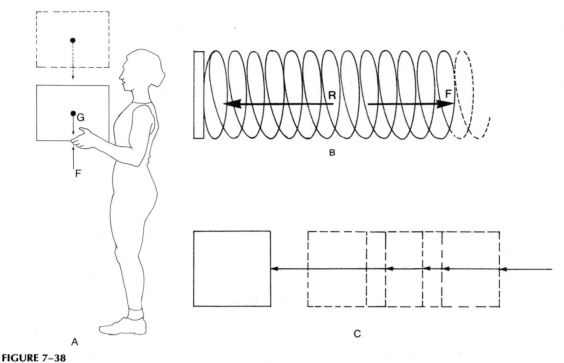

FIGURE 7–38

Negative work.

If the velocity changes as work is done the relationship may be found as follows:

$$W = \int_{s_1}^{s_2} F ds$$

since $F = ma$, then

$$W = \int_{s_1}^{s_2} ma\ ds$$

in terms of displacement $a = v\ dv/ds$. Then

$$W = \int_{s_1}^{s_2} mv \frac{dv}{ds} ds = \int_{v_1}^{v_2} mvdv$$

$$W = \tfrac{1}{2}mv_2^2 - \tfrac{1}{2}mv_1^2$$

The term $\tfrac{1}{2}mv^2$ is called the *kinetic energy* of the body. The kinetic energy possessed by the body is related to its velocity. Thus, kinetic energy may be defined as the energy of motion. The preceding equation shows that work done on an object equals the change in its kinetic energy. Any moving body must possess energy because a force must be exerted to stop it, and it cannot be stopped in zero distance. To start an object moving, force must be exerted over a distance. To look at the relationship another way, kinetic energy is the ability of a moving object to produce work. The work–kinetic energy formula may be written

$$W = \tfrac{1}{2}mv^2$$

where $\tfrac{1}{2}mv^2$ is the kinetic energy of the moving object.

Take, for example, the carnival strong man attraction in which the participant swings a large hammer, hits a lever, and tries to raise a block to ring a bell (Fig. 7–39). The kinetic energy of the hammer developed from gravitational and muscular force is transferred through the lever

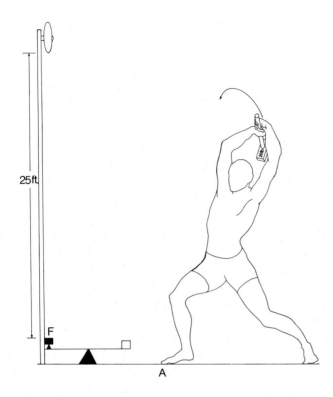

25ft

F

A

FIGURE 7–39

Energy used to produce work.

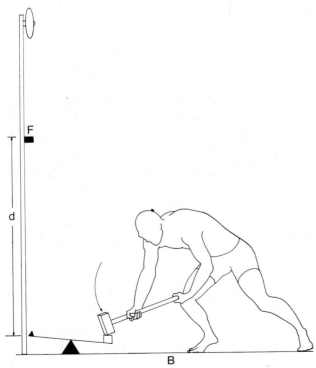

F

d

B

system to raise the block a certain height. If the system is frictionless, the product of the weight of the block and the distance the block is raised represents the work done by the kinetic energy. An increased velocity, which in turn increases the kinetic energy of the hammer, will produce a greater amount of work.

▶ **PROBLEM 7–26**

Suppose the head of a 10 Kg hammer is moving at a velocity of 5 m/sec. as it strikes the lever. The frictionless lever system is a simple first degree lever with a mechanical advantage of 1. The resisting block (F) to be raised is 2 Kg.

QUESTION:
How high will the block rise?

SOLUTION:
The diagram representing the action is shown in Figure 7–39B.
From the work-energy formula,

$$W = \tfrac{1}{2}mv^2$$
$$Fd = \tfrac{1}{2}mv^2$$
$$d = \frac{mv^2}{2F}$$
$$d = \frac{10 \text{ Kg} \times (5 \text{ m/sec.})^2}{2 \times 2 \text{ Kg} \times 9.8 \text{ m/sec.}^2}$$
$$d = 6.38 \text{ m}$$

The moving hammer moves the 2 Kg block 6.38 or produces 12.76 J of work. How fast must the hammer be moving to ring a bell 8 m high?

To solve problems in motion, we may need to use the law of *conservation of energy*. This law states that energy cannot be created or destroyed but may be transformed from one form to another. If we disregard the heat produced, the sum of potential energy and kinetic energy equals the total energy. This is written in the equation form

$$PE + KE = E \text{ (a constant), or}$$
$$mgh + \tfrac{1}{2}mv^2 = E$$

As potential energy decreases, the kinetic energy increases. This relationship is known as the principle of conservation of energy. If we hold a weight above the ground, it possesses potential energy, but no kinetic energy (Fig. 7–40A). If we let the weight fall, it loses potential energy, but gains an equal amount of kinetic energy. We then may state that the change in magnitude of kinetic energy equals the change of magnitude in potential energy, or

$$KE_1 - KE_2 = PE_1 - PE_2$$

When the weight hits the ground, it will have zero potential energy, and all the energy will have been converted to kinetic energy. Suppose a 5 Kg object is held 2 m above the ground (Fig. 7–40A). We may say that it has 98 J of potential energy. Since it is relatively motionless, it has no kinetic energy. As the object is allowed to fall with the force of gravity pulling on it (Fig. 7–40B), the object decreases in height. Hence, its potential energy decreases. On the other hand, the force of gravity is accelerating the object. Its velocity is being increased, which in turn, increases its kinetic energy. Just as the object reaches the ground (Fig. 7–40C), its potential energy is zero, and its kinetic energy is maximum.

▶ **PROBLEM 7–27**

QUESTIONS:
What is the amount of work needed to lift a 25 Kg mass to a height of 3 m? What is the potential energy at that point? What are its potential energy and kinetic energy every 0.5 m as it falls from its 3 m height?

SOLUTION:
Figure 7–41 shows the positions of the 25 Kg mass. To raise the mass at a constant velocity requires a force of 245 N. The distance (h) moved against the force of gravity is 3 m. Hence, the work done is

$$W = F \times h$$
$$= 245 \text{ N} \times 3 \text{ m}$$
$$= 735 \text{ J}$$

The work done to raise the 245 N weight 3 m is 735 J. Remember that the force of gravity (F) equals the product of the mass of the object and the acceleration due to gravity (g) or

$$F = mg$$

The object at this point has a potential energy (PE) equal to the work done to place it in that position. Then,

$$PE = mgh = 735 \text{ J}$$

The kinetic energy (KE) is obtained from the formula

$$KE = \tfrac{1}{2}mv^2$$

At this height, however, v = 0. Thus, the kinetic energy equals zero.

From the principle of conservation of energy, the total energy equals the potential energy plus the kinetic energy, or

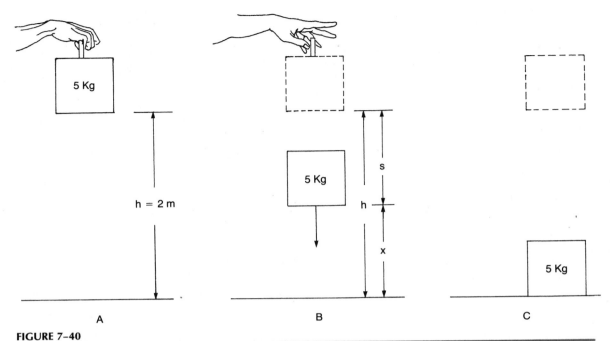

FIGURE 7–40

Relationship between kinetic and potential energy. *A,* The object is held motionless above a surface. *B,* The object is falling to the surface. *C,* The object is on the surface.

$$PE + KE = E$$
$$mgh + \tfrac{1}{2}mv^2 = E$$

Since the gravitational acceleration is constant, we may substitute for v^2 from the equation

$$v^2 = v_0^2 + 2\,gs$$

where s is the distance traveled. With v_0 equal to zero, the energy formula becomes

$$mgh + mgs = E$$

By using this equation, we may develop a table (Table 7–3) to show the potential and kinetic energy as the object falls.

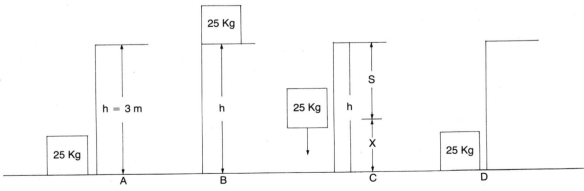

FIGURE 7–41

Relationship between kinetic and potential energy.

TABLE 7–3. RELATIONSHIP BETWEEN POTENTIAL ENERGY (PE), KINETIC ENERGY (KE), AND TOTAL ENERGY (TE)

		PE	KE	TE
h	*s*	*mgh*	*mgs*	*mgh* + *mgs*
3.0	0	735.0	0	735
2.5	0.5	122.5	245.0	735
2.0	1.0	490.0	245.0	735
1.5	1.5	367.5	367.5	735
1.0	2.0	245.0	490.0	735
0.5	2.5	122.5	612.5	735
0	3.0	0	735.0	735

A graph (Fig. 7–42) may be drawn from the data in Table 7–3 to represent the relative values of the potential and kinetic energy for this problem.

Frankel and Burstein (1970) suggested the use of the work-energy approach to determine the energy involved in trauma. The kinetic energy at the instant of impact may be determined from the potential energy of the body before the fall, and the height of the body's center of mass at impact. As shown in Figure 7–31,

$$KE = mgs = mg(h - x).$$

They presented the data for the energy involved when a 50 Kg woman fell on her hip. Her center of mass was located at 64 cm above the floor and 54

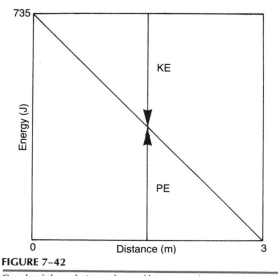

FIGURE 7–42

Graph of the relative values of kinetic and potential energy related to total energy.

cm. above a reference level similar to Figure 7–31. In relation to the reference level, her potential energy while standing was 270 J. Since her kinetic energy at impact would equal the potential energy at the beginning of the fall, they noted that the kinetic energy at impact would also be 270 J. Normally, this energy is dissipated by various bones, ligaments, muscles, and other soft tissues, keeping the energy absorption within tolerable limits. They stated that if the hip carries most of the impact, a fracture is likely to occur, since the femoral neck cannot absorb over 6 J. They concluded that sufficient energy is always present to fracture the neck of the femur when a person falls on the hip.

Frankel (1974) and Noyes (1974) discussed energy absorption related to the speed of loading a body tissue. Frankel found that with the fast loading of a bone, a greater load will be needed to fracture it. However, with a rapidly applied load, the bone will break with a high-energy explosion, while slow loading produces low-energy fractures. Noyes determined that the speed of loading affected the type of tissue damaged. A fast loading produced more ligament failures, whereas a slow rate resulted in more avulsion fractures.

SIMPLE PENDULUM

A simple pendulum may also be used to illustrate the principle of conservation of energy (Fig 7–43). The energy at the maximum displacement (*a*) is all potential energy. As the pendulum swings down through its arc, its potential energy decreases and its kinetic energy increases (*b*). At the bottom of the arc (*c*), its potential energy is zero and its kinetic energy is maximum. As the swing continues on an upward path, the kinetic energy decreases as its potential energy increases until the kinetic energy becomes zero and the maximum displacement is reached (*d*).

By experimentation, the laws of a simple pendulum have been determined for an arc of up to 16°. The gravitational effects on a limb in human motion resemble those on a pendulum, although the results are more complicated. Hence, these effects should be mentioned in the study of human motion. From experimental results, the laws governing a simple pendulum include:

1. Its period (time of complete cycle) is independent of the material or mass of the pendulum.

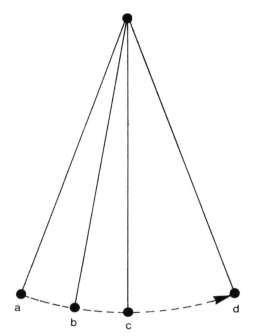

FIGURE 7–43

Simple pendulum.

2. The period is directly proportional to the square root of the length of the pendulum.

3. The period is inversely proportional to the square root of the acceleration due to gravity (g).

These laws may be put in equation form, so that:

$$T \text{ (period)} = 2\pi \sqrt{\frac{l}{g}}$$

where l = length to center of oscillation.

A shorter period means a more rapid angular velocity of the pendulum. Since g is constant, we can see that a shorter pendulum will have a shorter period. Can this be related to swing-through in running? How does the distribution of the mass of a prosthesis or brace affect the velocity of the limb?

Similar to a moving body in linear motion, a rotating body also has kinetic energy. The velocity of a particle moving in a rigid body rotating about an axis is

$$v = r\omega$$

where r is the distance of the particle from the axis, and ω is its angular velocity. The kinetic energy of a particle with a mass (m) is then

$$KE = \tfrac{1}{2}mv^2 = \tfrac{1}{2}mr^2\omega^2$$

The sum of the kinetic energy of all particles of the body yields the total kinetic energy of the body, or

$$KE = \Sigma\tfrac{1}{2}mr^2\omega^2$$

Since the body is rigid, all of its separate particles have the same angular velocity (ω). Hence,

$$KE = \tfrac{1}{2}\Sigma mr^2\omega^2$$

We have seen earlier that the term Σmr^2 equals the moment of inertia (I) of the body about the axis of rotation. Then, the rotational kinetic energy may be written as

$$KE = \tfrac{1}{2}I\omega^2$$

Since kinetic energy is the ability to produce work, the work-energy formula for rotation may be written as

$$W = \tfrac{1}{2}I\omega^2$$

The work done on a rotating body equals the change in its kinetic energy. Hence, if the torque is constant, the work-energy relationship in rotational motion may also be

$$T\theta = \tfrac{1}{2}I\omega_f^2 - \tfrac{1}{2}I\omega_i^2$$

The work done during rotational motion may also be determined in the following manner.

$$W = \int_{\theta_1}^{\theta_2} T d\theta$$

since $T = I\alpha$ and $\alpha = \omega\dfrac{d\omega}{d\theta}$. Then,

$$W = \int_{\theta_1}^{\theta_2} I\omega\frac{d\omega}{d\theta} d\theta = \int_{\omega_1}^{\omega_2} I\omega d\omega$$

$$W = \tfrac{1}{2}I\omega_2^2 - \tfrac{1}{2}I\omega_1^2$$

The change in angular displacement produced by a torque equals the change in rotational kinetic energy.

POWER

Power, another commonly misused term, also has a limited meaning in mechanics. Often the quantity of work done is not sufficient to meet our needs. In exercise programs, training muscular response can be quite specific, and the amount of time needed for the movement to take place can be important. In sports medicine programs, not only must many patients be trained to exert an increased force but also the rate of the movement must be considered. The same amount of work is done lifting 5 Kg 30 cm in height whether it takes 1 sec. or 1 min. However, the amount of power is different. *Power* is defined as the rate of doing work, or the rate at which energy is expended. Average power is the quantity of work done over a specific time interval and is calculated by the equation:

$$\overline{P} = \frac{W}{t}$$

The unit of power is the watt (1 W = 1 J/sec.). If work is expressed in terms of force times the distance moved, this equation becomes:

$$\overline{P} = \frac{Fs}{t}$$

and for the change of kinetic energy when the acceleration is constant,

$$a = \frac{v_f^2 - f_i^2}{2s}$$

then

$$\overline{P} = \frac{mas}{t} = \frac{m(v_f^2 - v_i^2)}{2t}$$

▶ PROBLEM 7–28

QUESTIONS:
Suppose a patient lifts a 45 N pulley weight a distance of 1 m in 2 sec. What is the work done? What is the rate of doing the work?

SOLUTION:
Figure 7–44 shows the movement involved in the exercise. We may use the work formula:

$$W = F \times s$$
$$= 45 \text{ N} \times 1 \text{ m}$$
$$= 45 \text{ J}$$

The work done is 45 J, which is done in 2 sec. The power formula provides for this answer.

$$P = \frac{W}{t}$$
$$= \frac{45 \text{ J}}{2 \text{ sec.}}$$
$$= 22.5 \text{ J/sec.} = 22.5 \text{ W}$$

The rate of doing work for this exercise repetition is 22.5 W. What would be the rate of work done if the patient took 5 sec. to lift the weight?

The formula for average power may also be expressed as $\overline{P} = F\overline{v}$.

The rate of doing work may not always be uniform. The quantity of power at any given instant may be desired. The instantaneous power is the amount of work done during the time interval. However, in this case, the time interval is extremely small. The formula for instantaneous power is

$$P = Fv$$

where v is an instantaneous value.

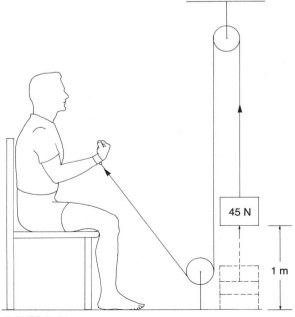

FIGURE 7–44

Patient moving a pulley weight.

Power may be determined for rotatory motion as well by using the formula

$$\overline{P} = \frac{W}{t} = \frac{T\theta}{t}$$

which may be changed to the form

$$\overline{P} = T\overline{\omega}$$

or, for instantaneous values,

$$P = T\omega$$

If the torque and angular velocity are known, the rotational power or rate of doing work, the rate of expenditure, or the development of rotational kinetic energy about an axis can be determined.

▶ **PROBLEM 7–29**

Suppose that during locomotion a constant torque is applied to the swinging leg over a 15° range for 0.09 sec., until it reaches a maximum velocity of 5.78 rad./sec. The moment of inertia of the foot and leg is 0.3332 Kgm².

QUESTIONS:
What is the work done on the leg? What is the magnitude of applied torque? What is the power involved?

SOLUTION:
Figure 7–45 shows the free body diagram of the motion. Since work may be defined as the change in kinetic energy, we may use the formula

$$W = \tfrac{1}{2}I\omega_f^2 - \tfrac{1}{2}I\omega_i^2$$

where $\omega_i = 0$.
Then

$$W = \tfrac{1}{2}I\omega_f^2$$
$$= \tfrac{1}{2} \times 0.3331 \text{ Kgm}^2 \times (5.78 \text{ rad./sec.})^2$$
$$= 5.56 \text{ J}$$

To determine the torque involved, we use the formula

$$\text{Work} = \text{Torque} \times \theta$$

Since θ equals 0.26 rad., then

$$W = T \times 0.26 \text{ rad.} = 5.56 \text{ J}$$
$$T = \frac{5.56 \text{ J}}{0.26}$$
$$T = 21.4 \text{ Nm}$$

The work done is 5.56 J by a torque of 21.4 Nm. Since the change of energy occurred in a time of

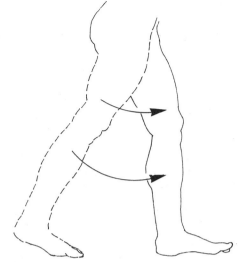

FIGURE 7–45

Kinetics of a swinging leg.

0.09 sec., the average power may be found from the formula

$$P = \frac{W}{t}$$
$$= \frac{5.56 \text{ J}}{0.09 \text{ sec.}}$$
$$= 61.8 \text{ W}$$

or, since we know the average velocity, we may use the formula

$$\overline{P} = T\overline{\omega},$$

where

$$\overline{\omega} = \frac{\omega_f - \omega_i}{2}$$
$$= \frac{5.78 \text{ rad./sec.} - 0 \text{ rad./sec.}}{2}$$
$$= 2.89 \text{ rad./sec.}$$

Then,

$$\overline{P} = 21.4 \text{ Nm} \times 2.89 \text{ rad./sec.}$$
$$= 61.8 \text{ W}$$

Power, calculated by the two different formulae, yields similar results. The proximity of the answers depends upon the precision of measurements used to obtain the data. The formula used depends upon the method used to obtain the data. In either approach to determine the power, it is necessary to know the value for angular velocity. The first formula, however, requires knowing the duration of the movement, while the amount of angular displacement is needed to find the torque used in the second formula.

You may desire to determine the instantaneous mechanical energy of each body segment during a given activity. The potential energy of the segment (mgh) and both the linear ($\frac{1}{2}mv^2$) and angular ($\frac{1}{2}I_c\omega^2$) kinetic energy component are needed. The equation for the energy of each segment would be

$$E = mgh + \tfrac{1}{2}mv^2 + \tfrac{1}{2}I_c\omega^2$$

The total energy of the body would be the sum of the energy of all the segments.

The work-energy formula is useful when the forces acting on the system are known according to the position of the body rather than time. To use the work-energy approach, it is necessary to know the amount of work done to move the object.

EXAMPLES FROM THE LITERATURE

Dynamic analysis of human motion can be cited by many examples. The following paragraphs present some of these, such as walking, running, and lifting.

Walking

The study of human locomotion has interested man since antiquity. Only recently, however, have we been able to record and measure the movement parameters objectively.

Saunders and associates (1953) described human locomotion as the translation of the body from one point to another and demonstrated that this simple concept requires an enormous collection of kinematic and kinetic data from the body segments. Although the body as a whole is moving in translation the limbs are moving in a rotatory fashion. Saunders and associates considered the synthesis of all the elements involved in locomotion a worthy task. At that time, however, because of the "magnitude and difficulty" of such a task, attainment of the dynamic information could not be expected at the clinical site. They therefore limited themselves to describing what they called the primary determinants of gait. Their purpose was to allow the clinician to analyze disorders of locomotion with greater precision than had previously existed.

The six major determinants of gait were presented as pelvic rotation, pelvic tilt, knee flexion in stance, foot and ankle motion, knee motion, and lateral shift of the pelvis. They are all either linear or angular displacements. In 1984 Sutherland introduced five determinants of gait which included temporal and velocity characteristics as well as displacements. These determinants are the duration of a single-limb stance, walking velocity, cadence, step length, and ratio of pelvic span to ankle spread. With the development of improved motion analysis equipment, evaluation of gait impairment was used more widely in the clinical environment.

Many investigators have studied the temporal patterns of walking, including detail of the various phases involved. Murray and associates, in a series of articles (1964, 1966a, 1966b, 1966c, and 1970), recorded displacements of the lower limb using intermittent light photography to relate the angular and linear displacements to the percent of the walking cycle. Four of these studies (1964, 1966a, 1966c, and 1970) were designed specifically to provide normative data of temporal and some kinematic values for both men and women. These also included a comparison of linear and angular displacement patterns for different walking speeds (1966c), for different ages (1964, 1966a, 1970), for different shoe styles (1970), and for the two sexes (1970). The fifth study (1966b) provided examples of lower limb displacement patterns and distorted pathways of the heel and toe for disabled patients. These included the gait patterns of a patient with an above-knee amputation, a patient with drop foot, and a patient with hemiplegia.

Sutherland and Hagy (1927) described a cinematographic approach to obtain kinematic patterns. Similar to the parameters studied by Murray and associates, their investigation presented angular displacements related to the percent of the walking cycle.

Other investigators, using electrogoniometers and speed calibrated recording paper, recorded the angular displacement of the lower limb. The parameters studied included the angular displacement related to the walking phases, step length, duration of phases, and cadence. Gollnick and Karpovich (1964) studied the changes in temporal and kinematic patterns during walking on the horizontal plane and on surfaces at various inclinations. A comparison of the patterns of different footwear and for different speeds of locomotion was done by Gollnick and associates (1964); and Finley and Karpovich (1964) investigated the patterns for normal and pathological gaits, including a patient with hemiplegia, one with an above-knee amputation, and one with cerebral palsy. The kinematic gait characteristics of patients with rheumatoid knee were studied by Kettlekamp and colleagues (1972).

Walking Kinetics

Many investigators have attempted to analyze the kinetics of walking.

Until 1938 the measurement of ground reaction forces that could lead to the calculation of joint forces and moments of force around the joint during the stance phase was inadequate. The equations and principles were defined by Newton, Euler, and d'Alembert, but the measurement technique was not available to add accurate ground reaction forces to the equations. Elftman (1938) developed a set of platforms which when photographed with cinematography provided displacement data. The data could then be converted mathematically to force data in the vertical and horizontal planes.

With the development of a system that allowed for the recording of the magnitude and location of the ground reaction force component, Elftman (1939) combined these force values with simultaneous limb position values to determine joint force, moments of force, and energy changes during walking. Cinematography provided the linear and angular position values with respect to time. Graphical differentiation of these data provided the velocity and acceleration information. By using the Newton-Euler equations and d'Alembert's principle, Elftman first calculated the joint forces and moments for the ankle. From these results he re-

peated the mathematical steps to determine the force and moment values at the knee and hip. The forces calculated at the joints were the result of the ground reaction, gravity, and inertia. The force in the joint did not include the forces resulting from muscle contractions. During the swing phase of gait the ground reaction components were zero. Thus, only gravity and inertia were used in the force equations at the ankle. For the more proximal segments, however, the distal joint forces were used. The moments of force were calculated using ground reaction and joint forces, gravity, and inertia times their appropriate lever arms. The resulting moment of force was caused by muscle activity. No muscle activity would be present if the moment was equal to zero. Such was not the case in Elftman's study. For example, he determined the maximum plantar flexor muscle force to be a value 3.7 times the weight of the individual.

Bresler and Frankel (1950) studied four normal subjects during the entire walking cycle. They used simultaneous cinematographic and force platform recordings to determine the joint forces and the moments of force around the joints for all three dimensions. This was an extension of Elftman's earlier work. The external forces during walking were presented as those of gravity (the weight of the limbs) and contact (the ground reaction force). The internal forces were inertia and contact at the joints. The inertia moments along with the external moments caused by gravity and reaction forces were used to determine the final moment around each joint. They presented in some detail the equations of motion used to calculate the forces and moments at each joint of the lower limb. Their study was one of the early studies that provided information related to ankle, knee, and hip joint forces during gait.

Paul (1965) extended the work done by Bresler and Frankel by calculating the muscle forces and total joint forces at the hip. The moment around the knee-hip joint was determined using the equations of motion. The peak moment value obtained was 180.8 Nm (1600 lb. in.). Electromyography was used to determine the relative activity of the muscles around the hip. From the preceding information and the estimation of the point of application and the line of application of three major muscle groups, Paul calculated the three muscle group forces. He then added the muscle force components to those force components calculated from the force equations of motion. When the muscle force components into the hip joint were added to the gravitational, inertial, and contact forces, the joint force was increased by about five times at peak force but affected very little during swing phase.

Paul (1966) found hip joint forces varying from 2.3 times body weight for a slow-walking woman to 5.8 times body weight for an energetic heavy male. The average of 12 subjects was five times body weight.

Morrison (1970), also using cinematography and a force platform, determined the joint reaction force on the knee. Electromyographic data provided information concerning the muscles that were active across the knee joint at any given time. Both compressive and shearing joint forces were considered. Ground reaction force was measured by the force plate, and accelerations were calculated from the film records. Summation of the effects of ground force reaction, acceleration, and muscle action provided the joint reaction force and its components of compression and shear. Calculation of muscle forces provided maximum magnitudes in the region of 400 lb. (1779 N). The maximum knee-joint reaction force during walking was about four times the body weight. The shearing forces through the range of motion indicated a mean maximum force of 35 lb. (156 N) carried by the anterior cruciate ligament and 74 lb. (329 N) on the posterior cruciate ligament.

Knowledge of joint reaction forces supplies needed information concerning further development in reconstructive joint surgery, partial or total joint replacement, and exercise programs. This type of study is only in its infancy, and much more work is necessary.

By using the joint forces calculated from the equations of motion at the hip and at the knee, Paul (1972) demonstrated how these values may be used to study the loads on a hip prosthesis and on a knee prosthesis. The results indicated that the likely mode of failure is by axial rotation.

The effects of speed on walking and variations of individual body segment parameters upon the forces and torque at the knee joint during the swing phase of walking were studied by Cavanagh and Gregor (1975). They set the foot and leg as a single rigid segment that rotated around a frictionless pin joint of the knee. They then applied the equations of motion to determine the forces at the joint and the moment of force around the knee joint, as described in Problem 7–21. They found a linear increase in peak flexor muscle moment of force just prior to the heel strike as the speed of walking increased. They determined that the angular inertial components ($I\alpha$) accounted for a much greater amount of torque around the knee (approximately 17.7 Nm) than that of the gravity component (approximately 4.8 Nm). The moment of inertia of the segment would be a major contributing factor among subjects if walking speeds were similar.

Calculations for joint and muscle forces during normal gait were done by Röhrle and coworkers (1984). The greatest joint forces for the hip joint (5437 N), tibiofemoral joint (4691 N), patellofemoral joint (1128 N), and ankle (3029 N) occurred at terminal stance. The largest muscle forces calculated were 2539 N for the rectus femoris and 1018 N for the gastrocnemius. They noted that joint forces seem to vary linearly with increase in gait speed. Their findings added to those of Paul (1970), who showed that joint force and muscular effort appear to depend upon body weight and stride length.

Elftman (1939a) also considered the impulse-momentum approach as he discussed the change in ground reaction related to the change in momentum of the body. The work-energy approach to walking was considered by Saunders and associates (1953), and Contini and colleagues (1965). Saunders and Contini and their associates discussed the attempts of the body to minimize the change in potential and kinetic energy by having the center of mass of the body maintain as constant an elevation and smooth a path as possible.

In fact, many early studies of work and energy during locomotion were concerned with displacements of the center of mass of the entire body (Cavagna et al., 1963, 1971, and 1976; Luhtanen and Komi, 1978). A weakness of this approach is that at any instant of the gait cycle some muscles of the body are performing negative work while others may be performing positive work (Luhtanen and Komi 1978).

Elftman (1966) elaborated on the idea of cooperation between muscular force and gravity to minimize the contribution of energy from the muscles.

Winter and co-workers (1976) calculated the energy of each body segment in the sagittal plane to show energy exchanges within segments and to demonstrate individual contributions to the total energy changes during the walking cycle. The instantaneous energy for each leg and thigh and the trunk were calculated from their two kinetic (rotational and translational) and potential components. The rotational and potential energy components of the leg appeared to remain fairly constant with a change of no more than 13 J. The translational change in energy was approximately 14 J. The rotational energy component showed no significant energy change, while the potential energy component changed by 4 J and the translational energy changed by 9 J. The kinetic energy was in opposite directions to the potential energy. The changes in kinetic and potential energy of the trunk are almost equal in magnitude (15 to 17 J) but opposite in direction. These authors did not assess the energy flow among segments since they did not calculate joint forces or moments of force.

Gordon and colleagues performed a power analysis of the swing and stance phases of gait over a range of walking speeds. An attempt to validate joint power and muscle power measures by comparing the total power supplied to the segments with the rates of change of mechanical energy of the segments. By combining joint reaction forces and moments with segmental and joint kinematics, they calculated the patterns of energy generation, absorption, and transfer by muscles and energy transfer through joints. Joint power was determined by the formula P = Fv, while muscle power was calculated from the formula P = Tw. Energy was obtained by using the work-energy approach. The total change in the energy of the foot was 11 J, which begins at heel off and reaches maximum by mid-swing. The leg has a pattern similar to

the foot and has an energy change value of 16 J. The thigh has a double-peaked energy change pattern with one peak of 12 J during swing and a second peak of 9 J at weight acceptance. All of these energy changes are dominated by translational kinetic energies. The authors traced the powers of the segments of the gait cycles and discussed the possible causes of power patterns and energy changes. Their results indicated that joint energy transfers may be as important as the muscle energy transfer in the causes of energy change among the lower limb segments.

Winter (1983) traced the power generated at the hip, knee, and ankle during fast, natural, and slow cadences. He described the various phases of work that occur at each joint. The knee was found to have two negative work phases for the extensor muscles and one for the flexor muscles. A positive work phase existed for the knee extensors during mid-stances. The ankle demonstrated two power phases, one small negative plantar flexor phase and one large positive phase at push off. The greatest negative power work values of the knee were −168 W and −17.3 J, respectively. The values for the large positive power and work phase for the ankle were 252 W and 24.6 J. This information can be useful for injury prevention and rehabilitation exercise programs. Winter (1983) suggested that the knee extensor should be exercised eccentrically and that a major strengthening exercise program should be directed toward the plantar flexors.

Several authors have used mechanical energy changes and the calculation of power to clinically evaluate gait. The results appear to be promising.

While studying the swing phase of normal gait, Cavanagh and Gregor (1975) found that a dissipation of power occurred just after toe-off as the knee continues to flex, halts, and then reverses direction. A major power dissipation occurred as the knee progressed toward extension. In this situation negative torques tended to resist the extension. The peak power dissipating was found to be up to 216.9 Nm/sec. in one of their subjects. They found a power output just prior to heel strike of about 135.6 Nm/sec. in one of their subjects. This output occurred as the knee flexed slightly with a net negative torque persisting. The authors believed that the power characteristics shown in this study are particularly relevant in defining performance criteria for the prosthetic knee. The knee at slow speeds appeared to be relatively passive, but as walking speeds increased, the knee became more involved in dissipation of power.

The mechanical energy of patients with hemiplegia was evaluated by Lowery (1980). She found that the hemiplegic patients had an average mechanical work cost of 3.11 J/Kg as compared with 1.1 J/Kg for normal subjects during level gait. The patients compensated by walking much slower. She determined that segmental energy analysis could expose the abnormal segment and allow for more appropriate treatment.

Mansour and co-workers (1982) assessed the exchange of kinetic and potential energy within a segment or group of segments, the energy transfer between segments, and the mechanical power needed for locomotion. They studied both normal subjects and subjects with impaired gait. To assess the exchange of energy, they used an energy correlation coefficient (ECC):

$$ECC = \tfrac{1}{2} - (\Delta PE)(\Delta KE)/(\Delta PE)^2 + (\Delta KE)^2$$

The ECC was found to be higher in normal subjects than in subjects with impaired gait. The authors noted changes in ECC when a subject walks with or without braces. They suggest the ECC can be used to assess improvement in gait abnormalities.

Mechanical energy changes in normal subjects and subjects with below-knee (BK) amputations during level walking were studied by Lanshammar (1982). The study was done to verify the procedure of energy analysis by Winter and colleagues (1976), who found that the energy changes in the normal leg of BK amputees were similar to those of normal subjects. The prosthetic limb, however, had considerably lower energy changes. When a 0.5 Kg mass was added to the prosthesis, the energy changes for this leg increased. No differences between groups existed in the magnitude of energy changes for the thighs; the addition of the extra mass did not affect the thigh values. Energy exchanges for the head, arms, and trunk were sim-

ilar for both groups. This investigation appeared to verify the results obtained by Winter and colleagues.

Tesio and associates (1985) evaluated the motion of the center of gravity of the body in patients with hemiplegia and patients with unilateral degenerative joint disease of the hip. From this data they determined that the transfer of energy during a step on a patient's normal limb was from 9 to 95 percent greater than that during a step on the impaired limb. The patients with hemiplegia demonstrated similar energy exchange patterns, while greater variability was present in patients with hip joint impairment.

Because of discrepancies in published data, major concerns related to the determination of power during locomotion were investigated by Williams and Cavanagh (1983). They calculated the magnitude of mechanical power of 31 distance runners using a variety of computational methods. Each method relied upon sometimes differing assumptions. The mechanical power may be studied by assuming energy transfer between segments, elastic storage of energy, eccentric muscle contraction, and relative metabolic differences. From the various computations of their data, they found a range of mechanical power values from 273 to 1775 W. Even with their increased restrictions on the assumptions, their values differed by 270 percent. These authors suggest that more research related to the role of energy transfer, negative work, and elastic storage of energy be done before we rely confidently on the measures of mechanical power.

The muscle and joint forces at the ankle and knee were calculated by Groh and Baumann (1976) for normal subjects and subjects with above-knee amputations. The muscle force was calculated after the moment of force was determined. Radiographs were used to determine the point of application and the line of application for the muscles. Following the calculation of the muscle force, they solved for the total joint force by adding the muscle force components to those of gravity, ground reaction, and inertia. They found that all the forces between the normal subjects and those with amputations were similar. The joint force values ranged between 3 and 6 times body weight. These results are similar to those found by other investigators (Paul, 1965; Morrison, 1968).

A two-dimensional quasi-static force analysis method was developed by Stauffer and co-workers (1977) to study forces and moments of force at the ankle joint in normal subjects and in patients with ankle joint disease before and after total ankle joint replacement. Their equipment included foot switches, a 16 mm high-speed camera and analyzer, and a force platform. Equations of motion were used to determine anterior tibial tendon force, Achilles tendon force, ankle joint normal force, and ankle joint tangential force. Their results generally showed that patients with ankle joint disease had less ankle motion and lower forces around the ankle than normal subjects. One year after ankle surgery, the patients' ankle range of motion and tangential force at the ankle were more than the normal subjects'. The Achilles tendon and compressive forces, however, remained near the presurgical values. They determined that compressive force in the ankle during normal level walking may exceed five times the body weight in the last half of the stance phase.

Similar results for patients with total ankle replacements were found by Demottoz and colleagues (1979). They found that the decreased ground reaction force and other abnormal gait patterns were likely related to plantar flexor muscle weakness. They recommended a greater emphasis be placed upon the postoperative physical therapy training program. Such gait analysis techniques appear to allow clinicians to recognize more precisely gait abnormalities. A follow-up of this study with an increased plantar flexor muscle strengthening program may reveal if their theory was correct.

Implications of studying the swing phase of gait were presented by Mena and co-workers (1981). Their study indicated that leg motion was less sensitive to increases in segment inertial properties than to decreases. A lightweight prosthesis would be less desirable than a heavy-weight prostheses during the swing phase. They proposed proper weight addition and distribution to the prosthesis or orthosis on an atrophied limb in order to obtain near normal mass and mass distribution.

A minicomputer system including optoelectronic methods to obtain kinematic data, and a force platform for the ground reaction force component was used by Oberg and Lanshammar (1982) to study gait characteristics of normal subjects and patients with lower-limb amputations (either above-knee or below-knee). The velocities and accelerations for the various joint and segment markings were numerically differentiated from the displacement data. The joint forces and moments of force of the segments were calculated using the equations of motion. They determined that their method of analysis was very useful in assessing gait dynamics. For example, they found that joint moments at the knee were quite different for the patients using a prosthesis compared to the normal subjects.

The analysis of various orthoses for the lower limb may be studied by using the procedures to obtain kinematic data and ground reaction forces followed by using equations of motion calculations. Lehmann and colleagues (1982) specifically studied the effect of a double-stopped ankle-foot orthosis on the moments of the knee during normal ambulation. Some of their findings showed that (1) if the orthosis was adjusted to have 5° flexion, the knee would be hyperextended and a marked knee extension moment would occur, and (2) if the orthosis was adjusted to 5° of dorsiflexion, the knee was thrust forward on heel strike and a marked increase in the flexion moment would result. Subjects altered the gait pattern to avoid the excessive increase in knee moments.

Analysis of stride kinematics and kinetics for children with lower-limb amputations was done by Hoy and co-workers (1982). Their study included the effects of different walking speeds and different prosthetic foot components. With increased speed compared to normal children, the children with an amputation had less out-toeing, greater knee extension and flexion during the swing phase, less knee flexion during the stance phase, and lower moments of force at the knee. The hip range of motion was greater in the prosthetic limb. A difference between the two foot components was evident. One type provided hip motion more nearly like normal than the other. The authors described the primary forces involved in producing the prosthetic motion.

Lewallen and associates (1983) praised the merits of the gait laboratory used to study pathological gait. One of their efforts was to compare the gait characteristics of patients having above knee (AK) or below knee (BK) amputations with normal subjects. Differences were not found between the adults and children. The step length-to-height ratio was 0.37 for AK amputees, 0.40 for BK amputees, and 0.45 for normal subjects. The stance phase lasted longer than in normal subjects by 12.4 percent in the AK group and by 4.0 percent in the BK group. The ground reaction forces for the prosthetic limb side, which was lower than that in normal subjects, was similar for both the AK and BK groups. The intact limbs of the amputees were similar to or slightly increased compared with those of normal subjects. The knee flexion moment and hip extension moment of the normal limb of the AK group were slightly above the normal range. The knee extensor moment and second-limb support moment peak was below the normal range for this group. The normal leg for the BK group had an increased ankle dorsiflexion moment. The joint moments for all amputated limbs were either in the low normal range or below normal.

Dysfunction of the ankle plantar flexion muscles during gait was studied by Lehmann and co-workers (1985). A tibial nerve block was performed on each of six normal subjects to obtain paralysis of the right gastronemius-soleus muscle group. Limb position data, ground reaction forces, step length, and event timing were measured during normal gait and during the nerve block situation. The results showed that, for the tibial block trials, the step length was reduced bilaterally, with the left step being shorter than the right. Certain timing patterns of right heel-off and left heel strike were altered. The change in gait pattern affected the moment of force around the ankle and knee as calculated by the equations of motion. The forward progression of the center of pressure occurred to avoid an unstable collapse of the foot into dorsiflexion. The result was a decrease in the ankle dorsiflex-

ion moment and an increase in the knee flexion moment. The knee became unstable. The authors suggested the use of an orthotic device to prevent excessive ankle dorsiflexion and to allow a more normal gait in subjects with tibial nerve paralysis.

Lehmann and colleagues (1987) discussed the use of objective gait assessment for patients with arthritis, first as a basis for corrective intervention then repeated as an aid in the assessment of therapy results. They used the joint force and the moment of force values computed from the equations of motion as a major basis of their analysis. They also included step and stride length, cadence, walking speed, and double support items in their analysis. The results of a patient with a knee flexion contracture caused by degenerative joint disease were presented.

Sutherland (1978) reviewed literature related to the analysis of the gait of children with cerebral palsy. His conclusion was that objective assessment was essential for progress in their treatment. Measurements should include kinematics, force-plate recordings, and electromyography.

Winter (1983) stated that the resultant moment of force provides powerful diagnostic information when patient gait analysis is compared with normal patterns. Winter presented a range of joint moments normalized to body mass. He found the ankle moment and support moment to be fairly consistent for normal subjects. The knee and hip moments of normal subjects, however, are quite variable. A patient must have a considerable amount of knee and hip moment of force deviation for these values to be abnormal. The moment of force patterns of two patients, one with a total knee replacement and one with a hip arthroplasty, were presented. The importance of determining the moment of force patterns to evaluate gait was discussed.

Examples of the information in this chapter are found in Elftman's (1939a) study of locomotion. By using cinematography and a force platform, Elftman determined the kinematic and kinetic values of the human leg in walking. Using methods similar to those we used to determine the velocity and acceleration of the forearm in elbow flexion, he determined the velocity and acceleration of the lower limb during walking. Measurements from a force platform and calculations from the acceleration approach (F = ma) provided the magnitude and direction of forces acting on the lower limb. With these forces determined and their point of application and line of direction known, he proceeded to calculate the torques applied to the limb by finding the product of force times the perpendicular distance to the axis of rotation. The effective countertorque was calculated from the formula T = 1α. The moment of inertia (I) was taken from Fischer's body segment parameter data (1906). The angular velocity was obtained from displacement, time, and velocity calculations, as we have shown earlier. From the momentum approach for both linear (mv) and angular (Iω) motion of the limb, Elftman determined the effects of change of momentum on the other parts of the system. Resultant forces for the muscles acting on a segment of the limb were calculated from the joint torque and lever arm length (F = T/d). Elftman's study ended with a discussion of energy transfer within the body, and the rate at which energy is transferred, or the rate at which work was being done by the various components of the system. The work-energy approach provided the basis for the explanation of energy change and rates of change of potential and kinetic energy. The rate of energy change or rate of doing work was calculated from the formulae for power, that is, P = Fv and P = Tω.

Running

The analysis of running has gained increased importance in relation to the medical field. Proper medical care is necessary for the injured athlete to return to his or her athletic endeavors, which quite often require running. More people are becoming actively involved in sporting events and may be injured in the process. For proper diagnosis, treatment, and rehabilitation, a thorough understanding of the basic skills and dynamic properties involved in running is nec-

essary. However, a thorough kinetic analysis of running has yet to be completed.

The joint forces during running in response to gravity, inertia, and contact forces were tabulated by Elftman (1940). He used the equations of motion to determine these values which did not include the forces at the joint from muscle components. He determined the moments for each segment from which muscle activity could be determined. The assumption, however, in calculating the muscle force production is that a minimum number of muscles are active at any one time, and that antagonistic muscle moments are not present.

James and Brubaker (1973) reviewed the dynamics of running and related the study to the medical field. They first described the temporal patterns of running. The running cycle was divided into two phases: support and recovery. Each of these was further subdivided into three periods. The review continued with brief kinematic and kinetic analysis of the lower limb during running. Some examples of the analysis are presented in the following paragraph. Note that the examples given do not represent a complete analysis and are meant only to illustrate the use of the dynamic principles mentioned in the text.

During running, the foot must change velocities in short periods of time as it accelerates and decelerates through the running cycle. As the hip of the recovery limb begins to flex, the angular knee flexion displacement increases to shorten the effective radius of the limb (r). This in turn reduces the limb's moment of inertia (I = Σmr^2), allowing more rapid recovery on swing-through with less muscular exertion. As the limb continues to swing forward, the flexing hip transfers angular momentum (Iω) to the leg and foot. The knee which has begun extension continues to extend until the foot reaches its most forward position.

Muscle torques (T = F $\times$ d) and muscle group activity about the lower limb during the recovery phase of running were calculated by Dillman (1970). His kinetic analysis of the recovery limb coincided well with the kinematic analysis of accelerations and decelerations of the limb. The muscular contractions near the extremes of motion provide an impulse (Ft) to the limb segments, which cause the limb to decelerate and reverse direction, and in turn supply the limb with sufficient momentum to swing through its range of motion without the aid of muscular action. From body segment parameter data, he used the equations of motion to determine joint reaction forces during the swing phase.

The moments of force and mechanical power of the hip, knee, and ankle during slow jogging were studied by Winter (1983). The support moment patterns for each joint were described. The peak moments for one of the subjects were approximately 180 Nm at the ankle, 210 Nm at the knee, and 85 Nm at the hip. From the moments of force found at each joint, power and work were analyzed at the ankle. The average peak power was 807 W, and the average peak work was 590 W. The knee demonstrated five distinct peak power values. The greatest average peak knee power occurs following heel strike as the knee extensor muscles absorb energy. The power value was 543 W, while the work was calculated to be 35.6 J. In general, the knee muscles absorbed 3.6 times as much energy as they produced. The ankles generated 2.9 times more than they absorbed. The ankles averaged three times the amount of positive power produced by the knee muscles.

The muscle moment of force patterns about the ankle, knee, hip, shoulder, and elbow during sprinting were studied by Mann (1981). He found that the magnitude of the moments for the lower limb joints indicated maximum exertion. The greatest moments occurred during eccentric contractions during the initial portion of foot strike. Some of the approximate maximum values were 225 Nm for plantar flexions, 190 Nm for knee flexors, 225 Nm for knee extensors, 425 Nm for hip extensors, and 300 Nm for hip flexors. The moment values for the upper limb were much lower. The shoulder values ranged between about 25 Nm for extensors and 30 Nm for flexors, and elbow values ranged from less than 10 Nm for extensors to about 20 Nm for flexors.

A biomechanical model of the ankle was developed by Burdett (1982) which was used to predict the forces at the ankle during the stance phase of running. From the leg, ankle, and foot, he analyzed the location of the muscles that cross the ankle to determine their point of application and line of application. He then had three subjects run across a force platform at a speed of approximately 4.4 m/sec. Cinematography was used to obtain the kinematic data. The ground reaction forces during the running trials were about 2.5 to 3.2 times body weight, which more than doubled the 1.0 to 1.2 times body weight values found during walking (Jacobs et al., 1972). These values in turn provided compressive ankle forces of 10 to 13 times body weight in running compared with about five times body weight in walking (Seirig and Arvikar, 1975; Stauffer et al., 1977). The maximum value of the plantar flexor muscle group force was calculated to be 10 times body weight or 6680 N (1502 lb.), which may be near the load that causes tendon injury. Models such as this in combination with strength of biological tissue studies may help us in predicting tissue injury.

During the support phase, the foot is placed under a great load as it takes the impact of foot strike, support of the body weight, and transmission of the thrust from the lower limb at toe-off. These forces are absorbed through the joints of the body. At mid-support, the center of mass of the body is carried over the foot by a combination of active hip extension and forward momentum (mv) of the body.

Undesirable moments are set up during the support phase that are counteracted by equal and opposite forces from arm swing and trunk rotation, as well as from the position and forces created by the recovery limb. The major factors that seem to limit the speed of running are the inertia of the lower limbs during recovery phase and the force that must be applied first to accelerate the recovery limb and then to decelerate it. (Note that injury to the hamstrings often occurs when this muscle group is attempting to decelerate the extending knee.)

An excellent review of kinematic and kinetic research was presented by Williams (1985). He cited the need for interdisciplinary research in the analysis of body movements. Mathematical modeling based upon the content of this chapter was included as being a necessary component of this research.

Steps

Ascending and descending curbs and steps are common gait activities. The typical patient with an orthosis or prosthesis, muscle weakness, or nerve damage often is expected to maneuver steps of some sort. Changes in joint range of motion, maximum joint forces, moments of force around the joint, and mechanical power occur in comparison to level walking. These gait characteristics should be considered when teaching patients various activities and in the design of orthoses and prostheses.

Andriacchi and co-workers (1980) used an optoelectric system to determine kinematic values, a force platform to obtain ground reaction forces, and electromyography to analyze muscle activity. They calculated these values for a series of three steps up and three steps down with and without using a handrail. They found maximum joint ranges of motion for the hip, knee, and ankle of 42°, 88°, and 27°, respectively. The maximum hip motion occurred during ascent from the floor to step two; while maximum knee and ankle motion occurred during descent from step two to the floor. The maximum moments of force around the joints occurred in different situations as well. They all were generally greater when the subject did not use the handrail. The greatest hip moment was present during ascent from step one to step three (123.9 Nm). The greatest knee moment occurred during descent from step three to step one (146.6 Nm). The greatest ankle moment was calculated during ascent from the floor to step two. The moments of force were also determined for joint motions outside the sagittal plane. These were all much lower than the moments in the sagittal plane. Abduction and adduction of the hip, however, produced a moment of 86 Nm.

A later study done by Andriacchi and co-workers (1982) used similar methods to compare differences in gait characteristics based upon five different prosthetic designs. During level walking the kinematic variables of stride length and knee flexion during stance appeared to be the major differences between normal subjects and patients with total knee replacement despite control of walking speed. They found that about 75 percent of the patients have abnormal patterns of flexion or extension during the stance phase of level walking. Stair-climbing provided greater differences between normal subjects and patients when compared with level walking. Patients with a total condylar prosthesis descended stairs more slowly than the others. Patients with the total condylar and Geomedic prosthesis had significantly smaller ranges of motion during stair descent. Differences were also found in knee flexion and extension, moment of force pattern, and magnitude.

McFadyen and Winter (1988) extended the study done by Andriacchi and co-workers (1980) by adding a series of five steps and studying muscle powers. Their range of motion values for ascending and descending were similar to those found by Andriacchi and co-workers. Their moments were reported as Newton-meters per body weight. During ascent the maximum support moment was approximately three times the body weight; the maximum hip moment was similar to body weight; the maximum knee and ankle moments were about 1.5 times the body weight. The calculated powers were approximately 120 W (hip), 220 W (knee), and 300 W (ankle). McFadyen and Winter (1988) believe that this type of analysis has direct application to rehabilitation and ergonomics.

Upper Limb During Gait

Dynamic studies of the upper limb during locomotion have not been made as extensively as those for the lower limb. However, Elftman (1939c) considered the function of the arms during walking. He questioned whether the arms reacted like pendulums, or whether they played an active integrated part in locomotion. From displacement data, he calculated the linear and angular velocities and accelerations for all parts of the body during stance phase on the right foot. He determined from further calculations of angular momentum that the arms played an important role in counteracting the rapid change in the trunk's angular momentum. Thus, arm movement makes the total momentum changes of the body more gradual as walking progresses. As the speed of locomotion increases, the elbows are flexed and the amplitude of the swing is enlarged to increase the needed angular momentum of the arm.

The forces and the moment of force involved during arm swing during gait was described by Elftman (1941). Graphic differentiation of cinematographic data for motion of the upper limb revealed horizontal acceleration (a_x) of the center of mass of the forearm to be -3600 cm/sec.^{2} and the vertical acceleration (a_y) of the center of mass of the forearm to be -3100 cm/sec.^{2} The mass of the forearm was estimated to be 2.0 Kg. He reported joint forces related to inertia as -7.2 Kg horizontally and -6.2 Kg vertically. These acceleration forces would be added to gravity and muscle forces. By using appropriate lever arms, he then calculated the moments of force around the elbow joint as -27 Kgcm from gravity, -29 Kgcm from horizontal accelerations, and 87 Kgcm from vertical acceleration. The angular acceleration (α) was found from cinematography to be 41 rad./sec.^{2} The moment of force as the result of angular momentum was calculated as -11 Kgcm. The muscle torque was then determined to be -42 Kgcm produced by the triceps brachii. With a lever arm of 2 cm, the muscle force was calculated to be 21 Kg. He then explained that by using the equations of motion as previously described, one could determine the forces and moments at the shoulder.

Inman and associates (1944) discussed the kinematic characteristics of angular displacement for joints of the upper limb during walking and added calculations of the muscle forces acting across the shoulder joint.

Although some dynamic studies of the upper limb have been done, Pearson (1967) emphasized a need for more knowledge of the kinematics and kinetics of the upper limb, which would represent essential and valuable data for the proper design, evaluation, and use of orthotic and prosthetic devices.

Kicking and Jumping

Analysis of body motion is not limited to gait activities. For example, the activities of jumping and kicking may be analyzed using the equations of motion.

Zernicke and Roberts (1976) reported the use of mathematical modeling to quantify the kinematic characteristics of the lower limb during toe-kicking activity, as in soccer. The hip was found to produce the greatest maximum moment of force (>28 Kgm) early in the kicking motion. The knee developed a moment of approximately 12 Kgm just prior to ball contact. The ankle moment of force was very low.

Gainor and associates (1978) compared the toe kick and the soccer-style kick. In the toe-kicking style a large knee extension moment of force of over 230 Nm (2000 in. lb.) was produced. After contact with the ball a large flexion moment of force about 280 Nm (2500 in. lb.) occurred. This motion is in a single plane of flexion and extension. The soccer-style kick had a varus moment of 230 Nm (2000 in. lb.) prior to ball contact and a large valgus moment of force of about 190 Nm (1700 in. lb.) just after contact with the ball. These moment values were higher than those found by Zernicke and Roberts (1976). The maximum kinetic energy of both styles was found to be 630 Nm (5600 in. lb.) for the toe style and 680 Nm (6000 in. lb.) for the soccer-style kick. They point out that the moment of force values are about five times greater than the flexion moment of force just prior to heel strike of an individual walking at 8 Km/hr (5 mph).

Huang and colleagues (1982) provided a detailed account of determining the joint forces and moment of force during kicking. They explained the modeling aspects of the equations of motion followed by experimental verification of their mathematical results.

The work-energy approach was used by Hubley and Wells (1983) to determine the work contributions of hip, knee, and ankle muscles during maximal vertical jumps. Two types of vertical jump were analyzed: the countermovement jump (CMJ) and the static squat jump (SJ). The positive mechanical work was calculated at each joint for the propulsive phase of the movement. The total body energy gain was determined from the sum of the potential, translational kinetic, and rotational kinetic energy values for all segments. Normalization of the absolute work values for the individual joints was performed by dividing these values by the total work done. They also calculated the ratio of energy gained to the work done (efficiency).

The dominant moments were found to be the hip and knee extensor and the plantar flexor muscles. The knee has the highest average absolute work output for both styles of jumping at approximately 330 J for CMJ and 336 J for SJ. The values for the hip were 188 J and 181 J, and the values for the ankle were 161 J and 151 J for CMJ and SJ, respectively.

The total body work was 679 J for CMJ and 668 J for SJ. The total body energy was calculated as 676 J for CMJ and 658 J for SJ.

The mean ratio of energy gained to work done was almost 1.0. The relative contributions of each joint to the total work done was approximately 28 percent for the hip, 49.7 percent for the knee, and 23 percent for the ankle. All three major extensor muscle groups appear to be important contributors to the work done in a maximal vertical jump. The hip and ankle joints should not be neglected in conditioning or rehabilitation exercise programs.

The maximal power output of plantar flexor muscles during maximal semisquat vertical jumps was calculated by Van Ingen Schenan and co-workers (1985) to be 2499 W. They determined that at the high angular velocities of 800°/sec. (14 rad./sec.) needed for the vertical jump, the high moments of force yield a power output of almost six times the power output of the isokinetic experiments done by Fugl-Meyer and colleagues (1982).

Joint moments, power, and work values were compared for one-legged and two-legged jumps (Van Soest et al., 1985). The peak moments of force were greater in all joints for the one-legged jump compared with those for each limb of the two-legged jump. The mean moments of force were also greater in the hip and ankle joints for the one-legged jump. Average peak moment values for the one-legged jump were 304.1 Nm for the hip, 196.0 Nm for the knee, and 243.7 Nm for the ankle. The average peak moments for the two-legged jump were 205.5 Nm for the hip, 179.4 Nm for the knee, and 152.7 Nm for the ankle. In the one-legged jump the ankle contributed the greatest amount of the total work at 41.7 percent, while the knees provided the greatest contribution of work at 37.7 percent during the two-legged jump. In the two-legged jumps, peak power was greater in the knee and smaller in the ankle than in the one-legged jump.

Bobbert and associates (1986) extended the work done by Hubley and Wells (1983) by comparing the variables of force, moments, power output, and amount of work done for the hip, knee, and ankle joints for the drop jump (DJ) and the countermovement (CMJ) jump. Their values for the maximum average absolute work output per body weight for the CMJ was 7.3 J/Kg (560 J) compared with 8.5 J/Kg (679 J total) found by Hubley and Wells. The ratio of total work done to total energy gain was approximately 1.0. The relative contributions of the work done at the joints were 38 percent (hip), 32 percent (knee), and 30 percent (ankle). The individual jumping variation of the subjects may account for these values being different from those found by Hubley and Wells. Two styles of the drop jump were observed. In the bounce type of drop jump, greater maximum moments at the ankles and knees (440 Nm and 414 Nm, respectively) than in the CMJ or counter movement type of drop jump. The hip moment was less in the bounce type. Greater force was needed in all joints in the DJ as compared with the CMJ. For example, the joint compressive force in the bounce group of DJ was 2785 N for the hips, 3393 N for the knees, and 3640 N for the ankles. The values for the CMJ were about 1586 N for the hips, 1779 N for the knees, and 1847 N for the ankles. The relative contributions of work done at each joint were different during the DJ compared with the CMJ. The two types of DJ also had different joint percent of work contribution. The bounce DJ had a reversed pattern, with the ankles (48 percent) greater than the knee (34 percent), which in turn, was greater than the hip (19 percent). The bounce DJ group had a percent work contribution very similar to those found in the two-legged jump by Van Soest and co-workers (1985). These were 33 percent for the hip, 37 percent for the knee, and 29 percent for the ankle. The Achilles tendon force for the DJ was calculated to be up to 7.0 times the body weight. The authors mentioned concern about using drop jumps greater than a drop of 40 cm since the tendon force value was nearing the value of ultimate tensile strength of the Achilles tendon.

Further study of the vertical jump (CMJ and SJ) plus hopping was done by Fukashiro and Komi (1987). They used the formula $P_j = Fv$ to determine joint power; the formula $P_m = T_w$ to calculate muscle power; and the formula $E_i = mgh + \frac{1}{2}mv^2 + \frac{1}{2}Iw^2$ to obtain the mechanical energy. The peak moments for all joints studied were greater in the CMJ than the SJ. The rank order of magnitudes in both cases was hip > knee > ankle. The hip extensors provided greater mechanical work in the CMJ than SJ, while the work done by the knee extensors and ankle plantar flexors were similar in the two types of jumps. The activity of hopping was different from the two styles of jumping. During the hop, the plantar flexor muscles demonstrated a large amount of mechanical work (71 percent) with very little in the hip joint muscles (−3 percent).

Lifting

The dynamics of lifting heavy objects has recently been investigated. Davis and associates (1965) studied the movement of the thoracic and lumbar spine when lifting. A major conclusion was that the process of overcoming the inertia of the object at the beginning of the lift provided the greatest stress to the back. This fact was confirmed by Grieve (1974), who found the highest stress values within the first 0.4 sec. of the lift. He used the momentum approach (Ft = mv) to compare the impulse patterns and resulting velocities of the stoop and crouch lifts. The peak forces in the hands always exceed the weight of the load. The acceleration approach (F = ma) shows that this must be true. The lift would be impossible, and acceleration would be zero, if the peak hand force merely reached the magnitude of the load.

The safety limits of lifting activities were the main concern of Ayoub and associates (1974). From displacement-time relationships they generated velocity and acceleration profiles for various lifting tasks. The linear accelerations of points on the body were calculated from these data, which in turn provided for force and torque calculations through use of the acceleration approach. They concluded that the determination of acceleration profiles plays an important role in the calculation of the stress components on the musculoskeletal system. Much more study is needed for greater understanding of these types of activities.

Bobet and Norman (1984) used the equations of motion combined with electromyography to investigate the effects of two different load distributions on the muscle activity of the back. They found that the muscle activity differences were related to the moments and forces responding to the angular and linear accelerations of the load and trunk.

More recently Freivalds and co-workers (1984) developed a dynamic model using segment motion to analyze lifting motions. The results included body position angles, angular velocities and accelerations, inertial moments and forces, and reactive moments and forces at each joint. Of major value from this study is the prediction of L5/S1 compressive forces for various lifting situations. The maximum estimated compression force at L5/S1 was approximately 7000 N (1574 lb.). Electromyography recording from the erector spinae muscles correlated significantly with the compression force.

Other

Amis and colleagues (1980) studied the movement of rapid elbow flexion to determine increased force at the elbow joint during dynamic effort as opposed to the static situation. They used cinematography to achieve position values and obtained time intervals of 0.02 sec. The angular velocity and acceleration were calculated from smoothed position time data. The angular accelerations revealed initial values of up to 500 rad./sec.^{2} and up to 1200 rad./sec.^{2} for deceleration at the end of the flexion movement. The typical values were about 200 rad./sec.^{2} for acceleration and 550 rad./sec.^{2} for deceleration. They treated the forearm and hand as a rigid system and calculated the joint forces using the equations of motion. They calculated the moment of force around the elbow joint using $I^0 = 0.0599$ Kgm^2. The forces at the elbow joint were calculated using the radial and tangential coordinates. The initial moment needed to overcome the gravity and inertia moments and to accelerate the limb was calculated to be 14.4 Nm. The humero-radial force (0.54 KN) and the humero-ulnar force (0.46 KN) were found to be much less than those found during maximal isometric flexion contraction at the same position. The moment for decelerating the forearm was 34.94 Nm was believed to be caused by the triceps brachii muscle. The joint forces for this situation were 0.97 KN (humero-radial) and 2.05 KN (humero-ulnar). These forces were much greater than those for the isometric contraction at this position but less than the maximum forces developed during an isometric contraction with the forearm 30° above the horizontal. Since the point of application, the line of application, and the magnitude of the muscle forces were not determined, the forces at the elbow joint only represented the forces related to the effects of gravity and inertia. Remember that the radial force component is directed away from the joint which would tend to reduce the joint force. Chaffin and Andersson (1984) suggested that if a weight were held in the hand the kinematic values would be less but the moments could be greater. Unpublished laboratory projects at the University of North Carolina at Chapel Hill (1976 to 1982) reveal that the velocity and acceleration of the hand and forearm as the subject held a 3.63 Kg mass in the hand was about 4.7 rad./sec. and 76.5 rad./sec.^{2}, respectively, at 20° of flexion above the horizontal. The moment needed by the muscle was about 55 Nm. These results support the prediction by Chaffin and Andersson that the kinematic values of the loaded limb would be less than the unloaded but that the moment of force

would be greater. The moment of force of the loaded limb (55 Nm) was similar to the maximum isometric values found by Amis and colleagues (1980) for the same position. The unpublished values for decelerating the loaded limb (140 Nm), however, were much greater than those found for maximal isometric extension (Amis et al., 1980). As predicted by Chaffin and Andersson (1984), the danger of rapidly decelerating a moving limb, especially a weighted limb, appears to be very real. From this study, they suggest that designers of elbow joint replacements should be aware that high-speed velocities are present near the end range of motions and that the components should not be made to impinge prematurely against each other.

Koozekanani and co-workers (1980 and 1983) used video analysis and the equations of motion as an alternative to force plate data to determine center of pressure movement. Their research may help improve the understanding of neural control mechanisms and evaluations of vestibular dysfunction and other neuromuscular diseases.

The ability to maintain balance in response to an accelerating base of support was studied by Romick-Allen and Schultz (1988). They investigated whole body response to unexpected disturbances using video cameras, electromyography, and equations of motion. Joint motions were seen as large as 92.8°. Maximum joint accelerations were determined to be as large as 29.7 rad./sec.^{2} The mean values of maximum joint moments were calculated to be 70 Nm at the ankle, 82 Nm at the knees, 73 Nm at the hips, and 19 Nm at the shoulders.

The studies by Koozekanani and co-workers (1980 and 1983) and Romick-Allen and Schultz (1988) demonstrate the use of equations of motion to evaluate joint forces and moments, although subjects did not move the feet in relation to the base of support.

Pandy and associates (1988) provide an example of the multitude of ways position information, a force platform, and equations of motion may be used to study motion. They used ground reaction and limb motion values to compute the intersegmental forces, moments of force, and power for three different gait patterns of a Nubian goat. The gait patterns included walking, running, and jumping. This study used the same procedures and equations used to study human motion. It demonstrates that a variety of activities may be analyzed in this manner. When studying activities, you are only limited by your imagination and certain assumptions that must be made in all activities.

The biomechanics of injury is an important topic that needs further research. Torg and co-workers (1990) used the acceleration approach and impulse-momentum approach to evaluate axial loading of the cervical spine. A common example of axial loading of the cervical spine is the use of the helmet to ram an opponent during a football game. The neck is slightly flexed straightening the cervical spine and converting it into a segmented column. Compression of the cervical vertebra occurs when the head strikes an object. The head is abruptly stopped as the remainder of the body keeps moving.

Films of 11 athletes who sustained severe injury were obtained. From these films the estimated force of the impact was up to 8133 N (1828 lb.). The maximum estimated force that resulted in quadriplegia of the athlete was 3608 N (811 lb.). The importance of rule changes, appropriate coaching techniques, and athlete attitudes can result in a decrease of serious injury. Continued biomechanical research is essential.

Optimization

Many of the studies have been based upon what may be called the reduction method, while a few have been based upon the optimization approach.

The reduction method makes several simplifications to make the problem solvable. For example, the muscles often are grouped and assumed to act at one point of application and to have one line of application. The simplification of this procedure is obvious when you consider the elbow flexors.

The optimization approach (Seirig and Arkivar, 1973 and 1975; Crowninshield 1978; Penrod et al., 1974; Patriarco et al., 1981; Hardy, 1978; Pedotti et al., 1978) is an attempt to reduce the inaccuracies apparent with the reduction approach. The procedure attempts to include the major contributing muscles involved in an activity, yet selects muscles in accordance to the minimization of energy and muscle force. Muscle models and often electromyography are involved in this process. Optimization techniques that assume muscle actions at any instant and are independent of their actions at other points of time are referred to as *static optimization* (Davy and Audu, 1987). The dynamic optimization approach described by Davy and Audu incorporates control and muscle force histories that have occurred during the motion.

A physiologic model for predicting individual muscle forces has been formulated by Pierrynowski and Morrison (1985a and 1985b). They stated that the optimization method in its present form is not physiologically viable and a better approach is needed. Their physiologic model is based upon neurologic, muscular, and anatomic data to determine the individual muscle forces. The neurologic level includes muscle synergies, antagonists, facilitation, and inhibition. The muscular level is based upon current kinematics and previous muscle activation. The anatomic level consists of muscle geometry, fiber type, and line of application. Pierrynowski and Morrison (1985b) presented data for one subject evaluated by their physiologic model, but they encouraged further rigorous testing of the model.

SUMMARY

With the basic procedures for the dynamic study of human motion presented in this chapter, the student should be prepared to apply these principles in clinical practice as well as in clinical research.

Numerous parameters of movement are interrelated, but none is capable of giving complete description of the movement alone. Velocity and acceleration come from time and displacement recordings, but they are not sufficient without relating them to force and moments. If the mass and its distribution for the various body parts are known, the kinematic and kinetic parameters can be deduced from each other. In gait, for example, rotations are transformed into a translational movement, and each movement can be analyzed in terms of time, displacement, velocity, acceleration, force, and moments.

Identification of movement parameters is essential for meaningful evaluation of distorted movement patterns of patients with movement disturbances and for their comparison with norms.

Quantitative analysis of the kinematic patterns in human motion is important in establishing normal limits and in determining status changes. Permanent recordings can be used to assess a patient's progress and to assist in the design or evaluation of devices used to control, support, or take the place of a natural limb. Objective data are amenable to statistical treatment for research, and clinically the recordings make comparisons easier and more reliable as well as being readily available as often as needed. Limited mobility, weakness, and lack of neuromuscular coordination might lead to abnormal range of motion and poor dynamic patterns which could be quantified.

With the development of recording and measuring devices capable of being utilized in the clinical setting, these movement parameters may become more universally applied, then Steindler's (1953) conjecture that the study of dynamics will be given equal status with anatomy and pathology will come true. With the advent of new and improved instrumentation to record and analyze human motion, better understanding of the kinetics of the human body should soon follow.

For a total understanding of dynamics, we must deal with both kinematics and kinetics. The data obtained only from kinematic analysis are no longer sufficient. For dynamic analysis, we first determine what parameters are needed, and what information is given. This process includes the selection of the mathematical approach that will be used to obtain the necessary parameters in which the forces are acting. Next, the system must be classified. Are we observing a moving particle, rigid body, or linked system? A free body diagram illustrates and helps to determine whether the motion is linear, angular, or a combination of the two. Finally, we apply the mathematical approach, which will provide the desired information.

This chapter presented the areas of kinematic and kinetic analysis of human motion. Although the precise analysis may involve more sophisticated mathematical calculations, the basic approach remains the same.

QUESTIONS

1. Define: displacement, velocity, acceleration, radian, momentum, work, energy, power.

2. How long will it take a runner to go 2 Km if he averages 5 m/sec.?

3. A runner changes speed from 5 m/sec. to 6 m/sec. in 4 sec.
   (a) What is his acceleration?
   (b) What is his average velocity during this time?
   (c) What total distance did he travel?

4. Find the angular velocity:
   (a) $\theta_1 = 300°$, $\theta_2 = 400°$, $t = 2$ sec.
   (b) $\theta_1 = 2$ radians, $\theta_2 = 0.4$ radian, $t = 0.4$ sec.
   (c) $\theta_1 = 30°$, $\theta_2 = 120°$, $t = 0.03$ sec.

5. Find the angular acceleration:
   (a) $w_1 = 90°$/sec., $w_2 = 180°$/sec., $t = 0.2$ sec.
   (b) $w_1 = 6$ rad./sec., $w_2 = 10$ rad./sec., $t = 2$ sec.
   (c) $w_1 = 16$ rad./sec., $w_2 = 2$ rad./sec., $t = 0.7$ sec.

6. A limb 1 m in length moves through an angle of 30° in 0.5 sec.
   (a) What is the angular velocity of:
      (1) The end point of the limb?
      (2) At a point 0.33 m from the point of rotation?
   (b) What is the average linear velocity of:
      (1) The end point of the limb?
      (2) The point one foot from the point of rotation?

7. A limb 60 cm in length moves through an angle of 90° in 0.5 sec.
   (a) What is the average angular velocity of a point 30 cm from the point of rotation?
   (b) What is the average linear velocity of the end point of the limb?
   (c) What is the average linear velocity of a point 15 cm from the point of rotation?

8. Is more muscle force needed at the beginning of a movement than at the middle of

the movement of elbow flexion starting from the horizontal position? Why?

9. Why would a fast movement tend to cause a muscle injury? Give two examples in which this often occurs.

10. Why is the radius of gyration so important in prosthetic designs?

11. Why are athletes taught to roll when they fall?

12. Can you relate head and neck injuries to Newton's laws of motion? Give at least three examples and explain each.

13. Does the speed of loading a tissue affect the type of injuries that result? Explain.

14. List examples in physical therapy that are based on principles of dynamics.

15. A greater force is needed to move an object rapidly. Discuss the importance of this principle in regard to resistive exercise programs.

16. A girl is sliding a 90 N box along a surface ($\mu = 0.3$). What force is needed to move the box at rest to a final velocity of 1 m/sec. after 0.5 sec.?

17. What is meant by "inverse dynamics"?

18. List the assumptions made when using the inverse dynamics approach.

19. What data are needed to solve equations of motion? How are these data obtained?

20. What is "plane motion"?

21. What are the forces that normally act on a moving limb?

22. Discuss how inertia affects the muscle force needed for at least five different exercises or activities.

23. Draw the acceleration components of a_x and a_y and $\omega^2 r$ and αr for the following situations:

(a) The upper limb at 20° of abduction as it is beginning to abduct toward 90°.

(b) The leg and foot just before heel strike in normal gait.

(c) The leg and foot at the very beginning of knee extension (90° to 0°) during an isokinetic exercise.

(d) The leg and foot in the mid-range of knee extension (90° to 0°) during an isokinetic exercise.

24. If a 3.63 Kg mass is added to the hand 0.36 m from the elbow joint, the kinematics is such that at a position of 20° to angular velocity of the limb is 4.7 rad./sec. with an instantaneous acceleration of 76.5 rad./sec². The mass of the forearm is 1.5 Kg. Its center of mass is 0.18 m from the elbow. Its moment of inertia around the elbow is 0.0589 Kgm².

(a) Find the muscle moment.

(b) If the elbow flexor muscle is attached 0.05 m from the elbow and acts at a 45° angle with the forearm, find the elbow flexor muscle force and the joint forces at the elbow.

25. In Figure 7–46, if the time to move from position 1 to position 2 takes 0.3 sec., what is the average linear velocity of points A, B, and C?

FIGURE 7–46

Two positions of the lower limb during the swing phase (Question 25).

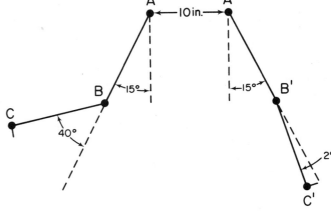

POSITION I   POSITION 2

REFERENCES

Amis AA, Dowson D, Wright V: Analysis of elbow forces due to high-speed forearm movements. J Biomech 13:824–831, 1980.

Andriacchi TP, Andersson GBJ, Fermier RW, et al.: A study of lower-limb mechanics during stair-climbing. J Bone Joint Surg (Am) 62:749–757, 1980.

Andriacchi TP, Galante JO, Fermier RW: The influence of total knee replacement design on walking and stair climbing. J Bone Joint Surg 64A:1328–1335, 1982.

Ayoub MM, Dryden RD, McDaniel JW: Models for lifting activities. In Nelson RC, Morehouse CA (Eds): Biomechanics IV. Baltimore, University Park Press, 1974, pp 30–36.

Benedek GB, Villars FMH: Physics with Illustrated Examples from Medicine and Biology, vol. I, Mechanics. Reading, MA, Addison-Wesley, 1973.

Bernstein N: The Coordination and Regulation of Movements. New York, Pergamon Press, 1967.

Bobbert MF, Mackay M, Schinkelshoek D, et al.: Biomechanical analysis of drop and countermovement jumps. Eur J Appl Physiol 54:566–573, 1986.

Bobet J, Norman RW: Effects of load placement on back muscle activity in load carriage. Eur J Appl Physiol 53:71–75, 1984.

Bouisset S, Pertugon E: Experimental determination of the moment of inertia of limb segments. In Wartenweiler J, Jokl E, Hebbelink M (Eds): Biomechanics I. New York, S. Karger, 1968, pp 106–109.

Bresler B, Frankel JP: The force and moments in the leg during level walking. Transactions of American Society of Mechanical Engineers 72:27–52, 1950.

Brinkerhoff RF, Cross JB, Lazarus A: Exploring Physics, rev. ed. New York, Harcourt, Brace, & World, 1959.

Broer M: Efficiency of Human Movement, 3rd ed. Philadelphia, W. B. Saunders Company, 1973.

Burdett RG: Forces predicted at the ankle during running. Med Sci Sports Exerc 14:308–316, 1982.

Cappozzo A, Figura F, Marchetti M: The interplay of muscular and external forces in human ambulation. J Biomech 9:35–43, 1976.

Carlsoo S, Dahllof A, Holm J: Kinetic analysis of the gait in patients with hemiparesis and in patients with intermittent claudication. Scand. J. Rehab. Med., 6:166–179, 1974.

Cavagna GA, Saibene FP, Margoria R: External work in walking. J Appl Physiol 18:1–9, 1963.

Cavagna GA, Komarek L, Mazzolenia S: The mechanics of sprint running. J Physiol 217:709–721, 1971.

Cavagna GA, Thys H, Zamboni A: The sources of external work in level walking and running. J Physiol 262:639–657m, 1976.

Cavanagh PR, Gregor RJ: Knee joint torque during the swing phase of normal treadmill walking. J Biomech 8:337–344, 1975.

Chaffin DB, Andersson GBJ: Occupational Biomechanics. New York, John Wiley and Sons, 1984.

Childs TF: Analysis of the swing-through crutch gait. Phys Ther 44:804–807, 1964.

Crowninshield RD: Use of optimization techniques to predict muscles forces. Transactions of American Society of Mechanical Engineers 100:88–92, 1978.

Contini R, Gage H, Drillis R: Human gait characteristics. In Kenedi RM (Ed): Biomechanics and Related Bioengineering Topics. Oxford, Pergamon Press, 1965, pp 413–431.

Dainty DA, Norman RW: Standardizing Biomechanical Testing in Sports. Champaign, IL, Human Kinetics Publishers, 1987.

Demottoz JD, Mazur JM, Thomas WH, et al.: Clinical study of total ankle replacement with gait analysis. J Bone Joint Surg (Am) 61:976–988, 1979.

Davis PR, Troup JDG, Burnard JH: Movements of the thoracic and lumbar spine when lifting: A chronocyclophotographic study. J Anat 99:13–26, 1965.

Davy DT, Audu ML: A dynamic optimization technique for predicting muscle forces in the swing phase of gait. J Biomech 20:187–201, 1987.

Dillman CJ: A kinetic analysis of the recovery leg during sprint running. In Casper JM (Ed): Biomechanics. Chicago, The Athletic Institute, 1970.

Drillis R: The use of gliding cyclograms in the biomechanical analysis of movement. Hum Factors 1:1–10, 1959.

Drillis R, Contini R, Bluestein M: Body segment parameters. Artif Limbs 8:44–68, 1964.

Eberhart HD, Inman VT, Bressler B: The principal elements in human locomotion. In Klopsteg PE, Wilson PD (Eds): Human Limbs and Their Substitutes. New York, McGraw-Hill, 1954, pp 437–471.

Elliott LP, Wilcox WF: Physics: A Modern Approach. New York. Macmillan, 1957.

Elftman H: Biomechanics of muscle. J Bone Joint Surg (Am) 48:363–377, 1966.

Elftman H: Forces and energy—changes in the leg during walking. Am J Physiol 125:339–356, 1939a.

Elftman H: The force exerted by the ground in walking. Arbeit Physiol 10:485–491, 1939b.

Elftman H: The function of the arms in walking. Hum Biol 11:529–534, 1939c.

Elftman H: The action of muscles in the body. Biol Symp 3:191–209, 1941.

Elftman H: The measurement of the external force in walking. Science 88:152–153, 1938.

Elftman H: The work done by muscles in running. Am J Physiol 129:672–684, 1940.

Elftman H: The functional structure of the lower limb. In Klopsteg PE, Wilson PD (Eds): Human Limbs and Their Substitutes. New York, McGraw-Hill, 1954, pp 411–436.

Finley FR, Karpovich PV: Electrogoniometric analysis of normal and pathological gaits. Res Q Am Assoc Health Phys Educ 35:379–384, 1964.

Fischer O: Theoretische Grundlagen für ein Mechanik der lebenden Körper, Leipzig, Teubner, 1906.

Fogiel M: The Essentials of Mechanics, vol. 2. Piscataway, NJ, Research and Education Association, 1987.

Fowler RG, Myer DI: Physics for Engineers and Scientists. Boston, Allyn and Bacon, 1958.

Frankel VH: Biomechanics of the knee. Orthop Clin North Am 2:175–190, 1971.

Frankel VH: Biomechanics of bone. Paper presented at the American Academy of Orthopaedic Surgeons. Buena Vista, FL, April 2–5, 1974.

Frankel VH, Burstein AH: Orthopedic Biomechanics, Philadelphia, Lea & Febiger, 1970.

Freivalds A, Chaffin DB, Garg A, et al.: A dynamic biomechanical evaluation of lifting maximum acceptable loads. J Biomech 17:251–262, 1984.

Fugl-Meyer AR, Mild KM, Hórnsten J: Output of skeletal muscle contractions. A study of isokinetic plantar flexion in athletes. Acta Physiol Scand 115:193–199, 1982.

Fukashiro S, Komi P: Joint moment and mechanical power flow of the lower limb during vertical jump. Int J Sports Med 8:15–21, 1987.

Gainor BJ, Piotrowski G, Puhl JJ, et al.: The kick: biomechanics and collision injury. Am J Sports Med 6:185–193, 1978.

Ghelman B, Walker PS, Shoji H, et al.: Kinematics of the knee after prosthetic replacements. Clin Orthop 108:149–157, 1975.

Gollnick PD, Karpovich PV: Electrogoniometric study of locomotion and some athletic movements. Res Q Am Assoc Health Phys Educ 35:357–369, 1964.

Gollnick PD, Tipton CM, Karpovich PV: Electrogoniometric study of walking on high heels. Res Q Am Assoc Health Phys Educ 35:370–378, 1964.

Gordon D, Robertson E, Winter DA: Mechanical energy generation, absorption and transfer amongst segments during walking. J Biomech 13:845–854, 1980.

Grieve DW: Dynamic characteristics of man during crouch- and stoop-lifting. *In* Nelson RC, Morehouse CA (Eds): Biomechanics IV. Baltimore, University Park Press, 1974, pp 19–29.

Grieve DW: The assessment of gait. Physiotherapy. 55:452–460, 1975.

Groh H, Baumann W: Joint and muscle forces acting in the leg during gait. *In* Komi PV (Ed): Biomechanics V. Baltimore, University Park Press, 1976, pp 328–333.

Halliday D, Resnick R: Fundamentals of Physics. New York, John Wiley & Sons, 1974.

Hardy DE: Determining muscles forces in the leg during normal human walking—an application and evaluation of optimization methods. Transactions of American Society of Mechanical Engineers 100:72–78, 1978.

Hof AL, Pronk CNA, Van Best JA: Comparison between EMG to force processing and kinetic analysis for the calf muscle moment in walking and stepping. Biomech 20:167–178, 1987.

Hooper BJ: The Mechanics of Human Movement. New York, American Elsevier Publishing Company, 1973.

Hoskikawa T, Matsui H, Miyashita M: Analysis of running pattern in relation to speed. *In* Biomechanics III (Medicine and Sport Series), vol. 8. Baltimore, University Park Press, 1973, pp 342–348.

Hoy MG, Whiting WC, Zernicke RF: Stride kinematics and knee joint kinetics of child amputee gait. Arch Phys Med Rehabil 63:74–82, 1982.

Huang TC, Roberts EM, Youm Y: Biomechanics of kicking. *In* Ghista DN (Ed): Human Body Dynamics: Impact, Occupational, and Athletic Aspects. Oxford, Clarendon Press, pp 409–443, 1982.

Hubley VL, Wells RP: A work-energy approach to determine individual joint contributions to vertical jump performance. Eur J Appl Physiol 50:247–254, 1983.

Inman VT, Saunders JB, Abbott LC: The function of the shoulder joint. J Bone Joint Surg 26A:1–30, 1944.

Jackson KM: Fitting of mathematical functions to biomechanical data. Transactions of Biomedical Engineering 26:122–124, 1979.

Jacobs NA, Skoracki J, Charnley J: Analysis of the vertical components of force in normal and pathological gait. J Biomech 5:11–34, 1972.

James SL, Brubaker CE: Biomechanics of running. Orthop Clin North Am 4:605–615, 1973.

Johnston RC: Mechanical considerations of the hip joint. Arch Surg 107:411–417, 1973.

Karpovich PV, Herden EL, Asa MM: Electrogoniometric study of joints. US Armed Forces Med J 11:424, 1960.

Karpovich PV, Karpovich GP: Electrogoniometer: A new device for the study of joint action. Fed. Proc., 18:79(310), 1959.

Kelley DL: Kinesiology. Englewood Cliffs, NJ, Prentice-Hall, 1971.

Kettlekamp DB: Clinical implications of knee biomechanics. Arch Surg 107:406–410, 1973.

Kettlekamp DB, Leaverton PE, Misol S: Gait characteristics of the rheumatoid knee. Arch Surg 104:30–34, 1972.

Koozekanani SH, Stockwell CW, McGhee RB, et al.: On the role of dynamic models in quantitative posturography. Transactions of Biomedical Engineering 27:10, 1980, pp 605–608.

Koozekanani SH, Barin K, McGhee RB, et al.: A recursive free-body approach to computer simulation of human postural dynamics. Transactions of Biomedical Engineering 30:12, 1983, pp 787–792.

Lanshammar H: Variation of mechanical energy levels for normal and prosthetic gait. Prosth Orth Int 6:97–102, 1982.

Lehmann JF, Condor SM, de Lateur BJ, et al.: Gait abnormalities in tibial nerve paralysis: A biomechanical study. Arch Phys Med Rehabil 66:80–85, 1985.

Lehmann JF, Ko MJ, de Lateur BJ: Knee moments: Origin in normal ambulation and their modifications by double-stopped ankle-foot orthoses. Arch Phys Med Rehabil 63:345–351, 1982.

Lehmann JF, Price R, Condon SM, et al.: The role of the biomechanics laboratory in the analysis of the gait of individuals with arthritis. J Rheumatol 14 (Suppl 15):46–52, 1987.

Lewallen R, Quanbury AO, Ross K, et al.: A biomechanical study of normal and amputee gait *In* Winter DA, et al. (Eds): Biomechanics IV. Baltimore, University Park Press, 1983, pp 587–591.

Lindgren SO: Experimental studies of mechanical effects in head injury. Acta Chir Scand Suppl 360:1, 1966.

Lowery LL: Mechanical energy analysis of hemiplegic gait: Monitoring and diagnosis in human locomotion I. Proceedings of the Special Conference of the Canadian Society for Biomechanics, London, Ontario, October 27–29, 1980, pp 56–57.

Luhtanen P, Komi PV: Mechanical energy states during running. Eur J Appl Physiol 38:41–48, 1978.

MacConaill MA, Basmajian JV: Muscles and Movements. Baltimore, Williams & Wilkins, 1969.

McKenzie JA: The dynamic behavior of the head and cervical spine during "whiplash." J Biomech 4:477–490, 1971.

Mann RV: Kinetic analysis of sprinting. Med Sci Sport Exerc 13:325–328, 1981.

Mansour JM, Lesh MD, Nowak MD, et al.: A three dimensional multisegmental analysis of the energetics of normal and pathological human gait. J Biomech 15:51–59, 1982.

McFadyen BJ, Winter DA: An integrated biomechanical analysis of normal stair ascent and descent. J Biomech 21:733–744, 1988.

McGill DJ, King WW: Engineering Mechanics: An Introduction to Dynamics, 2nd ed. Boston, PWS-Kent Publishing Co., 1989.

Mena D, Mansour JM, Simon SR: Analysis and synthesis of human swing leg motion during gait and its clinical application. J Biomech 14:823–832, 1981.

Miller DI, Nelson RC: Biomechanics of Sport. Philadelphia, Lea & Febiger, 1973.

Miller F Jr: College Physics. 3rd ed. New York, Harcourt, Brace, Jovanovich, 1974.

Miller NR, Shapiro R, McLaughlin TM: A technique for obtaining special kinematic parameters of segments of biomechanical systems from cinematographic data. J Biomech 13:535–547, 1980.

Morris JRW: Accelerometry—a technique for the measurement of human body movements. J Biomech 6:729–736, 1973.

Morrison JB: Bioengineering analysis of force actions transmitted by the knee joint. Biomed Engng 3:164–170, 1968.

Morrison JB: The mechanics of the knee joint in relation to normal walking. J Biomech 3:51–61, 1970.

Morton DJ, Fuller DD: Human Locomotion and Body Form. Baltimore, Williams & Wilkins, 1952.

Murray MP, Clarkson BH: The vertical pathways of the foot during level walking. I. Range variability in normal men. Phys Ther 46:585–589, 1966a.

Murray MP, Clarkson BH: The vertical pathways of the foot during level walking. II. Clinical examples of distorted pathways. Phys Ther 46:590–600, 1966b.

Murray MP, Drought AB, Kory RC: Walking patterns of normal men. J Bone Joint Surg (Am) 46:335–360, 1964.

Murray MP, Kory RC: Walking patterns of normal women. Arch Phys Med Rehabil 51:637–650, 1970.

Murray MP, Kory RC, Clarkson BH, et al.: Comparison of free and fast speed walking patterns of normal men. Am J Phys Med 45:8–24, 1966c.

Nelson RC, Petak KL, Pechar G: Use of stroboscopic-photographic techniques in biomechanics research. Res Q Am Assoc Health Phys Educ 40:424–426, 1969.

Noyes FR: Biomechanics of anterior cruciate ligament failure: An analysis of strain-rate sensitivity and mechanism of failure in primates. J Bone Joint Surg 56A:236–253, 1974.

Oberg K, Lanshammar H: An investigation of kinematic and kinetic variables for the description of prosthetic gait using the ENOCH system. Prosthet Orthot Int 6:43–47, 1982.

O'Connell AL, Gardner EB: Understanding the Scientific Bases of Human Movement. Baltimore, Williams & Wilkins, 1972.

Pandy MG, Kumar V, Berme N, et al.: The dynamics of quadrupedal locomotion. Transactions of American Society of Mechanical Engineering 110:230–237, 1988.

Patriarco AG, Mann RW, Simon SR: An evaluation of the approaches of optimization models in the prediction of muscle forces during human gait. J Biomech 14:513–525, 1981.

Paul JP: Design aspects of endo-prostheses for the lower limb. In Kenedi RM (Ed): Perspectives in Biomedical Engineering. Baltimore, University Park Press, 1972.

Paul JP: The effects of walking speed on the force actions transmitted at the hip and knee joints. Proc Roy Soc Med 63:200–202, 1970.

Paul JP: The biomechanics of the hip joint and its clinical relevance. Proc R Soc Med 59:943–947, 1966.

Paul JP: Bio-engineering studies of the forces transmitted by joints. In Kenedi RM (Ed): Biomechanics and Related Bioengineering Topics. Oxford, Pergamon Press, 1965, pp 351–357, 369–380.

Pearson JR: Need for research in fundamental biomechanical studies. Artif Limbs 11:24–27, 1967.

Pedotti A, Krishnan VV, Stark L: Optimization of muscle force sequencing in human locomotion. Math Biosci 38:57–76, 1978.

Penrod DD, Davy DT, Singh DP: An optimization approach to tendon force analysis. J Biomech 7:123–129, 1974.

Perry J: The mechanics of walking. In Perry J, Hislop H (Eds): Principles of Lower-Extremity Bracing. New York, American Physical Therapy Association, 1967, pp 9–32.

Petak KL: The acquisition and reduction of biomechanical data by minicomputer. In Cooper JM (Ed): Selected Topics on Biomechanics. Chicago. The Athletic Institute, 1971.

Pezzack JC, Norman RW, Winter DA: An assessment of derivative determining techniques used for motion analysis. J Biomech 10:377–382, 1977.

Pierrynowski MR, Morrison JB: A physiological model for the evaluation of muscle forces in human locomotion: theoretical aspects. Math Biosci 75:69–101, 1985a.

Pierrynowski MR, Morrison JB: Estimating the muscle forces generated in the human lower extremity when walking: A physiological solution. Math Biosci 75:43–68, 1985b.

Plagenhoef SC: Methods of obtaining kinetic data to analyze human motions. Res Q Am Assoc Health Phys Educ 37:103–112, 1966.

Plagenhoef S: Computer programs for obtaining kinetic data on human movement. J Biomech 1:221–234, 1968.

Plagenhoef S: Patterns of Human Motion: A Cinematographical Analysis. Englewood Cliffs, NJ, Prentice-Hall, 1971.

Röhrle H, Scholten R, Sigolotto C, et al.: Joint forces in the human pelvis-leg skeleton during walking. J Biomech 17:409–424, 1984.

Romick-Allen R, Schultz AB: Biomechanics of reactions to impending falls. J Biomech 21:591–600, 1988.

Salek M, Murdock G: In defense of gait analysis. J Bone Joint Surg (Br) 67:237–241, 1985.

Saunders JB de CM, Inman VT, Eberhart HW: The major determinants in normal and pathological gait. J Bone Joint Surg (Am): 35:543–558, 1953.

Sears FW, Zymanski MW: University Physics. Reading, MA, Addison-Wesley, 1949.

Seireg A, Arvikar RJ: The prediction of muscular load sharing and joint forces in the lower extremities during walking. J Biomech 8:89–102, 1975.

Seireg A, Arvikar RJ: A mathematical model for the evaluation of forces in lower extremities of the musculoskeletal system. J Biomech 6:313–326, 1973.

Slocum DB: The mechanics of some common injuries to the shoulder in sports. Am J Surg 98:394–400, 1959.

Smidt GL, Arora JS, Johnston RC: Accelerographic analysis of several types of walking. Am J Phys Med 50:285–300, 1971.

Stauffer RN, Chao EYS, Brewster RC: Force and motion analysis of the normal, diseased, and prosthetic ankle joint. Clin Orthop 127:189–196, 1977.

Steindler A: A historical review of the studies and investigations made in relation to human gait. J Bone Joint Surg (Am) 35:540–542, 728, 1953.

Straley JW: Basic Physics, Englewood Cliffs, NJ, Prentice-Hall, 1974.

Sutherland DH: An electromyographic study of plantar flexors of the ankle in normal walking on the level. J Bone Joint Surg (Am) 48:66–71, 1966.

Sutherland DH: Gait analysis in cerebral palsy. Devel Med Child Neurol 20:807–813, 1978.

Sutherland DH: Gait Disorders in Childhood and Adolescence. Baltimore, Williams and Wilkins, 1984.

Sutherland DH, Hagy JL: Measurement of gait movements from motion picture film. J Bone Joint Surg (Am) 54:787–797, 1972.

Tesio L, Civaschi P, Tessari L: Motion of the center of gravity of the body in clinical evaluation of gait. Am J Phys Med 64:57–70, 1985.

Torg JS, Vegso JJ, O'Neill MJ, et al.: The epidemiologic, pathologic, biomechanical and cinematographic analysis of football-induced cervical trauma. Am J Sports Med 18:50–57, 1990.

Tullos HS, King JW: Lesions of the pitching arm in adolescents. JAMA 220:264–271, 1972.

Tullos HS, King JW: Throwing mechanism in sports. Orthop Clin North Am 4:709–720, 1973.

van Faassen F, Molen NH: A new method in the treatment of gait disorders. In Biomechanics III (Medicine and Sport Series), vol. 8. Baltimore, University Park Press, 1973, pp 489–491.

van Faassen F, Molen NH, Boon W: Biomechanics of the normal and the pathological gait. In Biomechanics II (Medicine and Sport Series), vol. 6. Baltimore, University Park Press, 1971, pp 260–265.

Van Ingen Schenan GJ, Bobbert MF, Huijing PA, et al.: The instantaneous torque—angular velocity relation in plantar flexion during jumping. Med Sci Sports Exerc 17:422–426, 1985.

Van Soest AJ, Roebroeck ME, Bobbert MF, et al.: A comparison of one-legged and two-legged countermovement jumps. Med Sci Sports Exerc 17:635–639, 1985.

Wartenweiler J, Wettstein A: Basic kinetic rules for simple human movements. In Biomechanics II (Medicine and Sport Series), vol. 6. Baltimore, University Park Press, 1971, pp 134–145.

Wells KF: Kinesiology, 5th ed. Philadelphia, W. B. Saunders Company, 1971.

White AA: Kinematics of the normal spine as related to scoliosis. J Biomech 4:405–411, 1971.

Williams KR, Cavanagh PR: A model for the calculation of mechanical power during distance running. J Biomech 16:115–128, 1983.

Williams KR: Biomechanics of running. In Terjung (Ed): Exercise and Sport Sciences Reviews, vol. 13. New York, Macmillan, 1985, pp 390–440.

Winter DA: Biomechanics of Human Movement. New York, John Wiley and Sons, 1979.

Winter DA: Energy generation and absorption at the ankle and knee during fast, natural and slow cadences. Clin Orthop 175:147–154, 1983.

Winter DA: Moments of force and mechanicals power in jogging. J Biomech 16:91–97, 1983.

Winter DA: Overall principle of lower limb support during stance phase gait. J Biomech 13:923–927, 1980.

Winter DA: Use of normalized profiles in the assessment of the kinetics of pathological gait. In Winter DA, Norman RW, Wells RP, et al. (Eds): Biomechanics IX. Champaign IL, Human Kinetics Publishers, 1983, pp 520–524.

Winter DA, Greenlow RK, Hobson DA: Television-computer analysis of kinematics of human gait. Comput Biomed Res 5:498–504, 1972.

Winter DA, Quanbury AO, Reimer GD: Analysis of instantaneous energy in normal gait. J Biomech 9:253–257, 1976.

Winter DA, Sidwall HG, Hobson DA: Measurement and reduction of noise in kinematics of locomotion. J Biomech 7:157–159, 1974.

Woltring HT, Marsolais EB: Optoelectric gait measurement in two- and three-dimensional space—a preliminary report. Bull Prosth Res 17:46–52, 1980.

Younger JE: Advanced Dynamics. New York, Ronald Press Co., 1958.

Zernicke RF, Roberts EM: Human lower extremity kinetic relationships during systematic variations in resultant limb velocity. In Komi PV (Ed): Biomechanics V-B, Baltimore, University Park Press, 1976, pp 20–25.

Zernicke RF, Caldwell G, Roberts EM: Fitting biomechanical data with cubic spline functions. Res Quart 47:9–18, 1976.

8

Application

INTRODUCTION

When the infinite variety of postures of the human body is considered, along with the complexity of arrangement of the bones and muscles within the body, it is apparent that analysis of problems in biomechanics will involve forces in numerous types of configurations.

In the previous chapters we have seen how to approach examples of static and dynamic equilibrium. By using these basic techniques, an endless number of problems can be attacked.

In this chapter, a few selected examples and problems relating to body mechanics, exercise programs, and other clinical approaches are presented.

It must be remembered that when we select static positions for analysis, we are only approximating the precise forces accompanying actual movement. Analysis by this means ignores accelerations, momentum, and frictional effects, which require the techniques of dynamics. However, the conditions under which very slow, deliberate movements common in therapeutic exercises are carried out resemble those of static postures. Thus, analysis of a series of selected positions will give a minimum approximation of required muscle tension and articular forces.

In the human body, the rotational axis of the joint is not always stationary but changes position as motion occurs (Rolander, 1966; Frankel and Burstein, 1970; LeVeau, 1972; deDuca and Forrest, 1973; Sammarco et al., 1973). Also, soft tissue structures other than muscles offer resistance and support to the body parts involved. Thus, the problems presented in this chapter will not be exact but will be somewhat simplified to show the general procedures for biomechanical analysis.

MUSCULAR FORCES

When anatomic arrangements of muscles in relation to joint movement are analyzed, it is customary to place the arbitrary turning point about which moments are taken at the anatomic axis of the joint. When this is done, the moment of the joint force is zero, since its action line passes through this point. A theoretic set of axes and planes (see Figs. 2–14 to 2–17), such as utilized by Fick (1850), can then be visualized with the origin of the system at the anatomic joint. The action line of a muscle producing motion about a joint is determined by its anatomic position. Its lever arm is the perpendicular distance from the action line of the muscle or tendon to the axis of rotation of the joint (see Fig. 5–12). The moment may be determined by the muscle force component perpendicular to length of the bone times the distance from the point of at-

tachment to the joint axis (see Fig. 5–13A). From the definition of a moment we know that the farther a tendon lies from the axis of the joint, the better will be its turning effect on the segment about the joint.

The terms "shunt" and "spurt" muscles (coined by MacConaill, 1949) refer to a muscle's ability to exert rotatory force on a limb. Muscles that insert close to the joint and have their origin far from the joint are called "spurt" muscles (Fig. 8–1A). These tend to have a greater rotatory component compared to the stabilizing

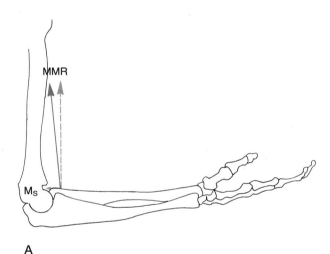

A

FIGURE 8–1

Spurt and shunt muscles. Compare the rotating and stabilizing components of the muscles in *A* and *B*.

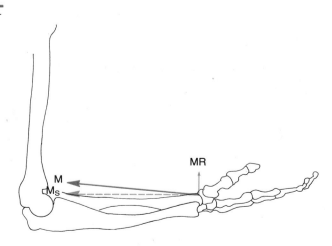

B

component. The "shunt" muscles have their origin close to the joint and their insertion far from the joint (Fig. 8–1B). Their action is more for stabilizing than for rotation. MacConaill and Basmajian (1969) present the biceps brachii as an example of a spurt muscle and the brachioradialis as an example of a shunt muscle. Although the shunt muscles have a greater stabilizing component and their rotatory component is less, their ability to produce a moment around the joint axis may not be less. We must consider the effective moment as the rotatory force component times its point of application from the joint. Stern (1971) questions the existence of shunt and spurt muscles, stating that the work done by the two muscles may be no different mechanically. A big difference lies in the greater activity found in the biceps muscle.

As demonstrated by Kaufer (1971), the interposition of the patella between the tendon of the quadriceps (Q) and the femur increased the lever arm of the knee extensor force (Fig. 8–2). Surgical removal of this bone (patellectomy) results in a decreased lever arm and hence in a decreased moment of quadriceps pull in knee extension. Thus, a greater amount of force must be applied by the quadriceps to obtain the same results with the patella intact. This may be compensated for by exercises designed to strengthen

the quadriceps muscle. Kaufer (1971) suggested building up the tibial tuberosity during the patellectomy to maintain the length of the lever arm.

EXTERNALLY APPLIED LOADS

Just as we think of a muscle pulling at its anatomic attachment on a segment, we can think of the force of gravity exerting a downward pull on the center of mass of the body parts. Gravity cannot be seen, as we can see muscles and tendons, but its effect is just as real. Since the center of mass moves in space as the part moves, the lever arm of gravitational pull (the perpendicular distance from the action line of gravitational force to the axis at the joint), or the gravitational component perpendicular to the body lever, changes according to the position of the part.

Since a rigid object behaves as if its entire mass were acting as its center of mass, it is at this point that we must locate the vector representing the weight of the segment (or total body, depending on what we are dealing with). Such a vector in a line diagram indicates the force of gravitational pull on the mass.

It is convenient to visualize the force of gravity acting on a moving part as a plumb line suspended from the center of mass of the part. In this way the action line and direction of the force will always be properly depicted—vertical and downward. The length of the line, considered as a vector, always represents the weight of the part. Figure 8–3 shows a line diagram of arm elevation with a vector representing gravitational pull acting at the center of mass. In this instance, as the arm moves upward, the angle it forms with the trunk constantly changes. The angle formed by the arm and the action line of gravity also changes. Therefore, the distance from the joint axis at the shoulder to the action line of gravitational pull constantly changes as the arm is elevated, and this distance is maximal when the arm is horizontal.

Analysis of posture and movement is based on an understanding of the leverage afforded gravitational force by body position. A segment is more difficult to lift when it is extended than when it is flexed. This knowledge enables us to

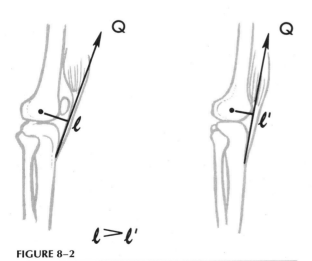

FIGURE 8–2

The patella increases the lever arm of the quadriceps force (Q) at the knee.

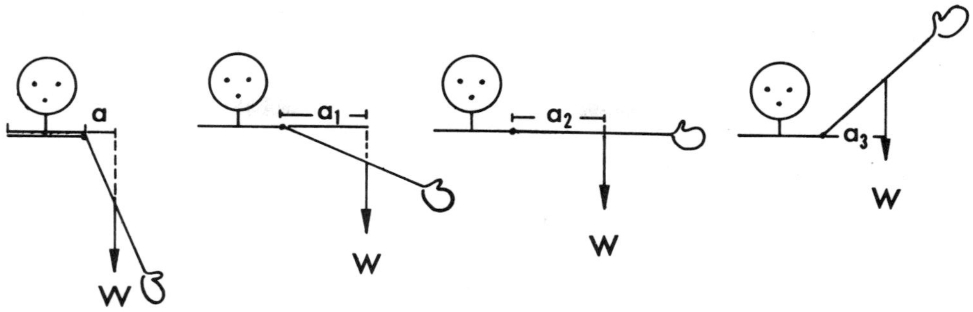

FIGURE 8-3

The action line of gravity does not change its direction as the arm is elevated or lowered. It does move outward or inward from the trunk but always remains vertical. (What are the four characteristics of gravitational force on the limb? Do any of them change as the arm is elevated and lowered?)

grade exercise effectively, but to minimize gravitational effects in everyday activity, everyone should know how to conserve energy and to prevent strain and injury to joint structures. Low back injury commonly results from ignorance of safe lifting techniques that minimize gravitational effects. Arm and shoulder strain may result from prolonged use of the hands away from the midline of the body. The change of body segment position away from the midline causing an increased need for muscle activity also increases the forces acting across the joints. This can aggravate damage and pain in arthritic hips and knees.

BALANCE

We learned in Chapter 2 that the center of mass of an object is a point about which the mass is equally distributed, and that gravity acts upon this point as though all the mass was concentrated at that spot. We have also learned in Chapter 5 that a motionless body is in static equilibrium. We can now use these ideas to study balance and body mechanics.

If a body in static equilibrium is slightly displaced, the characteristics of the forces acting on it may all change. If the object is displaced slightly and it tends to return to its original position, the equilibrium is stable. If after being displaced slightly, the object tends to increase its displacement, the equilibrium is unstable. A body is in a state of neutral equilibrium when upon being slightly displaced it remains in that displaced position. In Figure 8-4A, the cone resting on its base will return to its original position after being moved unless its line of gravity falls outside the base. The cone in Figure 8-4B, balancing on its apex, will tend to continue its displacement once it has been slightly displaced. The ball in Figure 8-4C will remain in the new position after being slightly displaced. It will not return to its original position, or continue its displacement. As was mentioned earlier, a body whose equilibrium is stable will return to its original position unless the line of gravity is made to fall outside its base of support. If the line falls outside this area, the object will topple over (Fig. 8-5). The object will be most stable when the line of gravity is in the geometric center of its base. Increasing the area of the base of support will also increase its stability.

The stability of an object is indirectly proportional to the height of its center of mass above its base. An object with a very low center of mass is more stable than one with a high center of mass. The punching doll in Figure 8-6 is an example. Because of the heavy weight located at the base of the doll, its center of mass is quite low. As you hit the doll it will be displaced, but it tends to return to its original position.

By increasing the weight of an object we also

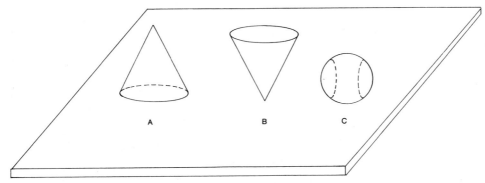

FIGURE 8–4

Stable, unstable, and neutral equilibrium: The cone in *A* is stable; the cone in *B* is unstable; and the ball in *C* is neutral.

increase its stability. Most of us have found that a heavy object of the same dimensions and configuration is more difficult to turn over than a light one.

▶ PROBLEM 8–1

To understand the previous concepts, we may utilize the principles of moments. First, let's look at the size of the base and the location of the line of gravity within this base (Fig. 8–7). Suppose each cone in Figure 8–7 weighs 100 N, the height of the center of mass is 10 cm above the base, and the line of gravity is located 5 cm from the base edge in *A*, 10 cm from the base edge in *B*, and 2.5 cm from the base in *C*.

QUESTION:
List in order of most to least stable to clockwise displacement using the principle of moments.
SOLUTION:
We may determine the object's resistance to displacement by multiplying its weight by the distance from the edge of its base. Thus, we would write:

$$\text{Weight} \times \text{Distance} = \text{Resisting Moment}$$
$$(A) \ 100\,\text{N} \times 5\,\text{cm} = 500\,\text{Ncm}$$
$$(B) \ 100\,\text{N} \times 10\,\text{cm} = 1000\,\text{Ncm}$$
$$(C) \ 100\,\text{N} \times 2.5\,\text{cm} = 250\,\text{Ncm}$$

From these answers the cones are listed in order from most to least stable as *B*, *A*, *C*. The cone with the larger base *B* offers the greatest resistance and is the most stable. The cone with its line of gravity near the edge of its base *C* is the least stable.

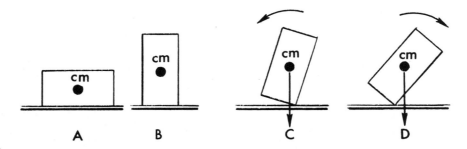

FIGURE 8–5

An object is most stable when its center of mass is low. *A* is more stable than *B*. The object in *C* will fall back into place and remain vertical. In *D*, where the center of mass is not over the base, the object will topple over.

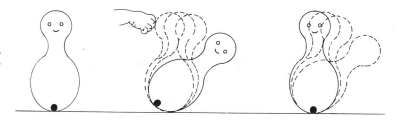

FIGURE 8–6

A punching doll with a low center of mass is difficult to tip over.

▶ **PROBLEM 8–2**

Now let's consider the height of the center of mass. Suppose that the cones in Figure 8–8 weigh 25 N each and the line of gravity for each is centered in the 12.5 cm radius base.

In *A* the center of mass is 25 cm high and in *B* it is 12.5 cm high.

QUESTION:

Which cone is more stable?

SOLUTION:

Since the line of gravity for each passes 12.5 cm from the edge of the base and each weighs 25 N, their resisting moments (25 N × 12.5 cm) would be the same. However, let's attempt to tip each cone over so that its line of gravity will fall outside its base. By using the formula for tangent we may find the angle formed by the base of the cone and the segment drawn from the supporting edge to its center of mass

(Fig. 8–8). For cone *A*, $\tan \theta_1 = \dfrac{25 \text{ cm}}{12.5 \text{ cm}} = 2.0$, and θ_1 equals about 63.6°. For cone *B*, $\tan \theta_2 = \dfrac{12.5 \text{ cm}}{12.5 \text{ cm}} = 1.0$, and θ_2 equals 45°. We may now determine the length of the segment from the edge of the cone to its center of mass by using either the cosine or sine functions of the angles. Thus, for cone *A*:

$$\cos 63.5° = \frac{12.5 \text{ cm}}{X_1} = 0.44620$$

$$X_1 = \frac{12.5 \text{ cm}}{0.44620}$$

$$= 28.0 \text{ cm}$$

and for cone *B*:

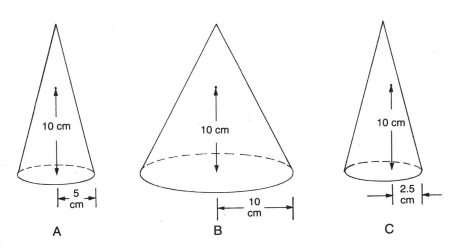

A B C

FIGURE 8–7

Three cones with the same mass and with identical location above the base: The line of gravity to the edge of cone is different for each.

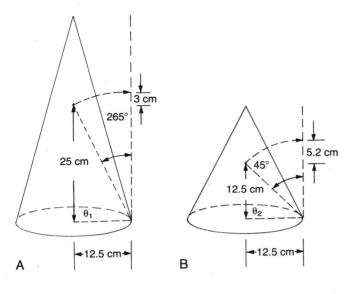

A   B

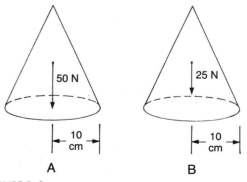

FIGURE 8–8

Two cones with the same mass and size of base. The center of mass of cone A is twice that of cone B.

$$\cos 45° = \frac{12.5 \text{ cm}}{X_2} = 0.707$$

$$X_2 = \frac{12.5 \text{ cm}}{0.707}$$

$$= 17.7 \text{ cm}$$

As shown in Figure 8–8, to tip cone A so that its center of mass lies outside its base, we must move the center of mass through an arc of at least 26.5° and raise it 3 cm. For cone B we must move the mass center through an arc of 45° and raise it 5.2 cm. This indicates that less movement and less work would be needed to tip cone A over. Thus, cone B, with the lower center of mass, is more stable. If the center of mass was approximately at the base, it would have to move through an arc of about 90° and be raised about 12.5 cm before toppling over.

▶ PROBLEM 8–3

Finally, let's consider the difference in weight of otherwise identical cones (Fig. 8–9). Let the bases have a 20 cm diameter and a center of mass 12.5 cm high. Cone A weighs 50 N and B weighs 25 N.

QUESTION:
Which cone is more stable?

SOLUTION:
We can approach this problem in a manner similar to the one related to the base size by multiplying the weight by the distance from the edge of the base size. By thus multiplying the weight by the distance

from the edge of the base, we may determine the resisting moment. Therefore,

Weight × Distance = Resisting Moment
(A) 50 N × 10 cm = 500 Ncm
(B) 25 N × 10 cm = 250 Ncm

Cone A offers twice the resisting moment to displacement than B. From the preceding examples, we can see that stability depends upon (1) the size of the base, (2) the location of the line of gravity related to the base, (3) the height of the center of mass, and (4) the weight of the object.

FIGURE 8–9

Two cones with their centers of mass at the same height and located the same distance from their edge. Cone A is twice as heavy as cone B.

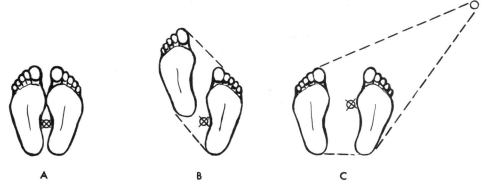

FIGURE 8–10

The position of the feet determines the size of the supporting area beneath the body. *B* has larger supporting area than *A*. Use of a cane greatly extends the base of support (*C*) and the area over which the body is stable.

The upright human body is least stable when the feet are parallel and close together. As the feet are moved apart and the base is broadened, the person becomes less likely to fall (Fig. 8–10). Recall the wide stance assumed by persons standing on a moving bus or on the deck of a ship that is pitching and tossing. In ordinary standing positions, the center of mass of the body is constantly shifting slightly, primarily in an anteroposterior direction (Hellebrandt and Fries, 1942). This postural sway, which normally

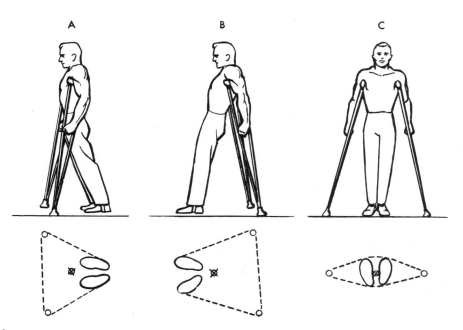

FIGURE 8–11

Bases of support with varying degrees of stability. Can you rank these from most stable to least stable? In *A* and *B* the subject is secure primarily in the anteroposterior direction. The position in *C* provides more stability in the frontal plane than in the sagittal plane.

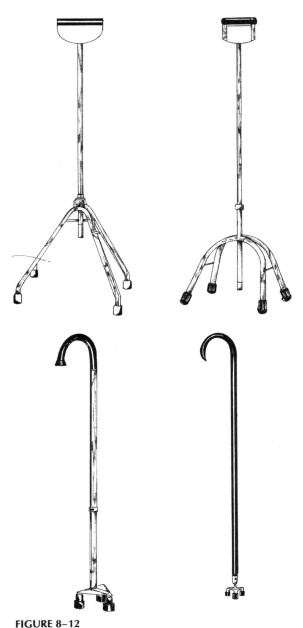

is under the control of automatic neuromuscular mechanisms, necessitates an adequate base area. The use of a crutch or cane will greatly increase the stability of a patient. In Figure 8–11 stable and unstable stance on crutches is illustrated. The tripod and quad canes and similar devices (Fig. 8–12) are designed to give a larger base of support for the cane. The hydraulic patient lifter (Fig. 8–13) is often used to move a patient from one place to another. When moving the patient, care should be taken to widen the base, keep the center of mass of the system in the center of the base, and have the patient raised only as high as necessary.

When a person stoops or reaches, he should advance one foot to broaden the supporting area. A broad base in the direction of body movement is essential in such activities as giving massage and in assistance and support of a patient who is walking or rising from or being seated in a chair (Williams and Worthingham, 1957). Stability of the therapist is vital to safety, as well as to ease of movement. In sup-

FIGURE 8–12

Various types of canes used to provide a larger base of support.

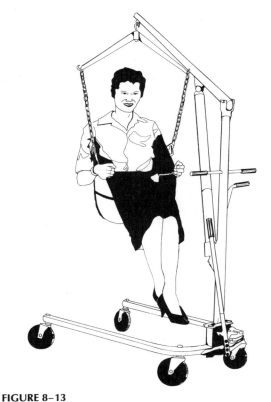

FIGURE 8–13

Hydraulic patient lifter.

porting or lifting a patient the therapist may add a considerable portion of the patient's weight to his own. In this case we must consider the center of mass of the combined mass of both persons.

Two familiar stunts illustrate how the center of mass shifts with a change in posture and how it is necessary to balance the weight over the feet. Ask a friend to stand with his back to a wall and his heels touching or as close to the wall as possible. Place a dollar on the floor in front of him and tell him that it is his if he can lean over and pick it up without moving his feet. Of course, this is impossible, since he must either move one foot forward to provide a base beneath his center of mass or he must shift his trunk backward to balance over his feet, which is prevented by the wall. A similar impossible feat is to stand facing the edge of a door that is ajar, place the forefeet on either side so that abdomen and nose are touching the door's edge, and try to rise on tiptoe. Why can this not be done?

When a person carries a heavy weight, the body shifts in the opposite direction in order to compensate; in this way the center of mass of the combined mass is maintained in a central position over the feet (Fig. 8–14). The opposite arm is automatically lifted to help counterbalance a very heavy load held in one hand. A load carried as near as possible to the midline of the body will minimize the necessary realignment of body segments and consequent muscle and ligament strain.

Balancing the center of mass of the body over the feet requires no conscious thought or effort for the ordinary person. However, for patients with spinal cord lesions and many other types of muscle weakness of the trunk and lower limbs, body balance becomes a critical problem. The slightest miscalculation may result in a fall. The paraplegic patient must learn to master the delicate interplay in position between his pelvis and his head and shoulders. When one of these segments moves forward the other must move backward to compensate, and vice versa. Since he retains muscular control of the head and shoulder position, he can move this mass to help place the pelvis where he wants it to go in ambulation, stair climbing, and so on. He throws his head backward or forward to assist in moving and placing the lower trunk mass. Control of this fine interplay of positions of these body segments is the key to basic posture and movement of the paraplegic. To assist and instruct the patient, the physical therapist must analyze the mechanics involved in segmental balance, in both resting and moving postures (Fig. 8–15). An excellent application of the interplay of head and pelvic positions in the movement of normal persons is in diving, where the position of the body "follows the lead" of the head.

Another type of motor disability in which body balance plays a critical role is muscular dystrophy. In the absence of strength in trunk muscles, the patient arches his spine in an exaggerated lordosis and balances in the upright position. Since the slightest touch may disturb this precarious position, it may be best for the therapist not to attempt to assist him. Walking is slow, requiring a new delicately centered position of balance over each supporting foot after it is swung forward. Here the patient often holds the therapist's arm for support (Wratney, 1958).

Speed of movement is closely associated with requirements for balance. It is easier to balance on a bicycle when it is moving fast than when it is traveling slowly. In the same fashion, patients with a precarious sense of balance may hurry along in order to decrease the requirements for lateral stability. It may be difficult for some patients to slow down their rate of ambulation, and it may even be helpful to some patients to move a little faster if this can be done with safety.

CENTER OF MASS

With a little practice it is not difficult to visualize the center of mass of objects, even if we have no need to work out problems mathematically. Balancing a loaded tray with one hand, for example, is a feat that requires that the carrier size up the load properly. Counterforce can best be

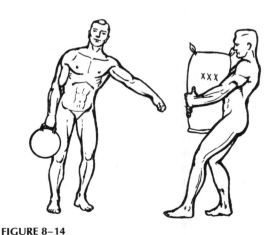

FIGURE 8–14

Automatic postural mechanisms normally center the total mass over the base of support when a load is carried.

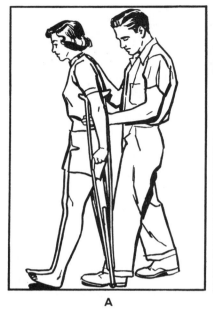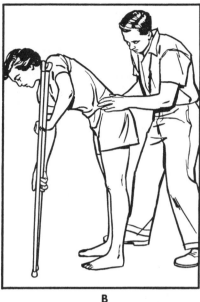

A   B

FIGURE 8–15

A, Manual control of pelvic and upper trunk alignment in ambulation training. Note the position of the therapist's feet. *B,* As the patient "climbs up" her crutches in rising to her feet, the therapist helps to keep her pelvis directly over her feet.

applied in lifting and carrying, pushing and pulling, and the like when the center of mass of the object is taken into consideration. Disaster has resulted from errors in judgment, such as removing eggs from an egg box from the wrong end first when the box is balanced over the edge of a table, or taking dishes off a partially supported cafeteria tray in the wrong order so that remaining items slide about or fall off completely.

The key to successful handling of patients who need assistance in walking and moving about is control and support at the pelvis, which is the center of the body's mass. In helping a patient to walk, the therapist may assist by grasping the patient's belt or steadying the pelvis (Fig. 8–15).

The force exerted by an object as a result of gravitational pull may be considered as a single force representing the sum of all the little individual weights within the object (Fig. 8–16). The magnitude of the single resultant force will equal the combined individual weights of the component units of the object. The action line of the resultant force will pass through a point about which all the moments of the individual

weights on one side will be exactly equal to the combined individual moments on the other side of the point. Thus, if the object is balanced on a "knife-edge" or suspended at this point, it will remain level since the clockwise and counterclockwise moments on either side of the bearing

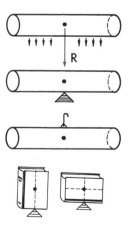

FIGURE 8–16

Locating the single resultant force of gravitational pull on a symmetrical object by balancing or suspending the object.

point or fulcrum are equal. If an object is not symmetric, the center of mass will be located toward the area of greater mass (or density), as in the baseball bat shown in Figure 8–17. This is because of the larger combined moments of the larger individual weights toward the heavier end of the object.

Suspending or balancing an object in one position locates the action line of the force of gravity with respect to that position. In order to find the exact position of the center of mass along this line, it is necessary to rotate the object through an angle, preferably 90°, and to suspend or balance it again in order to determine the action line of the resultant force in the new position. The intersection of this second action line of gravitational force with the original one gives us the location of the center of mass of an object in which the forces are acting in a single plane (Fig. 8–16).

This same principle has been utilized in finding the center of mass of the human body. As early as the seventeenth century, Borelli (1679), an Italian mathematician, used this method. He first balanced a plank over a wedge (Fig. 8–18), then placed the subject on the plank and adjusted the subject's position until he, too, was exactly balanced over the wedge. This indicated the height of the center of mass of the subject between the soles of the feet and the crown of the head. The same principle can be used to determine the anteroposterior "balance" of the subject (in the sagittal plane) and the lateral distribution of weight on right and left foot (in the frontal plane) (Fig. 8–18). The intersection of the three planes established by this technique

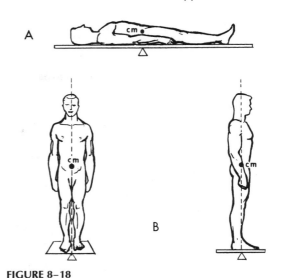

FIGURE 8–18

A, Method used by Borelli to locate the height of the center of mass of the body. *B,* Same principle applied to locate the center of mass with respect to the sagittal and coronal planes.

gives us the exact center of mass of the body. As mentioned earlier, this point has been found to lie within the pelvis and is frequently described as being located just anterior to the second sacral vertebra. A more practical means than Borelli's for determining the body's center of mass is by the well-known board and scale method, which will be studied later in this chapter.

In certain postures of the body, the center of mass may lie in space outside the body itself. If this seems strange to you, remember that the center of mass of a doughnut must lie in the middle of the hole. When a person leans forward to pick up an object from the floor, his or her center of mass may be displaced to a point anterior to the trunk (although it is still over the feet). The center of mass also moves forward when one is in a sitting position (Fig. 8–19). This explains why one is pitched forward if he or she sits too far out on the front of a folding chair seat. Compare the areas of floor support beneath a wheelchair (four wheels) and a conventional straight chair (four legs). Note that wheelchairs are designed for maximum stability. Patients with lower extremity amputations have a higher center of mass, and when they are on

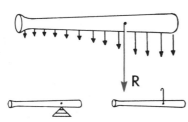

FIGURE 8–17

Locating the single resultant force of gravitational pull on an asymmetrical object by balancing or suspending the object.

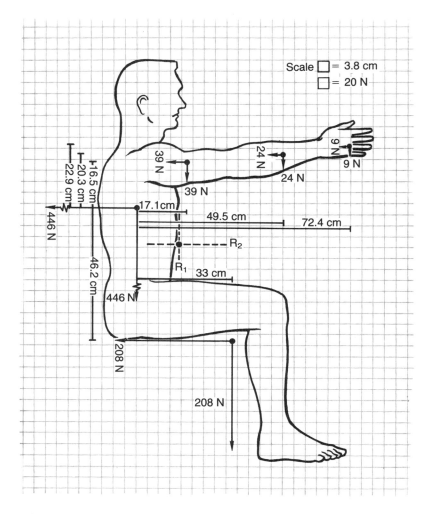

FIGURE 8–19

Locating the center of mass of a seated figure with arms flexed to horizontal.

crutches or in a wheelchair their balance will be less stable. In some cases adjustments to the wheelchair may be necessary.

In the case of a segmented or linked part, such as an upper or lower limb, the center of the entire part can be computed from the centers of the component segments. When a linked limb is flexed, the single center may be found outside the limb (Fig. 8–20). Here it is helpful to remember that this single center will always lie on a line joining the individual centers of two component segments and thus can be estimated

rather accurately. Note that the mass of a body or of a segmented part does not change with a change in its position; only the location of its center of mass changes. The only way the mass itself is altered is by amputation or by adding weight to the part, as with a shoe, cast, brace, or exercise load.

In solving problems involving the body and its parts, moments can be computed about any arbitrarily selected point. The moment center selected will ordinarily depend on the nature of the problem. In finding the single center of mass

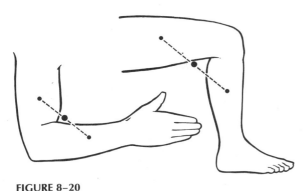

FIGURE 8–20

Location of the single center of mass of linked segments which are flexed.

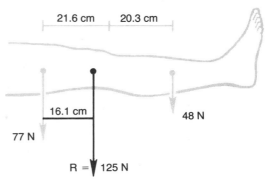

FIGURE 8–21

Computation of single resultant force of the lower limb and its position.

of the linked part in various positions, use of the center mass of the heaviest component part as origin or moment center is most convenient. This eliminates one large value from the computation. If pressure on a joint surface is being investigated, the point of application of force on the articular surface will probably best serve as origin of the system. Finally, if forces rotating a part are under investigation, such as muscle force, gravitational pull, or externally applied loads or manual forces, the axis of rotation of the part may be the most convenient moment center. In some cases the origin may be dictated by the forces that are known or unknown at the outset. Choice of the center will not alter the answer obtained in the solution of the problem.

A few problems are introduced now to help us become better acquainted with resistance offered by gravitational pull on the body segments in various positions. These will provide further practice in locating the action line of the resultant of a parallel force system.

▶ **PROBLEM 8–4**

Patient A weighs 780 N. The center of mass of his thigh lies 21.6 cm above the knee joint, and that of the leg and foot 20.3 cm below it (Fig. 8–21).

QUESTION:
Where does the center of mass of the entire lower limb lie in relation to the knee joint?

SOLUTION:
On the basis of Dempster's figures (1955) the thigh in this case weighs 77 N, and the combined leg and foot, 48 N. Thus, in our first equation for the resultant,

$$R = W_1 + W_2$$
$$= 77 \text{ N} + 48 \text{ N}$$
$$= 125 \text{ N}$$

Taking moments about the center of mass of the thigh (W_1), the resulting moment is

$$RX = \Sigma M$$
$$(125 \text{ N})X = 48 \text{ N} \times 41.9 \text{ cm} = 2011 \text{ Ncm}$$
$$X = \frac{2011 \text{ Ncm}}{125 \text{ N}}$$
$$= 16.1 \text{ cm}$$

Thus, the center of mass of the entire limb lies 16.1 cm distal to that of the thigh, or 5.6 cm proximal to the knee joint in this case.

▶ **PROBLEM 8–5**

QUESTION:
Find the center of mass of the lower limb with the knee flexed to a right angle. The person weighs 666 N. Distances are given in Figures 8–22 and 8–23, and the thigh, leg, and foot weigh 66 N, 31 N, and 9.5 N, respectively.

SOLUTION:
Here we will consider the three component units of thigh, leg, and foot. To find the center of mass of a linked segment that is flexed, it is necessary to de-

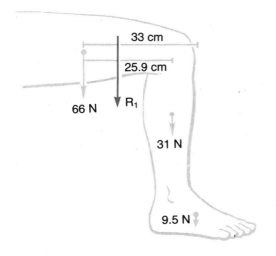

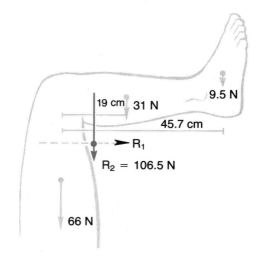

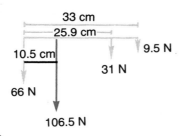

FIGURE 8–22

Center of mass computation.

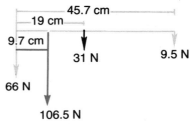

FIGURE 8–23

Second center of mass computation with part rotated 90°.

termine the resultant force with the object in two positions. As we begin with the thigh horizontal,

$$R = W_1 + W_2 + W_3$$
$$= 66\ N + 31\ N + 9.5\ N$$
$$= 106.5\ N$$

and by taking moments about the center of mass of the thigh, as a matter of convenience,

$$RX = (25.9\ cm \times 31\ N)$$
$$+ (33\ cm \times 9.5\ N)$$
$$(106.5\ N)X = 803\ Ncm + 313\ Ncm = 1116\ Ncm$$
$$X = \frac{1116\ Ncm}{106.5\ N}$$
$$X = 10.5\ cm$$

We must now find a second resultant in another position in order to locate the precise center of mass

point along the action line of the first resultant. To do this we turn the object through an arc of 90° and repeat our procedure (Fig. 8–23). The magnitude of the resultant has already been found. By taking moments about the thigh center,

$$RX = (31\ N \times 19.0\ cm)$$
$$+ (9.5\ N \times 45.7\ cm)$$
$$(106.5\ N)X = 589\ Ncm + 434\ Ncm = 1023\ Ncm$$
$$X = \frac{1023\ Ncm}{106.5\ N}$$
$$X = 9.7\ cm$$

Hence, the center of mass of the entire limb when flexed in this position is 10.5 cm distal to and 9.7 cm posterior to the center of mass of the thigh. Let us call this point "C." Notice that the point of application of the forces has no significance in taking mo-

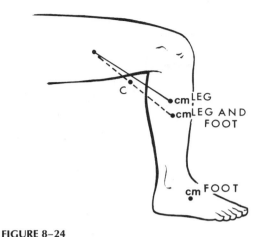

FIGURE 8–24

Locating the single center of mass of a flexed part (on a line between the respective centers of the component segments).

ments, since the moment arms to the action lines of all the forces lie along the same horizontal line.

Figure 8–24 shows that C lies just below a line drawn between the center of mass points of the thigh and leg. If a combined center for the leg and

foot had been used in these computations, C would lie on a line between these two initial points. This illustrates the observation made earlier that the center of mass of a linked part that is flexed will lie between the two centers of the component parts, and slightly closer to the heavier part if they are unequal in mass. The solution of the problem is diagrammed in Figure 8–25.

From the foregoing discussion, we may see that the center of the mass of the lower limb shifts backward as the knee is flexed and that of the upper limb shifts forward as the elbow is flexed. Since these limbs are suspended below the shoulder and hip axes like pendulums when the subject is upright, the lower limb will tend to move forward and the upper limb backward as the knee or elbow is flexed. In this way the center of mass remains directly below the supporting joint. If a load is carried on the hand, the arm moves still farther backward. These shifts in position lengthen important elbow and knee flexor muscles (biceps brachii, hamstrings) at their proximal ends so that they are better able to exert tension and maintain the next position of the joint.

In general, to determine the center of mass of a linked system, we may write:

$$X = \frac{W_1X_1 + W_2X_2 + \cdots W_nX_n}{W_1 + W_2 + \cdots W_n}$$

FIGURE 8–25

Locating the center of mass of the lower limb flexed to 90°.

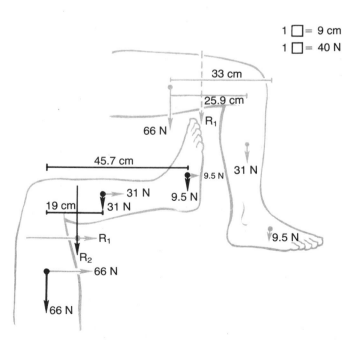

and

$$Y = \frac{W_1Y_1 + W_2Y_2 + \cdots W_nY_n}{W_1 + W_2 + \cdots W_n}$$

Often the center of mass of segments is obtained from photographs of the human body. Based on Dempster's work (1955), Walton (1970) devised a template that can be used to obtain the location of these segmental centers directly from the photograph. This saves considerable time in determining the X_n and Y_n values for each segment.

A method of tabulating data is suggested that will simplify the computations (Table 8–1); tabulation is useful whenever moments are found with the object in more than one position.

To simplify the procedure of finding a single center of mass for linked segments, moments are taken about the center of one of the parts, in this case the thigh. This eliminates a moment value for this part since its moment arm is zero. Data may be tabulated conveniently as follows: each part is listed in column 1; its weight is entered in column 2; the distance from its center of gravity to the moment center (origin of the system) appears in column 3. (Here we have chosen the thigh center.) Moments of each force are found by multiplying the weight in column 2 by the distance to the origin in column 3. This moment value is entered in column 4. Totaling column 4 gives the total moment acting about the origin when the limb is in the position shown. Totaling column 2 gives the magnitude and direction of the resultant force. The distance to the action line of the resultant, and therefore to the centroid, is obtained by dividing the sum of the moments in column 4 by the resultant force magnitude in column 2. If we have been careful with the signs of the forces and moments, we can now locate the action of the resultant (R_1).

In order to find the exact point of the center of mass along the action line we must rotate the limb 90° and repeat the process. We can extend the table to find the action line of the resultant (R_2), which lies at right angles to R_1. A fifth column shows the distances between the forces that are at right angles to the previous distances. Another moment column is obtained by multiplying these distances by the corresponding weights in column 2. Dividing the sum of the moments in column 6 by the total weight in column 2 again gives the position of the action line of the resultant force. The location of the center of mass of the entire limb at the juncture of these two vectors is now completely defined.

▶ **PROBLEM 8–6**

Let us consider another position of the body and again find the center of mass.

Mr. X is seated with both arms flexed to 90° (Fig. 8–19).

QUESTION:
Find the center of mass of the entire body when it is in this posture.

SOLUTION:
Table 8–2 gives weights, distances, and tabulation of data in the solution of the problem. Our subject weighs 726 N. Segment weights are shown in Figure 8–19. Since we are dealing with two limbs, we have doubled the weights. Drawing the figure on graph paper will help to give us the necessary distances to solve the problem. In Problem 8–5 we determined a single center of mass point for the lower limb in flexion, so we can make use of this point now. Remaining centers are for the three upper limb segments and the head and trunk.

Students should experiment for themselves with

TABLE 8–1. LOCATING THE CENTER OF GRAVITY OF A FLEXED LOWER LIMB

Segment	Weight (N)	R_1 Distance (cm)	R_1 Moment (Ncm)	R_2 Distance (cm)	R_2 Moment (Ncm)
Thigh	66	0	0	0	0
Leg	31	25.9	803	19.0	589
Foot	9.5	33.5	318	45.7	434
Total	106.5		1121		1023

$$R_1X = 1121 \text{ Ncm} \qquad R_2X = 1023 \text{ Ncm}$$
$$(106.5 \text{ N})X = 1121 \text{ Ncm} \qquad (106.5 \text{ N})X = 1023 \text{ Ncm}$$
$$X = 10.6 \text{ cm} \qquad X = 9.6 \text{ cm}$$

TABLE 8–2. LOCATING THE CENTER OF GRAVITY OF A SEATED SUBJECT

		R₁		R₂	
Segment	*Weight (N)*	*Distance (cm)*	*Moment (Ncm)*	*Distance (cm)*	*Moment (Ncm)*
Head and trunk	446	0	0	0	0
Arm	39	17.1	667	−16.5	−643
Forearm	24	49.5	1188	−20.3	−487
Hand	9	72.4	652	−22.9	−226
Lower limb	208	33.0	6864	+46.2	+9610
Total	726		9371		8254

$$R_1X = 9371 \text{ Ncm} \qquad R_2X = 8254 \text{ Ncm}$$
$$(726 \text{ N})X = 9371 \text{ Ncm} \qquad (726 \text{ N})X = 8254 \text{ Ncm}$$
$$X = 12.9 \text{ cm} \qquad X = 11.4 \text{ cm}$$

center of mass determinations of the body and its segments. Begin to look for variations in body build among people and to make visual estimates of resistances of parts in terms of their weight and lever arms. Notice differences in segmental proportions of children and adults, and estimate relative differences in gravitational moments corresponding to these variations in body size and shape.

▶ **PROBLEM 8–7**

Let us return to the problem of finding experimentally the location of the center of mass of the body (Fig. 8–26). We obtain a board long enough for the individual to lie on, and place it on two knife-edges at either end. (These may be triangular blocks of wood or pieces of angle iron.) One end of the apparatus rests on a platform scale and the other on a block. A zero reading on the scale can now be obtained which must be subtracted from subsequent readings to eliminate the effect of the weight of the board. Let's apply this to a man whose weight is 800

N and is lying on the board. We now have a parallel force system in equilibrium.
QUESTION:
Find the action line of gravitational force pulling on the subject (in other words, his center of mass with respect to this position).
SOLUTION:
We have determined that the distance between the board supports is 180 cm. For convenience we will compute moments around the support at "f." The scale reading is 400 N. By applying the equations of equilibrium, we have

$$\Sigma M = 0$$
$$(-800 \text{ N} \times X)$$
$$+ (400 \text{ N} \times 180 \text{ cm}) = 0$$
$$-800 \text{ N}X = 72000 \text{ Ncm}$$
$$X = \frac{-72000 \text{ Ncm}}{800 \text{ N}} = -90 \text{ cm}$$

The action line of gravitational force lies 90 cm to the right of the moment center (f). The position of this

FIGURE 8–26

Method of locating the body's center of mass between the soles of the feet and crown of the head.

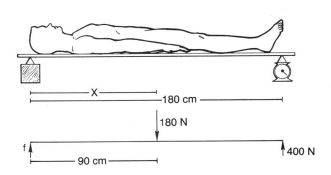

point as measured from the soles of the feet can be converted to a percentage of the total height of the individual for comparison with findings in the literature.

Although it may not particularly interest us in this case, we can easily find the reaction force under the board at *f*. (The same method will be used later on to determine forces in joints.) Since ΣF = 0, and two of the three forces are known, we can solve for the third. If downward forces are negative, then

$$-800 \text{ N} + 400 \text{ N} + f = 0$$
$$f = 400 \text{ N}$$

If the subject now stands on the board facing the scale, the action line of the force of gravity in the sagittal plane can be determined in the same manner. Finally, he makes a 90° turn and faces forward, so that we may establish the action line in the frontal plane. The three planes established by this procedure intersect at the center of mass of the body. The subject must be cautioned not to change his alignment in any of the three positions while measurements are being made, as this will shift the center of mass.

The vertical projection of the center of mass by the supporting surface can be determined by a simple experiment using the board and scale (Fig. 8–27). The subject, facing the scale, stands on a piece of paper and a tracing is made around the feet. The point at which the action line of gravitational force,

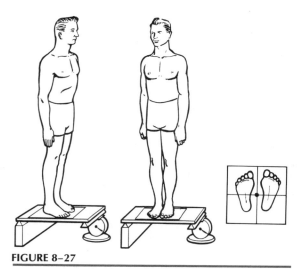

FIGURE 8–27

Locating the vertical projection of the gravity line in relation to the feet.

acting at the body's center of mass, falls in relation to the base is determined as before (from the body weight, the scale reading, and the distance between the knife-edge supports). A line is drawn across the paper to indicate this position. The paper is then turned as the subject turns to face forward, and the process is repeated. The intersection of the two lines indicates the point directly below the body's center of mass. The first cross-line indicates body balance in the anteroposterior direction and the second cross-line the balance in the lateral direction. Hellebrandt and Fries (1942) determined that this point commonly lies slightly forward and to the left of the center of the base of support (in women subjects).

In previous sections we have dealt with theoretical weights of body parts. A simple way of checking these values is possible since an object behaves as though its entire mass were acting at its center of mass. We can now estimate quite accurately the location of center of mass points in the segments of the limbs, and also center of mass of linked parts.

FIRST METHOD OF WEIGHING BODY PARTS. With the subject recumbent, place a sling around one limb at its center of mass and suspend the sling from a scale (Fig. 8–28). If moments are taken about the proximal joint center in each case, the lever arm of the supporting force is equal to that of gravitational force. Thus, the scale reading gives the weight of the part (ΣM = 0). (Some error probably results from the fact that the limb is attached to the body, but this error will be minimal if the subject is completely relaxed.)

Suppose the subject in Figure 8–28 is of average size, and his or her upper limb weighs 40 N. The center of mass of the limb is 25 cm from the axis of rotation at the shoulder. Thus, gravity is exerting a clockwise moment of 40 N × 25 cm = 1000 Ncm about the shoulder. If we place the test sling at the center of mass, the lever arm of the test force will also be 25 cm and the scale will read 40 N. The counterclockwise moment of the test force equals the clockwise moment of gravity about the shoulder, and if the lever arms of these opposing moments are kept the same (25 cm), the respective forces will also be the same (40 N).

Of course, in actual practice we do not know the weight of the limb at first. We apply the sling at the estimated center of mass and the scale reading gives us the weight of the part. If we place the sling and scale at some other point

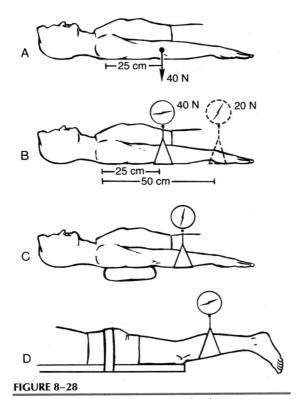

FIGURE 8–28

Method of weighing body segments by sling suspension.

along the part, we will expect a reading different from the true weight. If it is applied above the elbow where the lever arm is short, the scale reading will be higher; if the sling is applied to the forearm, the scale reading will be lower. At any point, the scale reading times the lever arm (distance to shoulder) will equal the gravitational force times its lever arm.

▶ **PROBLEM 8–8**

In the previous example (Fig. 8–28B), if the sling is placed at the wrist 50 cm from the shoulder, we will obtain a scale reading much lower than the previous one (20 N × 50 cm = 1000 Ncm). In this case, to find the weight of the part from our scale reading, we will fill in the known terms in our formula, $\Sigma M = 0$. We have estimated the lever arm of gravitational pull on the limb to be 25 cm. Then

$$(-20 \text{ N} \times 50 \text{ cm}) + (G \times 25 \text{ cm}) = 0$$
$$(-1000 \text{ Ncm}) + (25 \text{ cm} \times G) = 0$$
$$G = 40 \text{ N}$$

(weight of the limb)

In problems of this sort, three values are known so we can solve for the fourth. We have the scale reading and can measure the distances from moment center to action line of the test force and to the center of mass of the part; we can then solve for the part weight. In this weighing procedure the sling must support the full weight of the part. To obtain relaxation of the subject the segment proximal to the part involved must be completely supported (Fig. 8–28C). It is a good idea to stabilize the pelvis firmly before attempting to weigh the thigh or leg or entire lower limb (Fig. 8–28D).

SECOND METHOD OF WEIGHING BODY PARTS. We return to the board and scale apparatus to compute partial body weights. (The platform scale must be sensitive and accurate.) The principle here is that as a segment shifts its position, the scale reading will change proportionately.

▶ **PROBLEM 8–9**

Suppose we have a 700 N subject lying supine on a board resting on knife-edges that are 180 cm apart (Fig. 8–29).

QUESTION:
What is the weight of one lower limb?

SOLUTION:
Find on a yardstick along the edge of the board a point in line with the estimated center of mass of the limb. Have the subject flex the limb, find a second point in line with the new position of the center of mass, and take the new scale reading. Then,

$$WD = L (S_1 - S_2), \text{ and}$$
$$W = \frac{L (S_1 - S_2)}{D}$$

in which

W = weight of the limb

L = length of board between the supports

S_1 = first scale reading

S_2 = scale reading with the part in the second position

D = horizontal distance through which the center of mass traveled when the limb was moved.

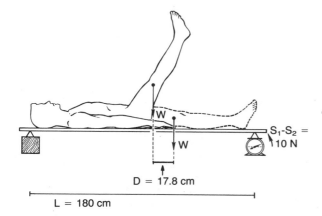

W

W

D = 17.8 cm

L = 180 cm

S_1-S_2 = 10 N

FIGURE 8-29

Method of weighing body segments with board and scale.

(For further explanation of the formula, see Appendix A.)

In this instance the first reading was 263 N and the new scale reading was 253 N (a difference of 10 N), and the center of mass shifted 17.8 cm. Applying these values to the formula,

$$W = \frac{180 \text{ cm } (263 \text{ N} - 253 \text{ N})}{17.8 \text{ cm}}$$

$$W = 101 \text{ N}$$

The second method above may be checked against the first one in finding experimentally the weights of the body segments. Finding the trunk weight is much easier by the second method. It is also of interest to weigh a part with the body in various positions, such as supine, side-lying, and prone, and to compare the values obtained. Values may be compared with the theoretical data of Dempster (1955) and of Clauser and associates (1969) in Appendix A.

POSTURE

According to Basmajian (1967), the balance of the human body over its several joints depends upon a fine neutralization of the forces of gravity by counterforces. In the standing posture, the least use of energy occurs when the vertical line of gravity falls through an inert supporting column of bones. The human body intermittently approaches this ideal situation. In humans the bones are a series of links connected by joints and held in the upright position by

muscles and ligaments. If these are stacked so that the line of gravity passes directly through the center of each joint, the least stress will be placed upon the muscles and ligaments. Steindler (1955) stated that complete passive equilibrium is impossible because the centers of mass of the links and the movement centers between them cannot all be brought to coincide perfectly with a common line of gravity.

Mechanically we can see what happens to the body in the upright posture in the sagittal plane. If the centers of mass of each body segment are lined up one above the other and these, in turn, are in line with the joints between the segments, the force needed to maintain this position is zero (Fig. 8–30A). With the superincumbent line of gravity falling through the supporting joint, the lever arm would be zero and no moment would be set up. There would only be a downward linear force. However, as soon as the center of mass of a segment moves out of line with the supporting joint, a moment is established. The further the segment's line of gravity moves away from the joint, the greater the moment becomes. To remain in equilibrium, a force must be exerted to create a moment equal in magnitude and opposite in direction. Notice the change in segment location in relation to the joints in Figure 8–30B. Muscles must contract actively, or ligaments are placed on stress in order to counteract the malposition of the segments. Remember that to maintain stability the line of gravity of the entire body must remain

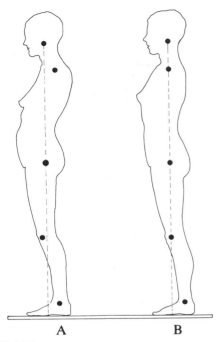

FIGURE 8–30

Alignment of body parts: *A*, Poor posture; joint centers out of alignment, requiring increased muscular activity. *B*, Good alignment; joint centers aligned for minimal muscle activity.

within the supporting base. Therefore, if one segment moves forward, another must move backward to compensate.

An important area that has been explored only recently is calculation of forces on joint surfaces in the body. With increased interest in arthritis, collagen diseases, degeneration of articular cartilage associated with the aging process, and joint replacement, the physician and therapist should be aware of joint pressure "dosages" resulting from various postural positions and types of therapeutic exercises.

Back

In the erect position with the erector spinae and abdominal muscles relaxed (Basmajian, 1967), the lumbosacral joint and trunk (Morris et al.,

1961) carry only the superincumbent weight of the body. However, Strait and associates (1947) demonstrated that tremendous low back strain may be involved in forward trunk flexion. According to their calculations, the compressive force in the fifth lumbar vertebra of an 800 N (180 lb) man with his trunk flexed 60° from vertical, arms hanging freely, is 2000 N (450 lb). If he holds a 220 N (50 lb) weight in his hands, the compression force on the fifth lumbar vertebra increases to nearly 3780 N (850 lb). Nachemson and Elfstrom (1970) substantiated this trend with direct disc pressure measurements. In Figure 8–31, the lumbosacral joint is considered to be a fixed fulcrum; P represents the spinal extensor muscle force necessary to counterbalance W, the weight of the head, arms, and trunk, acting at their combined center of mass; d increases as the trunk is flexed, and hence, the moment of the gravity force increases even though W does not change in magnitude. Thus, P must become very large, resulting in dangerous compression of the lumbar intervertebral discs and increased shearing force between the fifth lumbar vertebra and the sacrum.

Because of the high incidence of back pain in the population, therapists and educators must be aware of the effects of different postures on the low back. Many authors (Davis, 1959; Morris et al., 1962; Troupe, 1965; Nachemson and Elfstrom, 1970; Roozbazar, 1975; Chaffin and Andersson, 1984) have attacked this problem mathematically with electromyography and pressure transducers.

▶ PROBLEM 8–10

Let's take a look at what happens to the joint reaction at the lumbosacral joint in a few common postures of an 890 N man with 445 N of weight above the joint. Figure 8–32A shows the sacrum of a person standing erect with the line of gravity passing through the posterior edge of the lumbosacral joint. The normal sacral angle (the angle the top of the sacrum forms with the horizontal with the subject standing erect) is about 41° (Hellems and Keats, 1971). In this position no erector spinae muscle force is necessary to balance the superincumbent weight. Thus, 445 N of weight is the only force di-

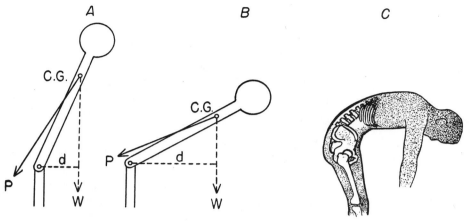

FIGURE 8–31

Comparative moment of gravitational pull on the trunk in two positions of trunk flexion: d' > d.

rected downward on the joint. This weight (W) is resolved into two components: one perpendicular to the surface of the sacrum (C) and one directed parallel to the surface of the sacrum (S) (Fig. 8–32B). C acts as a compressive force on the interposed disc, while S acts as a shearing force, tending to cause the fifth lumbar vertebra to slide forward on the top of the sacrum. Note that C and S are perpendicular to each other, so that a right triangle may be formed with C and S as the sides and W as the hypotenuse. By using the resolution of forces, we may determine the values of both C and S: $C = W \cos \theta$ and $S = W \sin \theta$. With W equaling 445 N and θ equaling 41°, we find that

$$C = 445 \text{ N} \times \cos 41°$$
$$= 445 \text{ N} \times 0.75471$$
$$= 336 \text{ N}$$

and

$$S = 445 \text{ N} \times \sin 41°$$
$$= 445 \text{ N} \times 0.65606$$
$$= 292 \text{ N}$$

Thus, an 890 N individual in the erect positon with a normal sacral angle has a joint compressive force of 336 N and shearing force of 292 N.

What would these forces be if this individual had an increased lordosis with a sacral angle of 60°? We again find the components of the superincumbent weight using 60° for θ.

$$C = 445 \text{ N} \times \cos \theta$$
$$= 445 \text{ N} \times 0.5$$
$$= 222.5 \text{ N}$$

and

$$S = 445 \text{ N} \times \sin \theta$$
$$= 385 \text{ N} \times 0.866$$
$$= 385 \text{ N}$$

If the lumbar spine is flatter than the average (for example, 30°), we find that the compression force is 385 N and the shearing force is 222.5 N. Note that the shearing force increases with the sine of the sacral angle. As the sacral angle increases, more weight must be carried by the articular processes and soft tissues to resist shearing, and less by the sacrum (Fig. 8–33). Ferguson (1934) indicated that an angle greater than 52° placed the lumbosacral joint under severe stress.

▶ **PROBLEM 8–11**

We have calculated what happens to the lumbosacral joint in the erect position. What changes take place when the individual bends forward? As soon as the trunk moves forward, the erector spinae muscles contract to balance the force of gravity. As was noted earlier, the greater the forward flexion, the greater the muscle force becomes. At full flexion, however, no erector spinae muscle action is present,

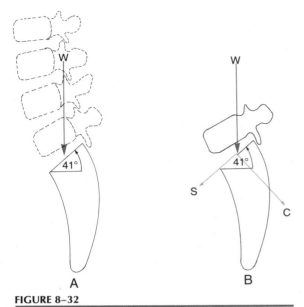

FIGURE 8–32

The position of the normal sacrum in erect standing. *A*, The superincumbent weight passing through the posterior edge of the lumbosacral joint. *B*, The compression (C) and shearing (S) components of the superincumbent weight.

and the ligaments must bear the full load (Mac-Conaill and Basmajian, 1969).

QUESTIONS:

What erector spinae muscle force is needed to support the trunk inclined to a 45° angle? What is the joint reaction force?

SOLUTION:

Assuming that the force arm perpendicular to the combined pull of the erector spinae muscles is 5 cm and the resistance arm perpendicular to the superincumbent weight is 21.25, we draw the free body diagram as shown in Figure 8–34. The X axis is placed along the spine and the center of motion at the lumbosacral joint. The muscle pull is acting at an angle of 8° with the X axis. Using the second condition of equilibrium ($\Sigma M = 0$), we may solve for the muscle force.

The joint reaction force (R) acts at the joint of rotation. Hence, it produces no moment of force. The moment created by the weight, W = 445 N, is counterclockwise and given a positive sign.

$$(-W \times d_W) + (M \times d_M) = 0$$
$$(445 \text{ N} \times 21.25 \text{ cm}) + (M \times 5 \text{ cm}) = 0$$
$$(9456 \text{ N}) + (5 \text{ cm} \times M) = 0$$
$$5 \text{ cm} \times M = -9456 \text{ N}$$
$$M = -1891 \text{ N}$$

Since the sign is negative, the muscle force is acting in a clockwise direction. The erector spinae muscle force to maintain a 45° trunk inclination of a 890 N man is 1891 N.

The first condition of equilibrium ($\Sigma F = 0$) will give us the joint reaction force. For its shearing component, $\Sigma F_y = 0$.

The rotatory Y component (W_y) of the superincumbent weight (W) is found by the equation

$$W_y = W \cos \theta$$

and the X component (W_x) is given by the equation

FIGURE 8–33

Change in the compression (C) and shearing (S) force components with the change in the sacral angle. *A*, At 30° C is greater than S. *B*, At 45° C is equal to S. *C*, at 60° C is less than S.

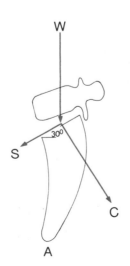

A

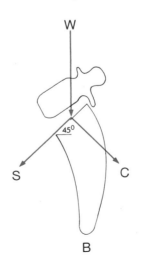

B

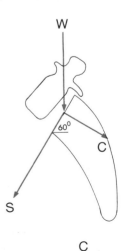

C

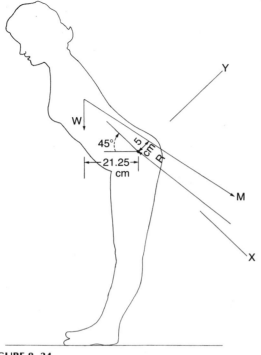

FIGURE 8–34

Forces on the low back when the trunk is inclined 45° from the vertical.

$$W_x = W \sin \theta$$

Since $W = 445$ N and $\theta = 45°$,

$$W_y = 445 \text{ N} \times \cos 45°$$
$$= 445 \text{ N} \times 0.707$$
$$= 314.6 \text{ N}$$

and

$$W_x = 445 \text{ N} \sin 45°$$
$$= 445 \text{ N} \times 0.707$$
$$= 314.6 \text{ N}$$

The components for the muscle force are

$$M_y = M \sin 8°$$
$$= 1891 \text{ N} \times 0.13917$$
$$= 263 \text{ N}$$
$$M_x = M \cos 8°$$
$$= 1891 \text{ N} \times 0.99027$$
$$= 1872 \text{ N}$$

and

$$W_y + M_y + R_y = 0$$

The value of W_y is given a negative sign since it is acting downward with respect to the X axis.

$$(-314.6 \text{ N}) + (263 \text{ N}) + R_y = 0$$
$$R_y = 51.6 \text{ N}$$

The shearing force on the sacrum would be about 51.6 N.

For the compression component

$$\Sigma F_x = 0$$
$$W_x + M_x + R_x = 0$$

Since W_x and M_x act toward the right with respect to the Y axis

$$(314.6 \text{ N}) + (1872 \text{ N}) + (R_x) = 0$$
$$2186.6 \text{ N} + R_x = 0$$
$$R_x = -2186.6 \text{ N}$$

Thus, the joint reaction to the compressive force is 2186.6 N toward the head. The magnitude of the reaction component (R) is found by the Pythagorean theorem.

$$\begin{aligned} R &= \sqrt{R_x{}^2 + R_y{}^2} \\ &= \sqrt{(2186.6)^2 + (51.6)^2} \\ &= \sqrt{4{,}781{,}219.6 + 2662.56} \\ &= \sqrt{4{,}783{,}882.1} \\ &= 2187.2 \text{ N} \end{aligned}$$

Its direction is found by using any one of the trigonometric functions.

$$\begin{aligned} \sin \phi &= \frac{R_y}{R_x} \\ &= \frac{51.6 \text{ N}}{2186.6 \text{ N}} \\ &= 0.0234 \\ \phi &= 1.4° \end{aligned}$$

The resultant acts at a 1.4° angle with the X axis, upward and to the left.

▶ **PROBLEM 8–12**

If a therapist bends the trunk forward in this manner to lift a patient, a mother to lift a child, or a worker to lift a container, the magnitude of forces increases. Let's consider the 890 N individual with the trunk inclined 45° lifting a 250 N load (Fig. 8–35). The load

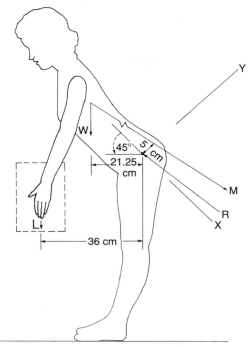

FIGURE 8–35

Forces on the low back when one lifts a 250 N weight while bending the trunk forward.

will have a resistance arm of 36 cm. The first step is to draw the free body diagram, placing the X axis along the trunk and the moment center at the lumbosacral joint. The position is the same as the previous problem. Hence, we need only to add the effects of the load (L). To find the muscle force we use the second condition of equilibrium ($\Sigma M = 0$). The force of the load and the weight both act counterclockwise and are positive.

$$(L \times d_L) + (W \times d_W) + (M \times d_M) = 0$$
$$(250 \text{ N} \times 36 \text{ cm})$$
$$+ (445 \text{ N} \times 21.25 \text{ cm})$$
$$+ (M \times 5 \text{ cm}) = 0$$
$$(9000 \text{ Ncm}) + (9456.25 \text{ Ncm})$$
$$+ (M \times 5 \text{ cm}) = 0$$
$$(18,456.25 \text{ Ncm})$$
$$+ (M \times 5 \text{ cm}) = 0$$
$$M \times 5 \text{ cm} = -18,456.25 \text{ Ncm}$$
$$M = -3691.25 \text{ N}$$

The muscle force to lift the 250 N load compared to lifting no weight has increased considerably in magnitude.

The shearing and compression effects on the lumbosacral joint are found by the first condition of equilibrium ($\Sigma F = 0$). For shearing,

$$\Sigma F_y = 0$$

For the Y components, L and W are acting downward, and we write

$$L_y = L \cos 45°$$
$$= -250 \text{ N} \times 0.707$$
$$= -176.75 \text{ N}$$
$$W_y = W \cos 45°$$
$$= -445 \text{ N} \times 0.707$$
$$= -314.6 \text{ N}$$
$$M_y = M \sin 8°$$
$$= 3691.25 \text{ N} \times 0.13917$$
$$= 513.7 \text{ N}$$

Thus,

$$L_y + W_y + M_y + R_y = 0$$
$$(-176.75 \text{ N}) + (-314.6 \text{ N})$$
$$+ (513.7 \text{ N}) + R_y = 0$$
$$22.35 \text{ N} + R_y = 0$$
$$R_y = -22.35 \text{ N}$$

For compression, $\Sigma F_x = 0$.

The X components, all acting to the right, are:

$$L_x = L \sin 45°$$
$$= 250 \text{ N} \times 0.707$$
$$= 176.75 \text{ N}$$
$$W_x = W \sin 45°$$
$$= 445 \text{ N} \times 0.707$$
$$= 314.6 \text{ N}$$
$$M_x = M \cos 8°$$
$$= 3691.25 \text{ N} \times 0.99027$$
$$= 3655.3 \text{ N}$$

Then

$$L_x + W_x + M_x + R_x = 0$$
$$(176.75 \text{ N}) + (314.6 \text{ N})$$
$$+ 3655.3 \text{ N} + R_x = 0$$
$$4146.65 \text{ N} + R_x = 0$$
$$R_x = -4146.65 \text{ N}$$

Compare these values with those found when no load was being carried in the previous example. To find the magnitude of the total reaction force, we again use the Pythagorean theorem.

$$R = \sqrt{R_x^2 + R_y^2}$$
$$= \sqrt{(4146.65)^2 + (22.35)^2}$$
$$= \sqrt{(17,194,706) + (499.5)}$$
$$= \sqrt{17,195,206}$$
$$= 4146.7 \text{ N}$$

Its direction is found by using a trigonometric function.

$$\tan \theta = \frac{R_y}{R_x}$$
$$= \frac{22.35 \text{ N}}{4146.7}$$
$$= 0.005$$
$$\theta = 0.3°$$

The reaction force of 3164 N is acting almost directly to the left along the X axis.

To maintain a certain amount of simplicity in the preceding problems, the columnar effect of the abdominal cavity was not included. However, Morris and colleagues (1961) calculated this supporting force to take about 30 percent of the compressive force.

The preceding problems illustrate some of the effects of body posture and lifting a load on the lumbar spine. Using these as a guide, the student should be able to determine the muscular force needed to support various trunk positions, and the lumbosacral joint reaction force, including its shearing and compression components.

Stooping by flexing the trunk forward gives gravitational force a fine lever arm with which to put strain on the low back structures, as does reaching by bending at the waist. Making beds is a daily chore that can easily lead to back injury if not done properly. Work involving the use of arms, such as carrying trays, typing, or peeling vegetables, should be done with the elbows close to the sides to minimize strain on supporting muscles.

Hip

The load on the femoral head varies with different body positions and with an added load in the hand. In the erect position, with the body weight balanced on both limbs, the superin-cumbent load acts in a purely vertical direction upon the head of the femur (Backman, 1957). The muscles around the hip are relatively inactive, and do not exert a force across the hip in this position.

▶ PROBLEM 8–13

QUESTION:
Find the joint reaction force on the hip joint of an 890 N man in the erect position with bilateral lower limb support.
SOLUTION:
The free body diagram as shown in Figure 8–36 is drawn passing the X axis through the joint axis of the femurs and perpendicular to the pull of gravity. The superincumbent weight (W) passes an equal distance of 15 cm between two hip joints. The value *l*

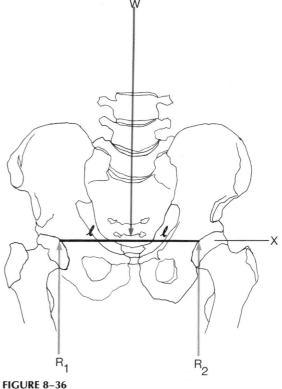

FIGURE 8–36

Static forces acting on the femoral heads in bilateral standing.

represents the distance from W to each hip joint. The value of W is determined by using the data from Appendix A. One lower limb weighs 15.6 percent of the total body weight. Both lower limbs would be 31.2 percent of the weight. Thus, W equals the total weight minus the weight of the lower limbs, or 68.8 percent of 890 N.

$$W = 0.688 \times 890 \text{ N}$$
$$= 612.3 \text{ N}$$

By using the second condition of equilibrium ($\Sigma M = 0$) and placing the moment center at the left hip joint (R_1), we may solve for the reaction force at the right hip joint (R_2). Note that this is a parallel force system.

$$(W \times l) + (R_2 \times 2l) = 0$$
$$(612.3 \text{ N} \times 15 \text{ cm}) +$$
$$(R_2 \times 30 \text{ cm}) = 0$$
$$9184.5 \text{ Ncm} + (R_2 \times 30 \text{ cm}) = 0$$
$$R_2 \times 30 \text{ cm} = 9184.5 \text{ Ncm}$$
$$R_2 = \frac{9184.5 \text{ Ncm}}{30 \text{ cm}}$$
$$= -306.15 \text{ N}$$

The reaction force on the right hip is 306.15 N acting clockwise.

To solve for R_1, we may repeat the above procedure using R_2 as the center of moments, or we may use the first condition of equilibrium, $\Sigma F = 0$, as follows:

$$\Sigma F_x = 0$$

All forces are vertical, so no forces are acting in the X direction.

$$\Sigma F_y = 0$$
$$W + R_1 + R_2 = 0$$

Since W is acting downward it is given a negative sign and R_2 is given a positive sign since it is acting upward.

$$-612.3 \text{ N} + R_1 + 306.15 \text{ N} = 0$$
$$-306.15 \text{ N} + R_1 = 0$$
$$R_1 = 306.15 \text{ N}$$

The joint reaction on the left hip is 306.15 N upward. Thus, each hip is carrying a load of 306.15 N. Note that the 306.15 N carried by the hip exerts a moment about the apex of the angle of inclination of the hip (Fig. 8–37). The greater the distance of this line of force to the angle apex, the greater the bending moment will be on the neck of the femur. This is increased in coxa varum or if the neck is surgically lengthened.

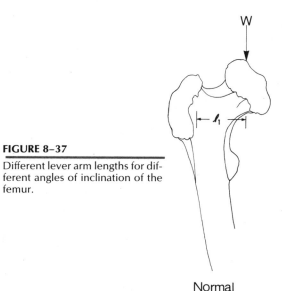
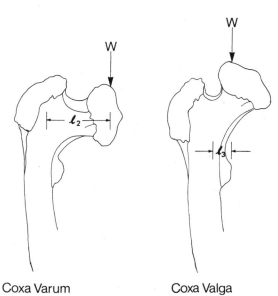

FIGURE 8–37

Different lever arm lengths for different angles of inclination of the femur.

Normal

Coxa Varum

$l_2 > l_1 > l_3$

Coxa Valga

$$R_c = \mathbf{R} \cos 50°$$
$$= 68.8 \text{ lb.} \times 0.64279$$
$$= 44.224 \text{ lb.}$$

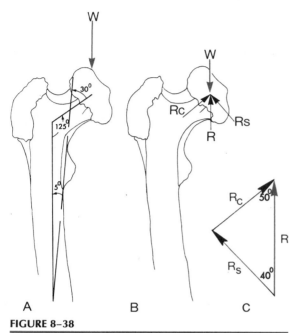

A **B** **C**

FIGURE 8–38

Forces acting on the femoral head in the normal adult: *A,* Normal angle of inclination. *B,* Forces on the femoral head. *C,* Graphic solution for the compression (R_c) and shearing (R_s) force components.

The normal angle of inclination of the femur is 125°, while the anatomical axis of the femur forms about a 5° angle with the vertical (Steindler, 1955). From these angles (Fig. 8–38A), we determine that the neck of the femur forms a 50° angle with the vertical. The compression, R_c, and shearing, R_s, components of the 306.15 N reaction force, R, of the hip as shown in Figure 8–38B can be found graphically (Fig. 8–38C) or by using trigonometric functions.

We may write

$$R_c = \mathbf{R} \cos 50°$$
$$= 306.15 \text{ N} \times 0.64279$$
$$= 196.8 \text{ N}$$
$$R_s = \mathbf{R} \sin 50°$$
$$= 306.15 \text{ N} \times 0.76604$$
$$= 234.5 \text{ N}$$

The compression reaction force is 196.8 N and the shearing reaction force is 234.5 N. In children, the shearing reaction may act along the epiphysis. An obese child with coxa varum will suffer a greater tendency toward slipping of the epiphysis.

When a subject stands on one limb, a different situation exists from that determined for standing on both limbs. To maintain balance, the line of gravity must fall over the supporting foot.

Normally, when one foot is lifted from the floor, the center of mass of the supported body weight resting on the stance hip lies medial to the head of the femur (W) (Fig. 8–39). This mass includes the head, arms, trunk, and opposite limb, which tend by their weight to force the pelvis to drop downward on the unsupported side. This drop is normally controlled by the hip abductor muscles on the stance side, which contract to stabilize the pelvis in the frontal plane. These two forces are opposed by the upward reacting force of the femoral head. Note in Figure 8–39B the similarity to the two boys on the teeter-totter in Figure 5–11. Remember that as one boy moved inward toward the fulcrum, the effectiveness of his body weight as a turning force decreased. Likewise, if a patient has weak hip abductor muscles, he leans his trunk toward the affected hip and walks with a so-called "abductor" gait (Fig. 8–40). Leaning the trunk sideways toward the affected hip moves the center of mass of the supported weight closer to the fulcrum at the femoral head, reducing the moment of the body weight about the stance hip, and consequently reducing the need for the hip abductor muscles to stabilize the pelvis. In the case of flail abductor muscles, the patient may shift the trunk so far to the side that the line of gravity falls lateral to the hip joint, stabilizing the joint in the frontal plane.

At first it may seem strange that the femoral head in walking must push upward with a force greater than the weight of the segments it supports. Figure 8–39B shows that this weight (W), acting at a considerable distance medial to the hip axis, must be counterbalanced by a downward force (M), acting on the lateral side of the joint with a relatively smaller lever arm.

Inman (1947) has estimated the forces W and M and their respective lever arms to be such that the static compression force on the head of the femur is 2.4 to 2.6 times the body weight in unilateral stance. Balancing the superincumbent weight over the head of the femur reduces this force to body weight alone (minus the mass of the supporting limb). For this reason persons with painful hip joints, as well as those with paralyzed hip abductor muscles, lean sharply

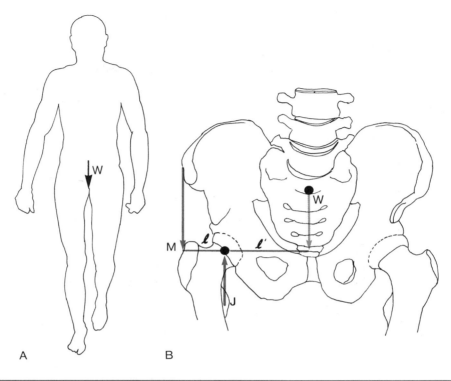

FIGURE 8–39

Static forces acting about the femoral head in the frontal plane in unilateral stance.

toward the affected side as they walk. This is often referred to as a "gluteus medius" limp, a term that ignores other important hip abductor muscles which also act to stabilize the pelvis in the frontal plane (gluteus minimus, tensor fasciae latae, upper fibers of gluteus maximus inserting into the iliotibial band).

Blount (1956) has pointed out the effectiveness of the lever arm of a cane carried in the contralateral hand in supporting the pelvis in the frontal plane (Fig. 8–41). The distance from the hip axis to the cane is vastly greater than the distance from the hip to the action line of the adjacent abductor muscles that normally prevent the pelvis from dropping downward on the unsupported side. Blount estimates that leaning with a force of 190 N on a cane held in the opposite hand will reduce the superincumbent force on the femoral head from 1930 N to 330 N in an "average" person. (Note that Blount's and Inman's figures compare favorably; if the superincumbent force on the femoral head is 2.5 times body weight, and 2.5X = 1930 N, then X, or body weight, would be 760 N.)

A cane held in the hand on the same side as the involved hip has a much less favorable lever arm, so that considerably more force on the hand would be required to relieve hip force to the same degree as if the cane were held on the opposite side.

In the following problems, the force applied to the femoral head under various conditions is considered. This is particularly important to know in the designing of hip prostheses. We have found that when the body weight is supported equally on both feet, half the suprafemoral weight falls on each hip joint. In walking, it is necessary for the entire supported mass to be distributed alternately on each hip joint. We will calculate hip joint compression forces in unilateral weight-bearing in the case of an 890 N man with no load, with a suitcase held in one hand, and with a suitcase held in each hand. (A body weight of 890 N has been selected for convenience. Results can be applied to persons of any weight by multiplying the results obtained here by W/890. Thus, for a 623 N person, results could be multiplied by $\frac{623}{890}$ or 0.7.)

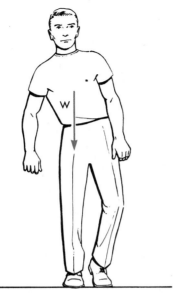

FIGURE 8–40

Method of walking when hip abductors are weak. The patient shifts his weight (W) over the supporting femoral head, *toward* the affected side.

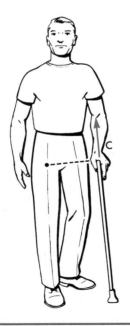

FIGURE 8–41

Correction of abductor gait with cane held in the opposite hand. The supporting force (C) is applied through a favorable lever arm.

▶ **PROBLEM 8–14**

An 890 N man is standing on one foot.
QUESTION:
Find the force on the head of the supporting femur.
SOLUTION:

We will make use of values based on Inman's study (1944), which determined that the direction of the resultant of the hip abductor muscle group acting at the greater trochanter made an angle of 71° with the horizontal. The other dimensions required have been obtained from measurements of x-ray films (Fig. 8–42).

From the consideration of a free body diagram of the entire body we determine the reaction of the ground on the foot to be 890 N. Adding the weight of the entire limb through its center of gravity, the X

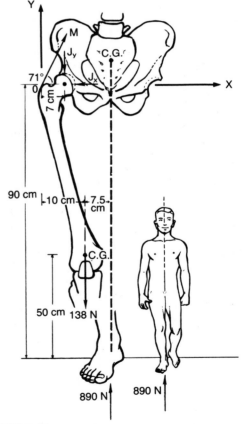

FIGURE 8–42

Determination of the compression force on the supporting femoral head in unilateral weight-bearing.

and Y components of the reaction at the hip joint, and the muscle force at the greater trochanter completes the free body diagram of the limb. In this problem we have a general force system, and the equations of equilibrium are

$$\Sigma F_x = 0$$
$$\Sigma F_3 = 0$$
$$\Sigma M = 0$$

Substituting in these equations, and taking the moment center (0) at the point where the muscle force is applied to the greater trochanter, we have

$$\Sigma F_x = 0$$
$$M \cos 71° + J_x = 0$$

Since the weight of the leg is downward, it is given a negative sign.

$$\Sigma F_y = 0$$
$$890 \text{ N} + M \sin 71° + (-138 \text{ N}) + J_y = 0$$

The ground reaction producing a counterclockwise moment is given a positive sign.

$$\Sigma M = 0$$
$$7 \text{ cm} \times J_y + (-138 \text{ N} \times 10 \text{ cm})$$
$$+ (890 \text{ N} \times 17.5 \text{ cm}) = 0$$
$$7 \text{ cm} \times J_y - (1380 \text{ Ncm})$$
$$+ (15575 \text{ Ncm}) = 0$$
$$7 \text{ cm} \times J_y + (14195 \text{ Ncm}) = 0$$
$$7 \text{ cm} \times J_y = -14195 \text{ Ncm}$$
$$J_y = -2027.8 \text{ N}$$

(clockwise, but downward)

Since J_y acts downward, in the first condition of equilibrium it is given a negative sign

From $\Sigma F_y = 0$
$$890 \text{ N} + M \sin 71° + (-138 \text{ N})$$
$$+ (-2027.8 \text{ N}) = 0$$
$$M = \frac{1275.8 \text{ N}}{\sin 71°} = \frac{1275.8 \text{ N}}{0.945}$$
$$M = 1349.3 \text{ N}$$

From $\Sigma F_x = 0$
$$M \cos 71° + J_x = 0$$
$$J_x = -M \cos 71°$$
$$= -1349.3 \text{ N} \times 0.326$$
$$J_x = -439.9 \text{ N} \text{ (to the left)}$$

$$J = \sqrt{J_x^2 + J_y^2} =$$
$$\sqrt{(439.9)^2 + (2027.8)^2}$$
$$J = 2075 \text{ N} \text{ (downward and to the left)}$$

$$\tan \Theta = \frac{J_y}{J_x} = \frac{2075 \text{ N}}{439.9 \text{ N}} = 4.72$$
$$\Theta_x = 78°$$

The femoral head supports a force of 2075 N (466.5 lb) acting at an angle of 78° from the horizontal.

The student may solve this problem by taking the hip joint as the center of moments instead of the point of muscle attachment on the trochanter. The results will be the same.

▶ **PROBLEM 8–15**

Another approach is by using the superincumbent weight as one moment around the hip joint being balanced by the muscle pull (Fig. 8–43). This approach appears to be more realistic, but the solution may be more involved. Using the measurements of the previous solution, we must locate the center of mass for the weight supported by the hip joint. We know the total body weight, its location with respect to the origin of the coordinate system, the weight of the lower limb, its location, and the superincumbent weight. Referring to the formula to locate the position of the resultant force we may write

$$X = \frac{\Sigma M}{\Sigma W}$$

where M = moments and W = segmental weights. Thus, the location of the line of gravity for the total body weight equals the weight of the supporting limb times its location from the origin of the coordinate system, plus the superincumbent weight times the location of its line of gravity (d) all divided by the sum of all the body parts. Note that the origin of the coordinate system in Figure 8–43 has been moved to the hip joint axis, 7 cm from that shown in Figure 8–42.

The distance of the line of gravity for the entire body is 10.75 cm from the hip joint. The following equation will then determine the value of d.

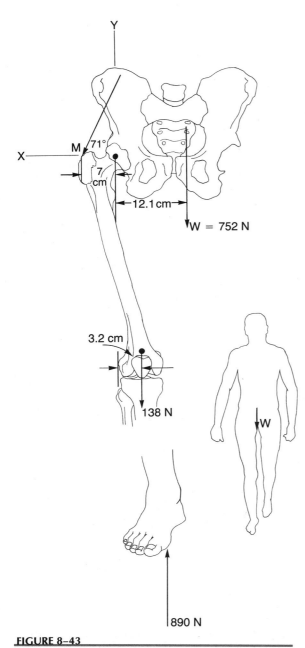

FIGURE 8–43

Forces acting about the hip joint in unilateral weight-bearing (alternate approach). Note the differences from Figure 8–42.

$$10.75 \text{ cm} = \frac{(138 \text{ N} \times 3.2 \text{ cm}) + (752 \text{ N} \times d)}{890 \text{ N}}$$

$$-(890 \text{ N} \times 10.75 \text{ cm}) + (138 \text{ N} \times 3.2 \text{ cm})$$
$$= 752 \text{ N} \times d$$

$$(-9567.5 \text{ Ncm}) + (441.6 \text{ Ncm}) = 752 \text{ N} \times d$$

$$\frac{(-9125 \text{ Ncm})}{752 \text{ N}} = d$$

$$d = 12.1 \text{ cm}$$

Then

$$-(752 \text{ N} \times 12.1 \text{ cm}) + (M \sin 71° \times 7 \text{ cm}) = 0$$
$$(-9099.2 \text{ Ncm})$$
$$+ (M \times 0.945 \times 7 \text{ cm}) = 0$$

$$M = \frac{9099.2 \text{ Ncm}}{6.6 \text{ cm}}$$

$$M = 1378.7 \text{ N}$$

The body weight supported by the hip is balanced by a counterclockwise muscle force of 1378.7 N, as also determined by the previous method.

You may extend this problem by having the man carry a 250 N weight in the left hand, or one in each hand.

The answers to these problems indicate that when a load is carried on one side of the body the force on the opposite supporting hip during walking is much greater than when the load is distributed on both sides. This is true even when the bilateral load is twice as great as the unilateral load. The demand on the hip abductor muscles varies in the same manner and is greatest when a load is carried on the contralateral side. Carrying loads in the midline of the body, as in a knapsack or on the head or shoulders, is effective in reducing required musculoskeletal force.

Knee

In the upright position the line of gravity falls approximately through the knee joint axis. With the knee in full extension, the moment arm of the line of gravity is zero (Fig. 8–44A). Hence, no muscular force is needed to maintain equilibrium at this point. The joint compression force is equal to half the superincumbent weight, or approximately 390 N for an 890 N person. As the knee is flexed, however, the line of gravity falls behind the joint axis (Fig. 8–44B).

In the next few problems we will consider the

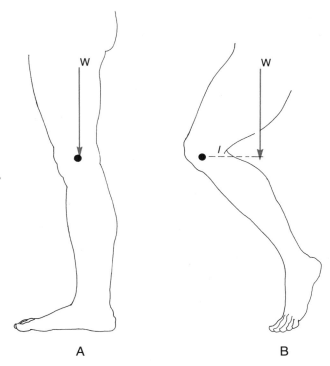

FIGURE 8–44

Moment arm of the superincumbent weight about the knee joint: *A*, Normal stance. *B*, Flexed knee stance.

A

B

knee extensor muscle force necessary to maintain the static knee position.

▶ **PROBLEM 8–16**

QUESTIONS:
For most of the stance phase, flexion is less than 20° (Morrison, 1970). What is the quadriceps muscle force needed to maintain knee flexion of 20° while standing on one limb? What are the tibiofemoral and patellofemoral joint reaction forces?

SOLUTION:
The free body diagram is drawn with the X axis perpendicular to the line of gravity and through the moment center at the joint axis (Fig. 8–45). The thigh and leg each form 80° angles with the horizontal. The superincumbent weight (W) is found to be 836 N, using the data from Appendix A. Suppose the perpendicular distance from the joint center to the line of gravity is 5 cm and the perpendicular distance from the joint center to the muscle line of pull is 5 cm. The angle of muscle pull is 60° with the horizontal. These values were determined from cinematographic and cinefluoroscopic analysis. We have

a force system established in which we can use the second condition of equilibrium ($\Sigma M = 0$) to solve for the muscle force. We may write

$$Wd_W + Md_M = 0$$
$$(836 \text{ N} \times 5 \text{ cm}) + (M \times 5 \text{ cm}) = 0$$
$$(4180 \text{ Ncm}) + (M \times 5 \text{ cm}) = 0$$
$$M \times 5 \text{ cm} = -4180 \text{ Ncm}$$
$$M = \frac{-4180 \text{ Ncm}}{5 \text{ cm}}$$
$$= -836 \text{ N}$$

The calculated quadriceps muscle force for maintaining this position in one-legged stance is 836 N (188 lb) acting clockwise. We must remember that in walking, other forces act as well. These calculated results, however, agree favorably with those of a more precise determination found by Reilly and Martens (1972). The highest value they calculated for the quadriceps muscle force during level walking was 804 N (180.7 lb).

For a graphic approach, the magnitude, direction, and line of application of the ground reaction force (G), the direction and line of application of the pa-

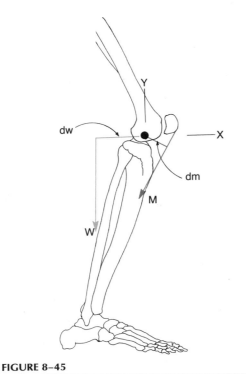

FIGURE 8–45

Moments of force about the knee joint in unilateral stance.

tellar tendon force, and the point of application of the joint reaction force must be known. Suppose the action line of the muscle force (M) intersects the action line of the reaction on the foot, as shown in the free body diagram (Fig. 8–46A). The action line of the reaction force must also pass through this point of intersection since three forces acting on a body in equilibrium are concurrent. The reaction force is drawn through this point and its point of application at the joint surface (Fig. 8–46B). A triangle of forces may be constructed by using vectors G, M, and R, as shown in Figure 8–46C. We first draw the ground reaction force vector (G). To the head of this vector, we draw the line of action for the muscle force (M). By drawing the line of action of the reaction force (R) through the tail of G, we close the triangle. This defines the magnitudes for both the muscle force and reaction force. The triangle may be scaled in terms of body weight, and the magnitude of the muscle force and joint reaction force may be determined. (The weight of the supporting leg was ignored in this solution.) The joint reaction force is 1.9 times the body weight, or 1690 N in a direction downward and to the left. Its angle with the horizontal (X axis) is measured as 74°.

The joint compression force (R_c) is found perpendicular to the tibial plateau and parallel to the long axis of the tibia, while the shearing force (R_s) is parallel to the tibial plateau (Fig. 8–46D). With the knee in 20° flexion, the thigh and leg each form an angle of 10° with the vertical (Y axis). Thus, the tibial plateau would form an angle of about 10° with the X axis. We may find the compression and shearing components by resolving the joint reaction into these two components. The angle formed by the reaction force with the long axis of the tibia is 16° minus 10°, or 6°. Thus,

$$R_c = R \cos \Theta, \text{ where } \Theta = 6°$$
$$= 1690 \text{ N} \times \cos 6°$$
$$= 1690 \text{ N} \times 0.99452$$
$$= 1680.7 \text{ N}$$

and

$$R_s = R \sin \Theta$$
$$= 1690 \text{ N} \times \sin 6°$$
$$= 1690 \text{ N} \times 0.10453$$
$$= 176.6 \text{ N}$$

The compression component is 1680.7 N and the shearing component is 176.6 N. Determine what happens to these forces as one climbs stairs with the knee angle at 90° (Shinno, 1971) and the tibia at a 60° angle with the horizontal.

The shearing reaction force in the normal knee is often supported by the cruciate ligaments. With injured or degenerated cruciates, the shearing load is shifted to the articulating surfaces and surrounding connective tissue. In prosthetic design that requires cruciate removal, the articulating surfaces must carry this load. Loads in this direction will tend to loosen the prosthesis. Hence, a secure method of fixation of the prosthesis is necessary (Shaw and Murray, 1973).

As a tendon changes direction upon passing over bone and joints, a force is applied to the underlying surface. In the case of the quadriceps, the patella has a force component directed as a compressive force toward the patellofemoral joint. The patellofemoral joint reaction force is the equilibrant to the force of the quadriceps muscle. We may consider the patella as a movable pulley, and the tendinous attachments to the patella as the two supporting strands (Fig. 8–47). Thus, M_1 and M_2 are equal in

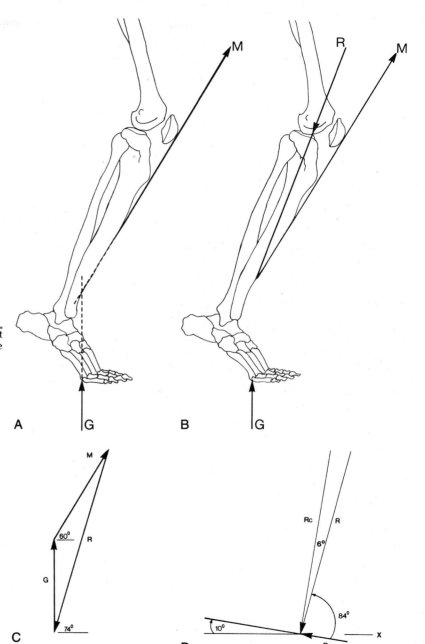

Static forces acting on the knee joint in unilateral stance (concurrent force system).

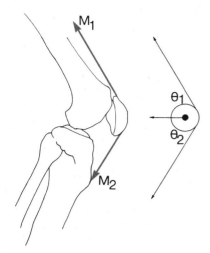

FIGURE 8–47

Tendinous attachments to the patella.

magnitude. By knowing the angle of approach of these tendinous attachments (θ_1 and θ_2) and the muscle force (M), we can calculate the patellofemoral joint reaction force.

The patellar tendon force was calculated as 836 N in a previous part of this problem. The action lines of the two tendinous attachments were traced from a cinefluoroscopic film, as shown in the free body diagram (Fig. 8–48). The X axis is horizontal. The first

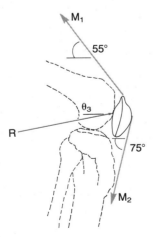

FIGURE 8–48

Static forces acting on the patellofemoral joint.

condition of equilibrium ($\Sigma F = 0$) is best used to solve this problem. The three forces are concurrent; hence, no moment center is necessary.

$$\Sigma F_x = 0$$
$$= M_1 \cos \theta_1 + M_2 \cos \theta_2 + R_x$$
$$= M_1 \cos 55° + M_2 \cos 75° + R_x$$

Since the X components of M_1 and M_2 are to the left, they are given negative signs.

$$= (-836 \text{ N} \times 0.57358)$$
$$+ (-836 \text{ N} \times 0.25882) + R_x$$
$$= (-479.5 \text{ N}) + (-216.4 \text{ N}) + R_x$$
$$R_x = 695.9 \text{ N}$$

Since M_1 with a 55° angle is upward in the Y direction, it will have a positive sign, while M_2 with the 75° angle is downward and will have a negative sign.

$$\Sigma F_y = 0$$
$$= M_1 \sin \theta_1 + M_2 \sin \theta_2 + R_y$$
$$= M_1 \sin 55° + M_2 \sin 75° + R_y$$
$$= (-836 \text{ N} \times 0.81915)$$
$$+ (-836 \text{ N} \times 0.96593) + R_y$$
$$= (684.8 \text{ N}) + (-807.5 \text{ N}) + R_y$$
$$R_y = 122.7 \text{ N}$$

The value of R is determined by the Pythagorean theorem.

$$R = \sqrt{R_x^2 + R_y^2}$$
$$= \sqrt{(695.9)^2 + (122.7)^2}$$
$$= \sqrt{484276.8 + 15055.3}$$
$$= \sqrt{499332.1}$$
$$= 706.6 \text{ N}$$

The angle formed by R with the horizontal is found by one of the trigonometric functions.

$$\tan \theta_3 = \frac{R_y}{R_x}$$
$$= \frac{122.7 \text{ N}}{695.9 \text{ N}}$$
$$= 0.1763$$
$$\theta = 10°$$

Thus, the patellofemoral joint reaction force is to the right and upward, with a magnitude of 706.6 N (158.9 lb). Note that the joint reaction force in this example bisects the angle formed by the two tendinous attachments. Can you see how a vector diagram giving the resultant forces of the tendons would also give us this information? By use of cine-fluoroscopic or x-ray films, patellofemoral reaction force at other angles of knee flexion can be determined.

Shoulder

During erect standing with the arms hanging at the side, the supraspinatus is active in order to resist downward dislocation of the humerus (Basmajian, 1967). Because of the slope of the glenoid fossa, the horizontal pull of the supraspinatus and the tightening of the superior part of the joint capsule prevent downward subluxation without the aid of the deltoid.

▶ PROBLEM 8–17

Let's see what force is needed to maintain the position of the upper limb. Suppose the slope of the glenoid fossa of a 890 N man is 80° with the horizontal.

QUESTIONS:
What is the force of the supraspinatus and joint capsule necessary to prevent subluxation of the humeral head? What is the joint reaction force?

SOLUTION:
A free body diagram is drawn (Fig. 8–49A) with the X axis perpendicular to the force of gravity. The weight of the upper limb from the data in Appendix A is 43.6 N.

By using the concurrent force system and vector analysis, we may determine the magnitude of muscle force and the direction and magnitude of the glenohumeral joint reaction force. We must know the magnitude, direction and line of action of the pull of gravity, the direction and the line of action of the supraspinatus muscle, and the point of glenohumeral joint contact. By drawing a line from the point of joint contact (R) to the point of intersection of the line of gravity (W) and muscle force (M) we have the action line of the joint reaction force (R) (Fig. 8–49B).

To determine its magnitude, we first draw the force vector for the weight of the limb (W). To the

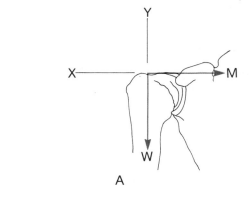

FIGURE 8–49

Static forces on the glenohumeral joint during erect standing.

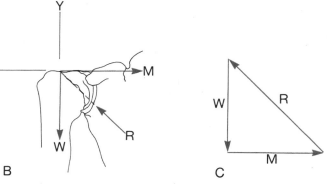

head of this vector, we add the line of action for the muscle force. By drawing the line of action of the joint reaction force, we enclose the triangle (Fig. 8–49C). The sense or direction of the joint reaction force is toward the tail of the limb weight vector. The magnitudes of the muscle and joint reaction force can now be scaled from the drawing.

The muscle force becomes 1.15 times the limb weight, or 50.1 N, and the reaction force is 1.52 times the limb weight, or 66.3 N, acting at a 40° angle with the horizontal.

Can you determine the shearing and compression reaction forces? What would happen if 110 N were added to the hand?

▶ **PROBLEM 8–18**

For another illustration of analysis of shoulder muscle and joint forces, let us look at the deltoid muscle supporting the arm in a horizontal position. We will assume the limb weighs 40 N and the deltoid alone represents the elevator muscle force. The angle of its action line with the long axis of the humerus is 15° (Fig. 8–50).

QUESTION:
What is the magnitude of the tension (M) in the deltoid muscle and the reacting force (R) necessary for equilibrium?

SOLUTION:
Force R, drawn from the point of concurrence of W and M to the glenohumeral joint, forms an angle of 6° with the horizontal. Then,

$$\Sigma F_x = (R \cos 6°) + (-M \cos 15°) = 0$$

$$\Sigma F_y = (M \sin 15°) + (-B \sin 6°) + (-W) = 0$$

(from $\Sigma F_x = 0$)

$$R = \frac{M \cos 15°}{\cos 6°}$$

(from $\Sigma F_y = 0$)

$$M \sin 15° - \frac{M \cos 15°}{\cos 6°} \sin 6° - W = 0$$

$$M \left(\sin 15° - \frac{\cos 15°}{\cos 6°} \sin 6° \right) = W$$

$$M \left(0.259 - \frac{0.966}{0.995} 0.105 \right) = 40 \text{ N}$$

$$M = \frac{40 \text{ N}}{\left(0.259 - \frac{0.966}{0.995} 0.105 \right)} = \frac{40 \text{ N}}{0.157}$$

$$M = 255 \text{ N}$$

Solving for R:

$$R = \frac{255 \text{ N} \times 0.966}{0.995}$$

$$R = 247 \text{ N}$$

As before, we may find the graphic solution relatively simple to support the algebraic findings. The student may find the compression and shearing components as the glenoid fossa forms an 80° angle with the horizontal.

It has been suggested that force R is the resultant of two components: active contraction of the infra-

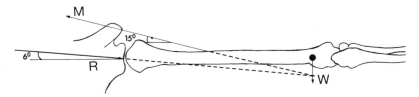

FIGURE 8–50

Forces involved in supporting the upper limb in a horizontal position.

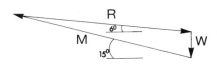

spinous muscles (teres minor, infraspinatus, subscapularis) and pressure and friction at the joint (Inman et al., 1944). It has been reported in the literature that the requirements for the downward pull of the cuff muscles, which "snub" the humeral head in the glenoid fossa, are greatest when the arm is elevated to 60°, and at this point the downward muscle force on the humeral head must be 9.6 times the weight of the extremity (Inman et al., 1944).

In analyzing gravitational forces in body movement, remember that the downward pull on the body is opposed by an equal upward push of the supporting surface, whether one is in a recumbent, sitting, or standing position. Frictional forces must be sufficient to stabilize the body. Adequate floor reactions are necessary, particularly for walking or running to be successful. The many joints of the body that support segments above them sustain compression forces. Both the superincumbent part and the supporting member on which it rests must resist equal and opposite forces applied to their respective articular surfaces. The shape of the joints and the arrangement of reinforcing ligaments and tendons are such that the upright posture is maintained with an economy of neuromuscular effort.

Another important aspect of gravitational force acting on the body is the effect that counterpressure of supporting surfaces has on neuromuscular mechanisms controlling posture and directing movement. For example, pressure on the soles of the feet activates the positive support reaction. Both exteroceptive and proprioceptive stimuli from skin, muscles, and joint structures contribute to the barrage of afferent impulses by which the central nervous system is able to maintain the delicate synergies of balance and movement. The vast importance of these mechanical and neurologic interactions is coming to be more fully appreciated in analysis of motor learning and body movements.

STRENGTH TESTING AND TRAINING

Procedures for strengthening muscles and the evaluation of muscle strength are based upon certain biomechanical factors. These factors should always be considered and, if possible, recorded for the exercise of a testing situation. A checklist could be devised to ensure that these important biomechanical factors are taken into account (Fig. 8–51).

When you are evaluating muscle strength, you must realize that you are not directly measuring the actual strength of the muscle or muscle group. You are only indirectly evaluating this muscle characteristic. What you are really doing is recording the effective force or torque being produced at the point of application of the resistance. You may determine that your client could (1) hold a 20 kg mass (44 lb) in the hand for 5 seconds, (2) resist 350 N (70 lb) before giving way, (3) produce 135 Nm (100 ft-lb) of torque at 30° per second, or (4) lower a 40 kg mass (88 lb) control. These values do not indicate what the actual force produced by the muscle group is.

The indirect evaluation of the force produced by a muscle or muscle group is influenced by several factors, which may be grouped into three major categories: body position, type of contraction, and other factors.

Body Position

The position of the body or body part can affect the amount of recorded muscle strength or exercise load by (1) the effective moment caused by gravity, (2) the effective length of the resistance arm, (3) the length of the effort arm, (4) the angle of muscle pull, (5) the length of the muscle, and (6) the stabilization of the body part.

The pull of gravity upon the body part used as the lever may either produce a resistive moment or assistive moment (Fig. 8–52), depending upon the muscle group involved. In Figure 8–52A and B, the weight of the forearm is providing a resisting moment to the elbow flexor muscles. In some instances this resisting moment may be the maximum load the muscle group may be able to support. In Figure 8–52C to E, however, the weight of the forearm is assisting the elbow extensors to extend the elbow. In Figure 8–52F and G, the weight of the limb is neither resisting nor assisting the muscle around the elbow.

If the body part moves through a range of motion, the effective component of weight or the effective resistance arm length will change. With the body part horizontal, the component of weight or the effective lever arm is maximal.

1. **WEIGHT OF THE TESTED PART:** _____
2. **RELATIONSHIP OF THE TESTED PART WITH THE HORIZONTAL:** _____
3. **ANGLE OF THE JOINT IF ONE-JOINT MUSCLES:** _____
4. **ANGLE OF JOINTS IF TWO-JOINT MUSCLES:** _____
5. **ANGLE OF RESISTANCE LINE OF FORCE WITH THE LIMB:** _____
6. **DISTANCE OF RESISTANCE POINT OF APPLICATION FROM JOINT:** _____
7. **STABILIZATION OF ADJACENT BODY PARTS:** _____
8. **TYPE OF CONTRACTION:** _____
9. **SPEED OF CONTRACTION:** _____
10. **DURATION OF CONTRACTION:** _____
11. **NUMBER OF WARM-UP AND LEARNING TRIALS:** _____
12. **TYPE OF MOTIVATION:** _____
13. **REST BETWEEN TRIALS:** _____
14. **AGE OF SUBJECT:** _____
15. **GENDER OF SUBJECT:** _____
16. **CONTROL OF CO-CONTRACTION:** _____
17. **JOINT LIMITATIONS:**   Yes   No

    a. Friction   _____   _____

    b. Bony mechanical block   _____   _____

    c. Soft tissue tightness   _____   _____

    d. Pain   _____   _____

FIGURE 8–51

Checklist of factors that may affect recorded strength values.

Thus, a greater amount of muscle force will be needed with the body part in this position. If the center of mass of the body part lies directly above or below the joint axis, the resisting lever arm would be zero; therefore, the resisting moment would be zero. As the body part moves from vertical to horizontal, the effective resisting moment of the body part gradually increases (see Fig. 8–31).

The point of application of the muscle is set anatomically. Unless surgically changed, the distance from the joint axis and the muscle attachment remains constant. Only the instantaneous joint axis changes will minimally affect this characteristic.

Although the anatomic effort lever arm length does not change, the effective length of the effort lever arm changes as the angle of the muscle (line of application) changes. As a joint changes from one position to another, often the muscles crossing the joint change their angle of pull. This angle of applied force may or may not be efficient. The most effective muscle angle of pull is when it is perpendicular to the lever,

while the least effective is when it is almost parallel to the lever (see Fig. 4–29).

As discussed in Chapter 3, the length of a contracting muscle makes a difference in the force it develops. The force of a muscle contraction is greater when it is in a lengthened position. A shortened muscle produces less effective force than the stretched muscle. The reasons may be related to the cross-bridge relationship or the series and parallel elastic components of the musculotendinous unit. A two-joint muscle may be in a position to enhance or to reduce the effectiveness of the muscle contraction.

When exercising or evaluating a specific muscle or muscle group, the segments adjacent to the lever system involved should be firmly secured to allow for a stable base from which the muscle can pull. Without a stable base, the muscles may not be able to produce their maximum effort. On the other hand, extraneous movement away from the involved lever system may provide unwanted effects. Substitution by other muscles and body parts may assist in applying force to the resistance.

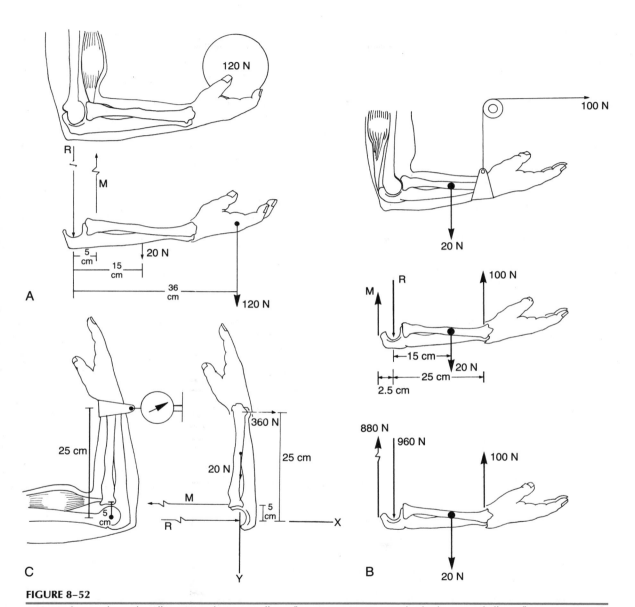

FIGURE 8–52

A, Static forces about the elbow joint during an elbow flexor exercise. *B*, Free body diagram of elbow flexor exercise. *C*, Static forces about the elbow joint during an elbow extensor exercise. *D*, Free body diagram of elbow extensor exercise. *E*, Muscle and joint forces for extensor exercise. *F*, Isometric contraction of the elbow flexors at 90° of elbow flexion. *G*, Free body diagram of isometric contraction.

Type of Muscle Contraction

The type of muscle contraction affects the resistance that can be controlled, held, or overcome. Eccentric or lengthening contractions allow for a greater resistance value to be controlled than isometric or concentric contractions. In turn, isometric contractions can hold a greater resistance than one can move with a concentric contraction. The reasons for this hierarchy of resistance values may relate to the elastic components of the muscle and to the contractile process.

Speed of Contraction

At higher movement speeds, the resistance recorded usually is lower. Although the muscle tension appears to be decreasing, it may not be less but similar or even greater. It is important to realize that the muscles must overcome inertia of the body part and the exercise device. An isokinetic muscle contraction is a special type of concentric contraction in which the angular velocity of the movement is held constant.

Other Factors

Several other factors can also influence the resistive values. These include the physiologic factors of muscle fatigue, movement coordination, and muscle co-contraction. Muscle viscosity and joint friction may reduce the ability to move a resistance. The individual's age, gender, motivation, and motor learning may also be important factors.

For evaluating muscle strength or providing an appropriate exercise program, you must account for all these factors. Otherwise, the results of your evaluation may not be valid or your exercise program may not be as effective as possible.

EXERCISE

Many different types of resisting force may be used when providing an exercise program.

These include, but are not limited to, the body part itself, manual resistance, free weights, pulley weights, and various other exercise machines.

Body Weight

Body weight may be used to offer resistance to exercise of various muscles. In this case, we must remember that gravity is acting on the body part only in a downward direction, and the mass of the part acts as though it were concentrated at its center of mass. The effectiveness of this weight for rotation can be changed by shifting its position in relation to the fulcrum. The further the line of gravity falling through the center of mass is from the axis of motion, the greater the moment arm will be; hence, the greater the moment will be. Thus, a greater muscle force will be needed to maintain equilibrium.

The action line of the gravitational force on a part can be moved nearer to or farther from the axis of the joint by changing the position of the part in space. For example, an exercise involving leg-raising can be performed with the knee straight or with it flexed (Fig. 8–53). The moment of the gravitational force is greater with the knee straight, not because the force (segment weight) has changed, but because the distance from the action line of the gravitational force to the hip axis has changed. This principle is used constantly in therapeutic exercises to vary the exercise load.

Another good example is the sit-up exercise, which is most easily performed with the arms at the sides (Fig. 8–54). Steps of increasing difficulty consist of moving the arms to various positions higher on the trunk (arms across the abdomen, over the chest, on the opposite shoulders). Most difficult is sitting up with the arms extended overhead, since in this case the center of mass of the trunk and arms is farthest from the axis at the hip joints.

The classic abdominal muscle strengthening exercise of flexing one knee toward the chest, straightening it toward the ceiling, and lowering the extended limb to the table demonstrates several stages of difficulty (Fig. 8–55). The action line of the gravitational force of the limb

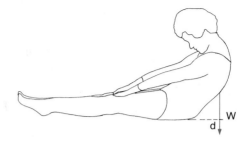

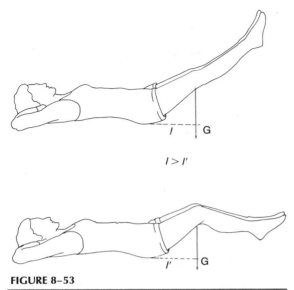

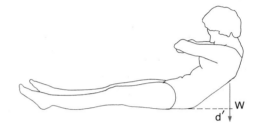

FIGURE 8-53

The movement of gravitational force (G) on the lower limb, exerting a clockwise turning effect about the hip, is decreased by flexing the knees: $l > l'$.

approaches the hip axis as the part is raised, passes through the joint during knee extension, and then moves away from the axis as the limb is lowered ($d'' > d' > d$). This final phase requires increasing effort of the abdominal muscles to stabilize the pelvis and prevent lordosis caused by tension of the iliopsoas and the other hip flexors pulling on their proximal attachments. Many patients must first lower the limb with the knee flexed and progress to lowering with full knee extension later on.

Various arm positions are used in exercises to strengthen back and shoulder muscles. Lifting the flexed arms requires less effort than lifting them extended. Of course, there are other factors to consider in evaluating the difficulty of specific exercises, such as the length of the antagonist muscles and the relative size of the various body segments of the patient.

Manual Resistance

Manual resistance exercises usually follow the same rule, with the therapist's hand a maximum

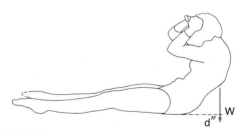

FIGURE 8-54

The lever arm of gravitational force (W) on the trunk is increased by moving the arms upward (lever arm $d'' > d' > d$).

distance from the axis of joint rotation—at the end of the segment. In this situation the patient must work hard to overcome relatively slight externally applied force. Manual assistance to movement may be given in a similar fashion, with a long lever arm.

In some instances the therapist purposely shortens the lever arm of the applied force, usu-

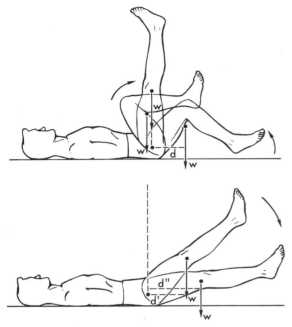

FIGURE 8-55

Variation in exercise load (moment of lower limb, W × d) with different phases of a posture exercise. W = gravitational pull acting at the center of mass of the limb; d = distance of action line to the hip axis: d″ > d′ > d (see text).

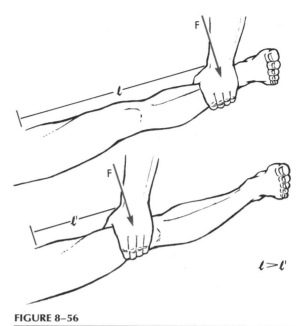

FIGURE 8-56

Two possible manual muscle test positions for hip adductors, with long and short lever arms (l and l') for manual force (F).

ally in order to obtain better control of the force. For example, in the manual muscle test for hip adduction, the examiner's hand might be placed at the ankle to obtain a maximum test force moment (Fig.8-56). However, manual force is usually given above the knee because it is easier to direct and grade the force opposing the adductors, and the therapist can more satisfactorily control the patient's position on the table and stabilize the pelvis with his other hand. By pressing at the knee he or she is required to push twice as hard as would be done at the ankle to obtain the same test force effectiveness (moment).

Loads applied by manual and mechanical means are used in physical therapy procedures, such as manual muscle testing, assistive and resistive exercises, and stretching and mobilization of joint structures. In manually applied forces all characteristics defining the force can be controlled—magnitude, action line, direc-

tion, and point of application on the body. In most situations, the lever arm of the force applied is made as long as possible; that is, force is applied to the distal end of the segment to obtain maximum effort.

In muscle testing, manual resistance is usually applied at the far end of the segment involved, just proximal to the next distal joint. This gives the applied force a much better lever arm than that of the muscles being tested (Fig. 8-57).

When manual force is applied in muscle stretching procedures, the hand may grasp the segment close to the joint involved (Fig. 8-58). Here again, an effective lever arm for the applied force is sacrificed in order to obtain better control of the movement. Also, the moment afforded the external force by a maximum lever arm might be sufficient to injure the joint structures; a shorter lever arm is safer.

Free Weights

As we have noted, therapists and physical educators use a variety of exercise devices, as well

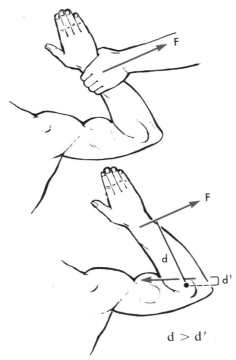

FIGURE 8-57

Manual force is applied far from the joint in muscle testing in order to obtain maximal rotational effect: F × d = moment. The lever arm of an elbow flexor muscle such as the brachialis is shown as d′, which illustrates the relative disadvantage in turning effect of the muscles being tested.

as body weight, to serve as resistance in exercise programs. Let's take a look at the way some of these devices offer resistance to the quadriceps acting across the knee joint.

▶ PROBLEM 8-19

Gravity is the most common force used to offer resistance. An exercise load of 100 N is placed on the patient's foot with its center of mass 60 cm from the knee axis. The patient extends his or her knee through 90° to exercise the quadriceps muscles. Assume that the weight of the patient's foot and leg is 30 N and their combined center of mass is located 20 cm distal to the knee axis. For simplicity, let's assume that the angle of the patellar tendon inserts at a constant 25° angle 10 cm from the knee axis.

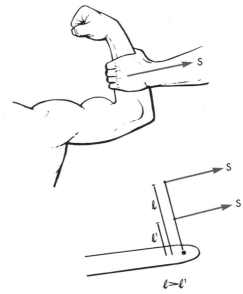

FIGURE 8-58

A short lever arm in applying manual pressure (S) sacrifices force for control. The moment of the force would be greater if it were applied at the wrist. (S × *l* > S × *l*′).

QUESTIONS:

What is the magnitude of force necessary for the quadriceps muscles to maintain the exercise load at 90°, 60°, 30°, and 0° of flexion? What is the joint reaction force that must be absorbed by the tissues around the joint? Solutions are presented for the 90° and 60° positions.

SOLUTION:

90° OF FLEXION. The free body diagram is shown in Figure 8–59A with the X axis passing through the knee joint center and perpendicular to the pull of gravity.

Substituting in the equations for the first condition of equilibrium ($\Sigma F = 0$), we find that

$$\Sigma F_x = 0$$

Since gravity pulls straight down, the resistance offers no X component (rotatory) in this position. The quadriceps will not contract, since their angle of pull will offer a rotatory component, and motion will take place.

$$\Sigma F_y = 0$$

Since the values of 30 N and 100 N are acting downward, they are given negative signs. Thus,

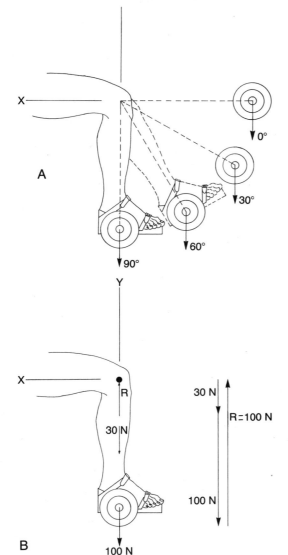

A

B

$$(-30 \text{ N}) + (-100 \text{ N}) + R = 0$$
$$(-130 \text{ N}) + R = 0$$
$$R = 130 \text{ N}$$

FIGURE 8–59

A, Static forces about the knee joint at four different positions while one uses a boot. *B to E,* Free body diagrams for limb at the four different positions shown in *A.*

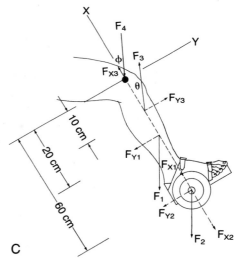

C

The reaction force supporting the foot, leg, and weights is 130 N (26 lb) in the upward direction. Since the quadriceps are not active, this tension stress must be borne by the passive elements across the knee joint. As far as the second condition of equilibrium is concerned in this position, the line of force application of the load passes through the knee joint axis. Hence, no moment is set up, and no muscle force would be necessary.

60° OF FLEXION. The free body diagram is shown in Figure 8–59B. We set the X axis along the length of the leg and the Y axis perpendicular to this. The next step is to find the X and Y components of the resisting loads. The resisting forces acting in the Y direction tend to cause rotation of the limb in the

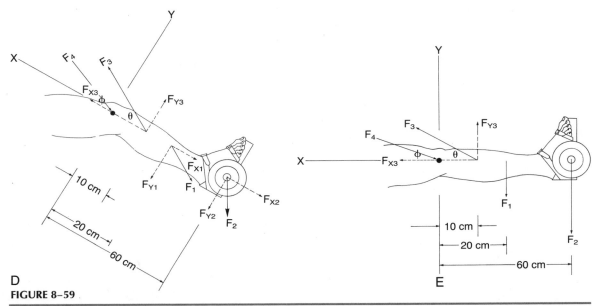

D

FIGURE 8–59

Continued

clockwise direction and to pull along the leg away from the knee joint (distraction). The rotatory component of the weight of the foot and leg (F_{y1}) may be found by the formula $F_{y1} = F_1 \cos \theta$, where $\theta = 60°$.

Thus,

$$F_{y1} = 30 \text{ N} \times \cos 60°$$
$$= 30 \text{ N} \times 0.5$$
$$= 15 \text{ N}$$

The rotatory force component for the foot and leg is 15 N (3 lb).

The distracting component along the length of the leg (F_{x1}) is found by the formula $F_{x1} = F_1 \sin \theta$, where $\theta = 60°$.

$$F_{x1} = 30 \text{ N} \times \sin 60°$$
$$= 30 \text{ N} \times 0.866$$
$$= 26 \text{ N}$$

Note: To keep the same point of application, we may use the $\cos \theta$ where $\theta = 30°$.

Similarly, for the weight on the foot for the rotatory component:

$$F_{y2} = F_2 \cos \theta, \text{ where } \theta = 60°$$
$$= 100 \text{ N} \cos 60°$$
$$= 100 \text{ N} \times 0.5$$
$$= 50 \text{ N}$$

and for the distracting component:

$$F_{x2} = F_2 \sin \theta, \text{ where } \theta = 60°$$
$$= 100 \text{ N} \sin 60°$$
$$= 100 \text{ N} \times 0.866$$
$$= 86.6 \text{ N}$$

The direction and magnitude of the reaction force and the magnitude of the quadriceps muscle force are unknown. However, the reaction force passes through the joint axis and will cause no rotation about the joint. Thus, for ease of calculation we will consider the second condition of equilibrium ($\Sigma M = 0$) as the next step. Since the quadriceps is pulling at a 25° angle, its components will be $F_{y3} = F_3 \sin \theta$ and $F_{x3} = F_3 \cos \theta$, where $\theta = 25°$. Note the use of sine and cosine as compared with the resisting loads. If you have trouble with this concept, review Chapter 4. In this case, since the force components of the loads are acting clockwise, we will give them negative signs.

$$\Sigma M = 0$$
$$\Sigma M_{cw} + \Sigma M_{ccw} = 0$$
$$(-15 \text{ N} \times 20.0 \text{ cm})$$
$$+ (-50 \text{ N} \times 60.0 \text{ cm})$$
$$+ (F_{y3} \times 10 \text{ cm}) = 0$$

$$(-300 \text{ Ncm}) + (-3000 \text{ Ncm})$$
$$+ (F_{y3} \times 10 \text{ cm}) = 0$$
$$-3300 \text{ Ncm} + (F_{y3} \times 10 \text{ cm}) = 0$$
$$F_{y3} \times 10 \text{ cm} = 3300 \text{ Ncm}$$
$$F_{y3} = 330 \text{ N}$$

Thus, the rotatory force produced by the quadriceps muscle is 330 N in the counterclockwise direction. To solve for the total quadriceps muscle force, we write:

$$F_{y3} = F_3 \sin \theta; \text{ where } \theta = 25°$$

$$F_3 = \frac{F_{y3}}{\sin 25°}$$
$$= \frac{330 \text{ N}}{\sin 25°}$$
$$= \frac{330 \text{ N}}{0.42262}$$
$$= 780.8 \text{ N}$$

The force along the X axis may be found two ways. Note that the angle θ position is in the second quadrant. Hence, the cosine and tangent are negative.

(1) $\quad \dfrac{F_{y3}}{F_{x3}} = \tan 25°$

$$F_{x3} = \frac{F_{y3}}{\tan 25°}$$
$$= \frac{330 \text{ N}}{-0.46631}$$
$$= -707.7 \text{ N}$$

(2) $\quad F_{x3} = F_3 \cos 25°$
$$= 780.8 \text{ N} \times -0.90631$$
$$= 707.6 \text{ N}$$

Thus, the force component acting toward the joint is 707.7 N. We now have the muscle components and load components acting in the X and Y directions. Using the first condition of equilibrium ($\Sigma F = 0$), we can determine the joint reaction force.

$$\Sigma F = 0; \Sigma F_x = 0; \Sigma F_y = 0$$
$$F_{y1} + F_{y2} + F_{y3} + F_{y4} = 0$$
$$(-15 \text{ N}) + (-50 \text{ N}) + (330 \text{ N}) + F_{y4} = 0$$
$$(-65 \text{ N}) + (330 \text{ N}) + F_{y4} = 0$$
$$265 \text{ N} + F_{y4} = 0$$
$$F_{y4} = -265 \text{ N}$$

and

$$F_{x1} + F_{x2} + F_{x3} + F_{x4} = 0$$
$$(26 \text{ N}) + (86.6 \text{ N}) + (-707.7 \text{ N}) + F_{x4} = 0$$
$$(112.6 \text{ N}) + (-707.7 \text{ N}) + F_{x4} = 0$$
$$F_{x4} = 595.1 \text{ N}$$

Using the Pythagorean theorem:

$$F_4 = \sqrt{(F_{y4})^2 + (F_{x4})^2}$$
$$= \sqrt{(265 \text{ N})^2 + (595.1)^2}$$
$$= 651.4 \text{ N}$$

The joint reaction force has a magnitude of 651.4 N. Its direction is found using one of the trigonometric functions:

$$\tan \phi = \frac{F_{y4}}{F_{x4}}$$
$$= \frac{-265 \text{ N}}{595.1 \text{ N}}$$
$$= -0.445303 \text{ in the second quadrant}$$
$$\phi = 24°$$

The joint reaction acts downward (note sign of F_{y4}) at a 24° angle with the axis.

Notice that as the amount of flexion in this exercise position decreases, the magnitude of muscle tone and tibiofemoral reaction force increases.

Pulley Weights

▶ PROBLEM 8–20

Let's analyze the resistance exercise using the application of gravity on weights transmitted to the leg by way of a pulley system. The pulley rope is attached at the patient's heel.

QUESTIONS:
What is the magnitude of force necessary for the quadriceps muscle to maintain the exercise load at 90° and at 0° of flexion? What is the joint reaction force that must be absorbed by the tissues around the joint?

SOLUTION:

AT **90°** OF FLEXION. The free body diagram is shown in Figure 8–60A with the X axis passing through the knee joint perpendicular to the pull of gravity. We will use the same body parameters as those in the boot exercise problem. The 100 N weight is transmitted to the patient's heel, forming a 90° angle with the leg. This problem has the same approach as the boot exercise problem using the general system of forces. The second condition of equilibrium ($\Sigma M = 0$) will help us solve for the quadriceps muscle force (M). We may write

$$\Sigma M_{cw} + \Sigma M_{ccw} = 0$$

In the position of 90° of knee flexion, the weight of the foot and leg pulls in the vertical direction through the center of the joint. Hence, it will not produce a moment around the joint center. The resistance offered by the pulley weight is acting clockwise and is given a negative sign. Thus,

$$\Sigma M = (-100 \text{ N} \times 60 \text{ cm})$$
$$+ (M_x \times 10 \text{ cm}) = 0$$
$$-6000 \text{ Ncm} + (M_x \times 10 \text{ cm}) = 0$$
$$M_x \times 10 \text{ cm} = 6000 \text{ Ncm}$$
$$M_x = 600 \text{ N}$$

The rotatory component of the muscle force is 600 N in the counterclockwise direction. The total muscle force (M) can now be determined.

$$M_x = M \sin \theta, \text{ where } \theta = 25°$$
$$M = \frac{M_x}{\sin 25°}$$
$$= \frac{600 \text{ N}}{0.42262}$$
$$= 1419.7 \text{ N}$$

The muscle component acting along the Y axis is

$$M_y = M \cos \theta$$
$$= 1419.7 \text{ N} \times \cos 25°$$
$$= 1419.7 \text{ N} \times 0.90631$$
$$= 1286.7 \text{ N}$$

The muscle force upward toward the joint is 1286.7 N, while the 30 N weight of the foot and leg pulls downward. The pulley weight has no component acting in the Y direction. To determine the joint reaction force, we use the first condition of equilibrium, $\Sigma F = 0$.

$$\Sigma F_y = 0$$
$$(-30 \text{ N}) + (1286.7 \text{ N}) + R_y = 0$$
$$1256.7 \text{ N} + R_y = 0$$
$$R_y = -1256.7 \text{ N}$$

Since the pulley weight acts toward the left, it is given a negative sign. The muscle force acting to the right is positive.

$$\Sigma F_x = 0$$
$$(-100 \text{ N}) + (600 \text{ N}) + R_x = 0$$
$$500 \text{ N} + R_x = 0$$
$$R_x = -500 \text{ N}$$

Using the Pythagorean theorem:

$$R = \sqrt{R_x{}^2 + R_y{}^2}$$
$$= \sqrt{(-500)^2 + (-1256.7)^2}$$
$$= \sqrt{1829294.9}$$
$$= 1352.5 \text{ N}$$

The direction of the joint reaction force is found using one of the trigonometric functions.

$$\tan \phi = \frac{R_y}{R_x}$$
$$= \frac{-1256.7}{-500}$$
$$= 2.5134$$
$$\phi = 68.5°$$

The magnitude of the joint reaction force is 1352.5 N (304 lb) acting downward and to the left, forming an angle of 68.5° with the X axis.

AT 0° FLEXION OR FULL EXTENSION. The free body diagram is shown in Figure 8–60D with the X axis at the knee joint center and along the leg that is perpendicular to the pull of gravity.

When the knee is in full extension, the pulley rope forms an angle of 19° with the leg. We again use the second condition of equilibrium, $\Sigma M = 0$, to solve for the quadriceps muscle force. To find the effective rotary components of the load, we must use trigonometric functions. For the weight of the foot and leg,

$$W_y = W \sin \theta_1, \text{ where } \theta = 90°$$
$$= 30 \text{ N} \times \sin 90°$$
$$= 30 \text{ N} \times 1.0$$
$$= 30 \text{ N}$$

For the 100 N load,

$$L_y = L \sin \theta_2, \text{ where } \theta_2 = 19°$$
$$= 100 \text{ N} \times \sin 19°$$
$$= 100 \text{ N} \times 0.32557$$
$$= 32.6 \text{ N}$$
$$\Sigma M_{cw} + \Sigma M_{ccw} = 0$$

The pulley and limb loads act clockwise and are given negative signs.

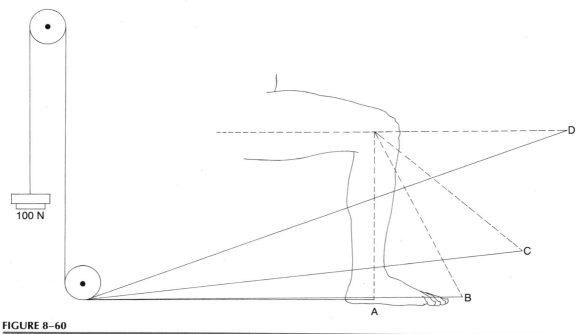

FIGURE 8–60

Static forces about the knees while one uses a pulley system.

$$(W_y \times 20 \text{ cm}) + (L_y \times 60 \text{ cm})$$
$$+ (M_y \times 10 \text{ cm}) = 0$$
$$(-30 \text{ N} \times 20 \text{ cm}) + (-32.6 \text{ N} \times 60 \text{ cm})$$
$$+ (M_y \times 10 \text{ cm}) = 0$$
$$(-600 \text{ Ncm}) + (-1956 \text{ Ncm})$$
$$+ (M_y \times 10 \text{ cm}) = 0$$
$$(-2556 \text{ Ncm}) + (M_y \times 10 \text{ cm}) = 0$$
$$M_y = 255.6 \text{ N}$$
$$M_y = M \sin \Theta, \text{ where } \Theta = 25°$$
$$M = \frac{M_y}{\sin 25°}$$
$$M = \frac{255.6 \text{ N}}{0.42262}$$
$$= 604.8 \text{ N}$$

The quadriceps muscle group is pulling with a force of 604.8 N (136 lb) in the counterclockwise direction.

To determine the joint reaction force, we apply the first condition of equilibrium ($\Sigma F = 0$) using the X and Y components of all the forces. The weight of the foot and leg has no force component (W) acting horizontally in the X direction. Its Y component (W_y) was determined earlier as 30 N.

The X component of the pulley weight is

$$L_x = L \cos \Theta_2, \text{ where } \Theta_2 = 19°$$
$$= 100 \text{ N} \times \cos 19°$$
$$= 100 \text{ N} \times 0.94552$$
$$= 94.55 \text{ N}$$

Its Y component (L_y) found earlier, is 32.6 N (7.3 lb). The X component for the muscle force is

$$M_x = M \cos \Theta, \text{ where } \Theta = 25°$$
$$= 604.8 \times \cos 25°$$
$$= 604.8 \times 0.90631$$
$$= 548.1 \text{ N}$$

For the sum of forces in the X direction, the muscle force and pulley force acting to the left are given negative signs.

$$\Sigma F_x = W_x + L_x + M_x + R_x = 0$$
$$0 + (-94.55 \text{ N}) + (-548.1 \text{ N}) + R_x = 0$$
$$(-642.65 \text{ N}) + R_x = 0$$
$$R_x = 642.65 \text{ N}$$

For the sum of force in the Y direction, the weight of the foot and ankle and the pulley force acting downward are given negative signs. The muscle force acts upward and is positive.

$$\Sigma F_y = W_y + L_y + M_y + R_y = 0$$

$$(-30\ N) + (-32.6\ N) + (255.6\ N) + R_y = 0$$

$$193\ N + R_y = 0$$

$$R_y = -193\ N$$

The total joint reaction force is found by using the Pythagorean theorem:

$$R = \sqrt{R_x^2 + R_y^2}$$

$$= \sqrt{(642.65)^2 + (-193)^2}$$

$$= \sqrt{450248}$$

$$= 671\ N$$

The direction of the joint reaction force is found using one of the trigonometric functions.

$$\tan \phi = \frac{R_y}{R_x}$$

$$= \frac{-193\ N}{642.65}$$

$$= -0.300319 \text{ in the second quadrant}$$

$$\phi = 17°$$

Thus, the joint reaction force of 671 N (150.8 lb) acts downward and to the right at a 17° angle with the X axis.

A comparison of the muscle force and joint reaction force for the boot and pulley exercise devices are presented in Table 8–3. The student may fill in the missing values.

TABLE 8–3. COMPARISON OF BOOT AND PULLEY EXERCISE DEVICES ON THE MUSCLE FORCE (M) AND JOINT REACTION FORCE (R) AT FIVE DIFFERENT POSITIONS

Knee Angle	Boot		Pulley	
	M	R	M	R
90°	0	26.0 t	283.94	270.50 c
60°	156.17	130.29 c	?	?
45°	?	?	?	?
30°	?	?	?	?
0°	?	?	120.84	134.20 c

t = tension.
c = compression.

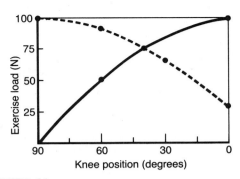

FIGURE 8–61

Graph showing quadriceps exercise resistance pattern applied by free weight (solid line) and pulley system (dashed line) through the range of knee extension.

The pattern of exercise force supplied by pulley system is quite different from that of a weight hanging on the foot. The contrast in these resistance patterns may be seen in the curves plotted in Figure 8–61. The maximum load is applied at opposite ends of the range of movement in these two exercise methods.

It would appear that the boot method is appropriate if the physical therapist wishes to apply a highly variable load that is maximal when the knee is fully extended. The pulley method provides an exercise load that offers less variation of the exercise resistance, and the maximal resistance is applied when the knee is at a 90° angle.

The muscle force and compression force in the knee joint increase rapidly with knee bending. In the relaxed standing position, no activity is necessary in the quadriceps muscle since the line of the supported body weight falls slightly anterior to the axis of rotation at the knee. In this position, the force compressing the femoral and tibial surfaces and the shearing of the femur on the tibia is due to the supratibial body weight and to tension in the posterior knee structures that stabilize the joint (prevent hyperextension). As the knees flex as in squatting or knee bending, the moment caused by the superincumbent weight rapidly increases. This necessitates an increased muscular force to maintain equilibrium, which in turn produces a greater joint reaction force. The ligaments of the knee joint must bear the increased shearing load, while the menisci and joint surfaces carry the increased compression load.

Some exercise devices have been designed to provide a more constant resistance to the muscles

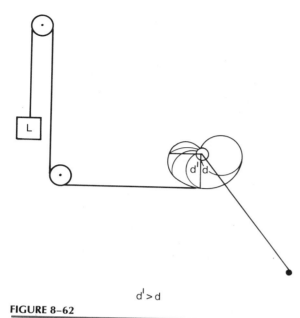

$$d^I > d$$

FIGURE 8–62

Exercise pulley system with cam of variable radius.

throughout the range of motion. A chain pulley system using cams with varying radii (Fig. 8–62) can adjust the resisting moment as movement progresses. Note that as the cam rotates around its axis, the effective radius at which the chain attaches changes. A long radius (resistance lever arm) would provide a greater resisting moment than a short radius. Adjustment in the radius could be made to negate the effect of the weight of the body part. Such a cam could be designed so that a nearly constant resistance could be maintained during the entire exercise movement. The exercise load in Figure 8–62 would be a straight horizontal line. This type of device can offer resistance for concentric, isometric, and eccentric contractions. However, in general use only the concentric muscle contraction would be loaded maximally.

Friction

Other exercise devices have friction as the resisting force. The friction may offer a constant resisting moment or may provide a variable resistance depending upon the speed of the movement. This resisting moment throughout the motion would be a factor added to the resisting moment provided by the weight of the body part. Their combined resisting moments would give the total resisting moment to the muscle groups being exercised. Note that such a device would offer resistance in both directions of movement (e.g., flexion and extension), so no eccentric contraction would occur in this type of device. The antagonist muscle groups may be exercised at the same resistance level.

Isokinetic

Some popular exercise devices set the exercise movement at a constant speed. Resistance is offered from the device when the moving limb reaches the set speed of the device. At that point the faster the client attempts to move the limb, the greater the resistance will be. This type of device does not provide resistance for eccentric contractions but will exercise antagonist muscle groups at the resistance the specific muscle group can overcome. Remember that accelerations and decelerations must occur to reach the set speed. In some devices, adjustments may be made to compensate for the resistance related to the weight of the body part.

Selection

Each exercise device has its advantages and disadvantages. With knowledge of biomechanical principles and an understanding of the mechanisms of the exercise method, you may more readily determine these advantages and disadvantages. To select an exercise mode, you must understand the purpose of the exercise. From this beginning you need to determine where in the range of motion you want the greatest resistance, what type of contraction is wanted, and what speed should be used. If you understand the resisting moments and the exercise effects being provided, you can better select the exercise procedure that will best serve your client.

Selected Application

One purpose of exercise is to strengthen the knee extensors sufficiently to go up and down stairs or step up on a curb. How much quadriceps muscle force is needed for an individual to climb a step? You must first analyze the activity. What is the body position during performance of this activity? Where is the center of mass of the body's superincumbent body parts? What is the angle of the knee? How fast is the motion?

If the motion is slow, the inertia properties presented in Chapter 7 may have little effect on the force needed. You may set up a free body diagram similar to Figure 8–45. The problem would be solved similarly to Problem 8–16. In the situation of stair-climbing the resistance lever arm (dW) would be increased because of the increased angle of the knee (perhaps 80°). If dW is doubled, the muscle force (M) required to lift the body would be doubled. Depending upon the height of the steps and the individual's leg length, the resistance of the lever arm may be tripled. This would triple the muscle force. If the force needed in a stance with 20° of knee flexion is 836 N, then the tripled amount would be 2508 N (564 lb). What amount of resistance would be needed to obtain this muscle force with the boot exercise? With the pulley exercise? If you calculate for this value using the knee flexion value of 80° (see Problems 8–19 and 8–20), the weight on the boot would need to be 1010 N (227 lb). The weight on the pulley system would be 178 N (40 lb).

Is the muscle-strengthening angle specific? If so, and if your purpose is to exercise the knee extensor muscles for climbing stairs, which exercise method should be used?

Upper Limb Exercise

Dumbbells make use of the force of gravity to offer resistance to a muscle group. These are often used for strengthening the muscles of the upper limbs.

▶ **PROBLEM 8–21**

Suppose a paraplegic patient is strengthening his shoulder muscles by means of dumbbell exercises. The arm is abducted to horizontal and the weight of 50 N is held in the hand 66 cm from the shoulder joint axis. Assume that the deltoid is carrying the full load with its line of action forming an angle of 15° with the humerus, and with its point of attachment to the humerus 12.5 cm from the shoulder axis. The weight of the upper limb is 35 N, centered 30 cm from the shoulder axis.

QUESTIONS:
What force must the deltoid muscle exert to keep the limb and weight abducted? What is the joint reaction force?

SOLUTION:
Draw the free body diagram as shown in Figure 8–63, with the X axis drawn along the upper limb, perpendicular to the pull of gravity and through the shoulder joint axis. We may use the second condition of equilibrium, $\Sigma M = 0$, to solve for the rotatory component of muscle force. This sets up a general force system, in which the muscle rotatory component is $M \sin 15°$.

$$\Sigma M_{cw} + \Sigma M_{ccw} = 0$$
$$(-35 \text{ N} \times 30 \text{ cm}) + (-50 \text{ N} \times 66 \text{ cm})$$
$$+ (M \sin 15° \times 12.5 \text{ cm} = 0$$
$$(-1050 \text{ Ncm}) + (-3300 \text{ Ncm})$$
$$+ (M \times 0.25882 \times 12.5 \text{ cm}) = 0$$
$$(-4350 \text{ Ncm}) + (M \times 3.24 \text{ cm}) = 0$$
$$M \times 3.24 \text{ cm} = 4350 \text{ Ncm}$$
$$M = \frac{4350 \text{ Ncm}}{3.24 \text{ cm}} = 1342.6 \text{ N}$$

The muscle force is acting counterclockwise with 1342.6 N (302 lb) of force. The joint reaction force is determined by the first condition of equilibrium, $\Sigma F = 0$. With the limb horizontal, its weight and that of the dumbbell provide no force components in the X direction. Their combined effect acts downward in the Y direction and in our equation, ΣF_y, they are given negative signs. The X component of the deltoid muscle force (M_x) is $M \cos 15°$. The muscle force acts to the left along the X axis and is given a negative value. Its Y component acting upward is positive. Thus,

$$\Sigma F_x = W_x + L_x + M_x + R_x = 0$$
$$0 + 0 + M \cos 15° + R_x = 0$$
$$(-1342.6 \text{ N} \times 0.96593) + R_x = 0$$
$$R_x = 1296.8 \text{ N}$$

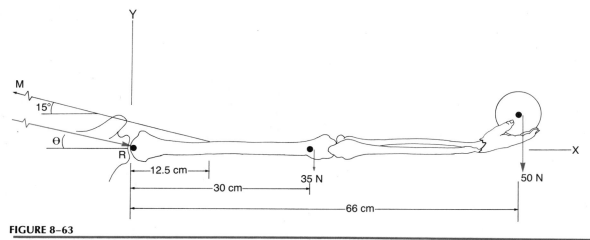

FIGURE 8–63

Static forces about the shoulder joint involved during abduction of the loaded upper limb.

$$F_y = W_y + L_y + M_y + R_y = 0$$
$$= (-35\ N) + (-50\ N)$$
$$+ M \sin 15° + R_y = 0$$
$$= (-85\ N) + (1342.6\ N \times 0.25882)$$
$$+ R_y = 0$$
$$= (-85\ N) + (347.5\ N) + R_y = 0$$
$$262.5\ N + R_y = 0$$
$$R_y = -262.5\ N$$

To find the resulting magnitude of joint reaction force we use the Pythagorean theorem:

$$R = \sqrt{(1296.8)^2 + (262.5)^2}$$
$$= \sqrt{1681690.2 + 68906.2}$$
$$= \sqrt{1750596.5}$$
$$= 1323.1\ N$$

The direction of the reaction force is found by using one of the trigonometric functions.

$$\tan \Theta = \frac{R_y}{R_x}$$
$$= \frac{-262.5\ N}{1296.8\ N}$$
$$= -0.20242 \text{ in the second quadrant}$$
$$\Theta = 11.5 \text{ degrees}$$

Thus, for this exercise the shoulder joint reaction force has a magnitude of 1323.1 N (297.5 lb) acting

to the right and downward at a 11.5° angle with the horizontal (X axis).

Let us consider an exercise device for muscles controlling the forearm.

▶ PROBLEM 8–22

Suppose a patient with his elbow at 90° is pushing his forearm downward against a sling to oppose a 100 N exercise weight attached to the wrist 25 cm from the elbow joint center. The forearm and hand weigh 20 N with their combined center of mass located 15 cm from the elbow joint. The triceps muscle attaches 2.5 cm from the joint at a 90° angle to the ulna.

QUESTIONS:

What is the contraction force of the triceps muscle (M) and the joint reaction force (R) on the distal end of the humerus?

SOLUTION:

A free body diagram of the forearm is shown in Figure 8–52B, with the X axis passing through the joint center and lying along the forearm perpendicular to the pull of gravity and the line of pulley force.

Now, by applying the second condition of equilibrium ($\Sigma M = 0$) for this parallel force system, the magnitude of the triceps muscle force can be found.

The sling exerts a counterclockwise force of 100 N on the forearm and is given a negative sign. The weight of the forearm and hand acting clockwise is negative. We may write

$$\Sigma M_{CW} + \Sigma M_{CCW} = 0$$
$$(-20 \text{ N} \times 15 \text{ cm})$$
$$+ (100 \text{ N} \times 25 \text{ cm}) + (M \times 2.5 \text{ cm}) = 0$$
$$(-300 \text{ Ncm}) + (2500 \text{ Ncm})$$
$$+ (M \times 2.5 \text{ cm}) = 0$$
$$(2200 \text{ Ncm}) + (M \times 2.5 \text{ cm}) = 0$$
$$M = -880 \text{ N}$$

The triceps muscle exerts a force of 880 N (198 lb) upward toward the elbow joint. The joint reaction force can now be calculated with the equation for the first condition of equilibrium, $\Sigma F = 0$.

The pulley force and triceps muscle force act upward and are positive, while the combined weight of the forearm and hand acts downward and is given a negative sign. In this situation no forces are acting in the X direction. Thus,

$$\Sigma F_y = (-20 \text{ N}) + (100 \text{ N}) + (880 \text{ N})$$
$$+ R_y = 0$$
$$960 \text{ N} + R_y = 0$$
$$R_y = -960 \text{ N}$$

The joint reaction R equals R_y since there is no X reaction component. Thus, the joint reaction force acts downward with a force of 960 N (215.8 lb).

Another Application

Another clinical area of application of external forces in body movement is in the use of canes and crutches. Here, ground reaction forces are applied to the trunk in walking not only through the lower limbs but also through the assistive device (Fig. 8–64). Some degree of elbow flexion is common when a cane is used. The upward thrust of the cane with weight-bearing tends to flex the elbow joint and to elevate and extend the shoulder, requiring strong stabilizing activity of the triceps, latissimus dorsi, and pectoral muscles in particular. The greater the flexion of the elbow, the greater are the moments around the elbow and shoulder resulting from ground reaction forces. The same principle applies to the use of crutches where the weight is borne on the hands.

When the cane is used, "locking" the elbow in full extension spares the triceps muscle, just as keeping the knees straight in walking spares

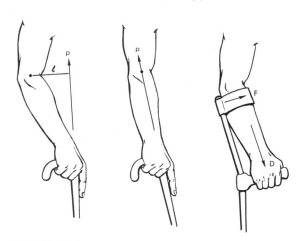

FIGURE 8–64

Moments related to use of a cane. As the hand pushes downward, the elbow is forced into flexion and the shoulder tends to extend. The moment about the elbow axis is P × l. If the elbow is fully extended, the torque is reduced, or it is absent if the lever arm becomes zero. Pressure (D) downward against the handrest of Canadian crutches provides force (F) forward against the forearm to stabilize the elbow joint and to prevent elbow flexion.

the quadriceps. Canadian crutches, which have a posterior band around the forearm, help to oppose elbow flexion. The upright is angled in such a way that downward pressure on the hand bar pushes the forearm cuff forward, forcing the elbow into extension.

▶ **PROBLEM 8–23**

A patient is leaning on a cane with a force of 190 N, with the elbow flexed 30° (Fig. 8–65A). The axis of the elbow joint is 36 cm to the hand, and 2.5 cm to the triceps brachii muscle attachment.
QUESTION:

What muscle force is needed to maintain this force on the cane? (What is the elbow joint reaction force?)
SOLUTION:

We first draw a free body diagram showing the forces involved (Fig. 8–65B). The X axis is drawn through the joint axis along the forearm. We then use the second condition of equilibrium to solve for the muscle force. The Y component (rotatory force) and X component (stabilizing force) of the cane are determined using trigonometric functions.

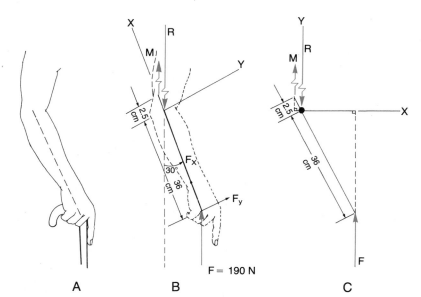

FIGURE 8–65

Static forces about the elbow joint while one is using a cane.

$F_x = F \cos \theta$; $F_y = F \sin \theta$, where $\theta = 30°$

$F_x = 190 \text{ N} \times 0.866$

$= 165 \text{ N}$

$F_y = 190 \text{ N} \times 0.5$

$= 95 \text{ N}$

The force of the cane, acting in a counterclockwise direction, is given a positive sign.

$(F \sin \theta \times 36 \text{ cm}) + (M_y \times 2.5 \text{ cm}) = 0$

$(95 \text{ N} \times 36 \text{ cm}) + (M_y \times 2.5 \text{ cm}) = 0$

$(3420 \text{ Ncm}) + (M_y \times 2.5 \text{ cm}) = 0$

$M_y = -1368 \text{ N}$

Since

$$M_y = M \sin \theta,$$

then

$$M = \frac{M_y}{\sin \theta}$$

$$= \frac{-1368 \text{ N}}{0.5}$$

$$= -2736 \text{ N}$$

The triceps brachii muscle force is 2736 N acting clockwise. An alternate approach in this case may simplify the calculation of the muscle force. If we used the horizontal as the X axis instead of the forearm (Fig. 8–64C), the lever arms in the second condition of equilibrium would be applied as follows:

$(190 \text{ N} \times 36 \text{ cm} \times \sin 30°)$

$+ (M \times 2.5 \text{ cm} \times \sin 30°) = 0$

$(190 \text{ N} \times 36 \text{ cm} \times 0.5)$

$+ (M \times 2.5 \text{ cm} \times 0.5) = 0$

$(3420 \text{ Ncm}) + (1.25 \text{ cm} \times M) = 0$

$1.25 \text{ cm} \times M = -3420 \text{ Ncm}$

$M = -2736 \text{ N}$

The joint reaction force is determined using the first condition of equilibrium, $\Sigma F = 0$. In Figure 8–65B, the cane force and muscle force both act to the left and are given negative signs.

$\Sigma F_x = F \cos 30° + M \cos 30° + R_y = 0$

$(-190 \text{ N} \times 0.866)$

$+ (-2736 \text{ N} \times 0.866) + R_x = 0$

$(-164.5 \text{ N}) + (-2369.4 \text{ N}) + R_x = 0$

$(-2533.9 \text{ N}) + R_x = 0$

$R_x = 2533.9 \text{ N}$

The cane and muscle force both act upward and are positive.

$$\Sigma F_y = F \sin 30° + M \sin 30° + R_y = 0$$
$$(190 \text{ N} \times 0.5) + (2736 \text{ N} \times 0.5) + R_y = 0$$
$$(95 \text{ N}) + (1368 \text{ N}) + R_y = 0$$
$$(1463 \text{ N}) + R_y = 0$$
$$R_y = -1463 \text{ N}$$

By using the Pythagorean theorem:

$$R = \sqrt{R_x^2 + R_y^2}$$
$$= \sqrt{(2533.9)^2 + (-1463)^2}$$
$$= \sqrt{6,420,649.2 + 2,140,369}$$
$$= 8,561,018.2$$
$$= 2925.9 \text{ N}$$

The direction of the joint reaction force is found by using one of the trigonometric functions.

$$\tan \theta = \frac{R_y}{R_x}$$
$$= \frac{-1463 \text{ N}}{2533.9 \text{ N}}$$
$$= 0.57739$$
$$\theta = 30°$$

Thus, a joint reaction force in the elbow acting downward and to the right at 30° with the forearm is 2925.9 N (657.8 lb). Compare this triceps brachii muscle force and joint reaction force to those when the elbow is locked in extension.

How much weight would need to be placed on the sling apparatus as shown in Figure 8–52B to equal this load on the triceps brachii? Calculate with the forearm in the 30° flexion position.

Calculate the triceps muscle force needed by a 890 N man as he swings between two crutches with the weight distributed evenly on both crutches. Place the crutches vertical and the elbow position at 30° of flexion. Use data from Appendix A.

Occasionally, the triceps muscle and elbow joint must bear a considerable amount of force when using assistive walking devices. The therapist should be well aware of this and his or her approach to the patient should be guided accordingly.

We have seen in this chapter how forces involved in many body postures as well as the effects of external forces and force systems applied to the body can be calculated.

By knowing what minimum forces are required of certain muscle groups during selected activities (for example, the quadriceps in stair-climbing; triceps and latissimus dorsi in crutch-walking; and anterior tibialis for prevention of drop foot), the therapist may have guidelines for judging when the patient is ready to attempt these activities or for judging whether assistive devices are necessary.

A given problem may become more complex as more factors are considered, as in adding the weight of the part, which may be a minor consideration in some instances. The choice of procedure will depend on how precise an answer is desired.

QUESTIONS

1. Does the center of mass of a patient always lie within the body no matter what his or her position? Explain.

2. Upon what factors does the stability of an object depend?

3. How does changing the position of the limb with respect to the horizontal affect the muscle force necessary to support the resistance?

4. List three ways to determine body segment parameters and tell what assumptions are necessary for each.

Use the body parameter data from Appendix A and your own body size to answer the following problems.

5. Calculate the magnitude of force needed by your quadriceps to lift 100 N on the N–K table at 90°, 60°, 45°, 30°, and 0° of flexion. What happens to the joint reaction force? Compare this with the boot. What happens if the resistance arm of the N–K table is set at a 45° angle forward from the force arm?

6. Discuss the difference in erector spinae muscle force and joint reaction when a 670 N individual arises from sitting (1) with the trunk inclined 60° and (2) with the trunk inclined 15°.

7. Compare your erector spinae muscle force and joint reaction when lifting a 250 N weight (1) with your trunk flexed to 90° and (2) with your back straight and hips and knees flexed.

8. The patient you are treating has a possible medial meniscus tear in the left knee with limited range of motion and pain past 60° of

flexion. You are asked to strengthen the left quadriceps muscle group in the last 30° of extension.

(a) How would you position the patient and what exercise device, if any, would you use (pulleys, N–K table, sandbags, etc.) to get the patient's left quadriceps muscles to have an equal moment of force as the right quadriceps muscle group (2600 Ncm in full extension)?

(b) How much resistance would you add 37.5 cm from the knee axis if the leg weighs 50 N, with its center of mass 12 cm from the knee axis?

(c) How much force is the muscle group exerting at full extension if the patellar tendon inserts at a 30° angle 5 cm from the knee axis?

9. A patient with chondromalacia of the patella needs a strengthening program for the quadriceps muscles. How much weight may be added to the ankle (37 cm from the knee joint) with the knee of the sitting patient in 30° of flexion to maintain less than 500 N of compression force on the patellofemoral joint? Assume the leg and foot weigh 40 N with their combined center of mass located 25 cm from the knee joint, that the patellar tendon inserts at a 25° angle with the tibia 5 cm from the knee joint, and that the quadriceps muscle pulls horizontally along the femur. What would happen to the patellofemoral force as the knee was extended? If it were flexed further? Estimate how far a 1000 N patient could squat without exceeding the 500 N compression force.

10. Analyze the strengthening effect of the different knee exercise devices that are on the market.

11. A patient has a painful right hip owing to arthritis.

(a) The pain increases as she walks slowly, attempting a normal gait. Explain why.

(b) How may the patient attempt to decrease the pain without using a cane? Why does this work?

(c) A physical therapist may help reduce this pain by giving the patient a cane. Explain why this would help, based on the laws of equilibrium.

(d) Should the cane be used in the opposite hand for all joint problems involving the lower limb?

12. A paraplegic patient strengthens his shoulders by raising a 70 N dumbbell to shoulder level with his arm straight.

(a) Find the effective "exercise force" (rotatory component of gravitational pull on the weight) when the arm is abducted 40° from the side of the trunk.

(b) Find the force in the deltoid muscle necessary to maintain the arm in a horizontal position. (Consider the angle of deltoid force application on the arm to be 20°, and estimate the distances you need in solving the problem.)

13. (a) Diagram the rotational component of gravitational force acting on the head, trunk, and arms (considered as a unit) during a sit-up exercise when the patient's trunk is halfway to vertical and (1) the arms are at the sides; (2) the arms are overhead.

(b) Estimate distances you need and determine the moment exerted about the hip joints by gravitational force on the trunk in Question 13a (1) and (2).

14. Find the single resultant force for one upper limb in Figure 8–19. What moment must the shoulder flexor muscles exert to maintain this position of the limb?

15. Using the three component segments (arm, forearm, hand) find the center of mass of the upper limb when it is in an extended position and when the elbow is flexed to various angles. Repeat the preceding problem, using different moment centers.

16. During leg-raising, the abdominal muscles must stabilize the pelvis against anterior rotation caused by reverse action of the hip flexors (pulling on their origins). What moment must be exerted by the hip flexor muscles in order to lift:

(a) One flexed lower limb.

(b) One extended limb.

(c) Two flexed limbs.

(d) Two extended limbs.

17. Why is the center of mass of a 1 m pipe located at its midpoint, while this is not true of either the upper or lower limb of the body?

18. Where is the center of mass of the human body in the anatomic position, and how does it shift when the subject sits down? Account for this shift.

19. How would the location of the center of mass in the body be changed after an above-knee amputation? How does this affect a patient's stability in a wheelchair or on crutches?

20. According to Dempster's data, how much does one of your own upper limbs weigh? One lower limb? Your head?

21. Locate on yourself and then show by a line diagram where the center of mass of the upper extremity might be expected to lie:
(a) With the limb fully extended.
(b) With the elbow flexed to 90°.
 (1) On each diagram draw a vector representing the pull of gravity on the arm.
 (2) Draw vectors representing the pull of the deltoid and supraspinatus muscles.
Would making a fist or extending the fingers affect the location of the center of mass of the extremity? How?

22. In a center of mass experiment using the board and scale method, the gravity line of a 600 N subject bisects a 3 m board.
(a) What is the scale reading?
(b) What would be the scale reading if the subject moved 0.3 m closer to the scale?
(c) Would the scale reading increase or decrease if the subject faced the scale in this spot and flexed both arms to horizontal (toward the scale)?

23. Why is it not possible to sit upright in a chair and rise to one's feet without first leaning forward? What implications has this fact for the design of chairs? For the handling of patients with trunk and lower limb muscle weakness?

24. Compare the relative pressure on the hands when crutches are used as shown in Figure 8–14. Why does the hand pressure differ?

25. Explain why pressure against the joint surfaces may be great when relatively light loads are supported by the body parts.

26. Review some of the problems in this chapter in which "mean" action lines of muscle forces have been estimated. Apply slightly different action lines in order to observe the magnitude of error introduced by such estimates.

27. Assume the forearm weighs 20 N and its center of mass is located 12.5 cm from the elbow. The brachialis muscle, pulling at a 90° angle, is inserted 5 cm distal to the elbow.
(a) Find the muscular force required to keep the forearm in a horizontal position. How much of the force is rotatory? How much of the force is directed toward the elbow joint?
(b) In the above situation, what would the muscle force be if we added 100 N to the hand 37.5 cm from the elbow?
(c) Calculate the muscle force and its rotatory and linear components for the following situations. The 20 N limb and 100 N weight are the same as above. Determine the joint reaction force in each case.
 (1) The limb is horizontal, the angle of muscle pull is 60°.
 (2) The limb is horizontal, the angle of muscle pull is 15°.
 (3) The forearm is held 30° below the horizontal, the muscle is inserted at 45°.
 (4) The forearm is held 30° above the horizontal, the muscle is inserted at 45°.
(d) What changes take place in the muscle force as the angle of insertion changes?
(e) What difference does the position of the arm with the horizontal make? Why?
(f) Are there any other factors which would influence the muscle force being exerted?

28. List the biomechanical factors that affect the recorded force produced by a muscle.

29. Using the values in Problem 7–21, determine the hamstring muscle force values if a person had a 1 kg mass attached to his or her ankles.

REFERENCES

Aglielti P, Insoll JN, Walker PS, et al.: A new patella prosthesis. Clin Orthop *107*:175–187, 1975.

Backman S: The proximal end of the femur. Acta Radiol Suppl *146*:1–166, 1957.

Basmajian JV: Muscles Alive, 2nd ed. Baltimore, Williams & Wilkins, 1967.

Bearn JG: Function of shoulder muscles in posture and in holding weights. Ann Phys Med *6*:100–104, 1961.

Bernstein N: The Coordination and Regulation of Movements. New York, Pergamon Press, 1967.

Blount W: Don't throw away the cane. J Bone Joint Surg 38A:695–708, 1956.

Borelli GA: De Motu Animalium. Lugdundi Batavorum. 1679. Reprint with English translation: On the Motion of Animals. New York, Springer-Verlag, 1989.

Brunnstrom S: Muscle group testing. Physiol Rev 21:3–22, 1941.

Cailliet R: Low Back Pain Syndrome, 2nd ed. Philadelphia. F. A. Davis, 1968.

Chaffin DB, Andersson GBJ: Occupational Biomechanics. New York, John Wiley & Sons, 1984, pp 147–232.

Clauser CE, McConville JJ, Young JW: Weight, volume, and center of mass of segments of the human body. Wright-Patterson Air Force Base, Ohio, 1969 (AMRL-TR-69-70).

Davis PR: Posture of the trunk during lifting of weights. Br Med J 1:87–89, 1959.

DeDuca CJ, Forrest WJ: Force analysis of individual muscles acting simultaneously on the shoulder during isometric abduction. J Biomechanics 6:385–393, 1973.

Dempster W: Space requirements of the seated operator. WADC Technical Report 55:159, 1955.

Dempster WT: The anthropometry of body action. Ann NY Acad Sci 63:559–585, 1955.

Elftman H: Biomechanics of muscle. J Bone Joint Surg 48A:363–377, 1966.

Farfan HF: Muscular mechanism of the lumbar spine and the position of power and efficiency. Orthop Clin North Am 6:135–144, 1975.

Fenlin JM: Total glenohumeral joint replacement. Orthop Clin North Am 6:565–583, 1975.

Ferguson AB: The clinical and roentgenographic interpretation of lumbosacral anomalies. Radiology 22:548–558, 1934.

Fick A: Statische Berachtung der Muskulature des Oberschenkels. Zeitschrift für Rationelle Medicin 9:94–106, 1850.

Ford WR, Perry J: Analysis of knee joint forces during flexed knee stance. J Bone Joint Surg 54A:1118, 1972.

Frankel VH: Biomechanics of the knee. Orthop Clin North Am 2:175–190, 1971.

Frankel VH, Burstein AH: Orthopaedic Biomechanics. Philadelphia, Lea & Febiger, 1970.

Frankel VH, Burstein AH, Brooks DB: Biomechanics of internal derangement of the knee. J Bone Joint Surg 53A:945–962, 1971.

Hellebrandt FA, Fries EC: The constancy of oscillograph stance patterns. Physiol Rev 23:220–225, 1942.

Hellems HK, Keats TE: Measurement of the normal lumbosacral angle. Am J Roentgenol Radium Ther Nucl Med 113:642–645, 1971.

Inman VT: Functional aspects of the abductor muscles of the hip. J Bone Joint Surg 29A:607–619, 1947.

Inman VT, Saunders JBM, Abbott LC: Observations on the function of the shoulder joint. J Bone Joint Surg 26A:1–30, 1944.

Johnston RC: Mechanical considerations of the hip joint. Arch Surg 107:411–417, 1973.

Johnston RC, Larson CB: Biomechanics of cup arthroplasty. Clin Orthop 66:56–69, 1969.

Jones CL: The damaging effects of a disaligned musculoskeletal system. J Am Podiatr Assoc 61:369–381, 1971.

Jørgensen K, Bankov S: Maximum strength of elbow flexors with pronated and supinated forearm. In Biomechanics II (Medicine and Sport Series), vol. 6. Baltimore, University Park Press, 1971, pp 174–180.

Kaufer H: Mechanical functions of the patella. J Bone Joint Surg 53A:1551–1560, 1971.

Kettlekamp DB: Clinical implications of knee biomechanics. Arch Surg 107:406–410, 1973.

Kostuik JP, Schmidt O, Harris WR, et al.: A study of weight transmission through the knee joint with applied varus and valgus loads. Clin Orthop 109:95–98, 1975.

LeVeau BF: Axis of joint rotation of the lumbar vertebra during abdominal strengthening exercises. In Nelson RC, Morehouse CA (Eds): Biomechanics IV. Baltimore, University Park Press, 1974, pp 361–364.

MacConaill MA: 1. The movements of bones and joints. 2. Function of the musculature. J Bone Joint Surg 31B:100–104, 1949.

MacConaill MA, Basmajian JV: Muscles and Movements. Baltimore, Williams & Wilkins, 1969.

McCusker H: Cervical traction sling. Phys Ther Rev 36:763–764, 1956.

Merchant AC: Hip abductor muscle force. J Bone Joint Surg 47A:462–476, 1965.

Moeller FA: Biomechanics and its relationship to foot surgery. J Am Podiatr Assoc 63:383–389, 1973.

Morris JM: Biomechanics of the spine. Arch Surg 107:418–423, 1973.

Morris JM, Brenner G, Lucas DB: An electromyographic study of the intrinsic muscles of the back in man. J Anat 96:509–520, 1962.

Morris JM, Lucas DB, Bressler B: Role of the trunk in stability of the spine. J Bone Joint Surg 43A:327–351, 1961.

Morrison JB: The mechanics of the knee joint in relation to normal walking. J Biomechanics 3:51–61, 1970.

Nachemson A, Elfstrom G: Intravital dynamic pressure measurements in lumbar discs. Scand J Rehab Med, Suppl. 1, 1970, pp 1–40.

O'Connell AL: An estimate of tension exerted by hip extensors during two different balance poses on the right lower extremity. In Cerquiglini S, Venerando A, Wartenweiler J (Eds): Biomechanics III (Medicine and Sport Series), vol. 8. Baltimore, University Park Press, 1973, pp 172–174.

Ogden JA, Gossling HR: Slipped capital femoral epiphysis following ipsilateral femoral fracture. Clin Orthop 111:167–170, 1975.

Outerbridge KE, Dunlop JAY: The problem of chondromalacia patellae. Clin Orthop 111:177–196, 1975.

Reilly DT: Experimental analysis of the quadriceps muscles force and patello-femoral joint reaction force for various activities. Acta Orthop Scand 43:126–137, 1972.

Reilly DT, Martens M: Experimental analysis of the quadriceps muscle force and the patello-femoral joint reaction force for various activities. Acta Orthop Scand 43:126–137, 1972.

Rolander SD: Motion of the lumbar spine with special reference to the stabilizing effect of posterior fusion. Acta Orthop Scand, Suppl. 90, 1966.

Roozbazar A: Biomechanics of lifting. In Nelson RC, Morehouse CA (Eds): Biomechanics IV. Baltimore, University Park Press, 1975, pp 37–43.

Sammarco GT, Burstein AH, Frankel VH: Biomechanics of the ankle: A kinematic study. Orthop Clin North Am 4:75–96, 1973.

Seireg A, Arvikar RJ: A mathematical model for evaluation of forces in lower extremities of the musculo-skeletal system. J Biomech 6:313–326, 1973.

Shaw JA, Murray DG: Knee simulator. Clin Orthop 94:15–23, 1973.

Shinno N: Analysis of knee function in ascending and descending stairs. *In* Vredenbregt J, Wortenweiler J (Eds): Biomechanics II. (Medicine and Sport Series), vol. 6. Baltimore, University Park Press, 1971, pp 202–207.

Smidt GL: Biomechanical analysis of knee flexion and extension. J Biomech 6:79–92, 1973.

Steen B: The functions of certain neck muscles in different positions with and without loading of the cervical spine. Acta Morphol Neerl Scand 6:301–310, 1966.

Steindler A: Kinesiology. Springfield, IL, Charles C Thomas, 1955.

Stern JT: Investigations concerning the theory of "spurt" and "shunt" muscles. J Biomech 4:437–453, 1971.

Strait LA, Inman VT, Ralston HJ: Sample illustrations of physical principles selected from physiology and medicine. Am J Physics 15:375–382, 1947.

Troupe JDG: Relation of lumbar spine disorders to heavy manual work and lifting. Lancet 1:857–861, 1965.

Walker PS, Erkman MJ: The role of the menisci in force transmission across the knee. Clin Orthop 109:184–192, 1975.

Walton JS: A template for locating segmental centers of gravity. Am Assoc Health Phys Ed 41:615–618, 1970.

Weis EB: Stresses at the lumbosacral junction. Orthop Clin North Am 6:83–91, 1975.

Weiss M, Bentkowski Z: Biomechanical study in dynamic spondylodesis of the spine. Clin Orthop 103:199–203, 1974.

Williams M, Worthingham C: Therapeutic Exercise for Body Alignment and Function. Philadelphia, W. B. Saunders Co. 1957, p 101.

Woolson ST, Meeks LW: A method of balanced skeletal traction for femoral fractures. J Bone Joint Surg 56A:1288–1289, 1974.

Wratney MJ: Physical therapy for muscular dystrophy children. Phys Ther Rev 38:26–32, 1958.

Yamakawa J: A study concerning the center of gravity in the infant. Ann Rep Phys Ed 1:61–69, 1967.

Appendix A

Body Segment Parameters

SUMMARY OF DEMPSTER'S DATA

In much of the literature on locations of centers of mass of the limbs and trunk, the classic work of Braune and Fischer (1889) has been cited. Studies by Dempster (1955) and Clauser and associates (1969) provide more comprehensive data. Excerpts pertinent to the present text are included here through the courtesy of Dr. W. T. Dempster, Department of Anatomy, University of Michigan, and the Office of Technical Services, U.S. Department of Commerce. The following sections are based primarily on the report of this work.

METHOD OF INVESTIGATION

Eight male cadavers of "more or less medium" build were selected to be dismembered. Seven were embalmed. They ranged in age from 52 to 83 years (two ages unknown). Heights (supine) were 155.3 to 186.6 cm (61.1 to 73.5 in) and weights were 486 N to 709 N (109 to 195.5 lb). After initial anthropometric measurements were made, the hips and shoulders of the cadavers were frozen in a semiflexed position. This was considered most favorable for apportionment of the tissue to the respective segments on either side of the joint axis. After the limbs were separated from the trunk, the head and trunk segment and the four limb segments were weighed, and the center of mass of each was determined on a balance-plate (segments straight). The limbs were then frozen in a semiflexed position (elbows 70°, knees 62°) and saw cuts were made through the joint centers. The resulting eight limb segments were weighed and centers of mass found. The ankle and wrist joints were frozen in a midposition. The wrist was divided through the head of the capitate bone, at the dorsal wrist crease. The saw cut through the ankle passed from the upper border of the calcaneus to the tip of the fibular malleolus, just proximal to the head of the talus. Three remaining masses were divided: shoulder girdle, including attaching muscles; head and neck, separated along the upper border of the first rib; and thorax and abdominopelvic complex, divided between the last thoracic and first lumbar vertebrae.

After centers of mass for the parts were determined, distances were measured from these points to the ends of the segments. In order to locate the center of mass of the various segments in three dimensions, each part was suspended from various points or balanced on the balance-plate. Drill holes were aimed at the center of mass, dowel sticks inserted in the holes, and saw cuts made in the plane of the sticks. Specific loci as described by Dempster are shown in Figure A–1 and detailed in Table A–1.

The surface landmarks associated with joint centers and percentage distance of center of mass points from joint axes are also given in Figure A–1 and Table A–2. Additional observations made by Dempster on living subjects included measurement of strength, range of joint motion, and body dimensions, including limb volume.

CONCEPT OF BODY LINKS

In kinematic analysis of human motion, the important moving units are not the various bones, which support the surrounding soft tissue structures, but rather the total mass of the segments that turn about the joint axes. The rotational axes are not located at the junctures of the bones. For example, the axis at the hip lies

TABLE A–1. AVERAGE WEIGHT OF BODY SEGMENTS FOR 670 N (68.4 Kg) MAN, PERCENTAGE OF TOTAL BODY WEIGHT AND LOCATION OF CENTERS OF MASS*

Segment Weights and Percentage of Total Body Weight for 670 N Man	Location of Centers of Mass
Head: 46.2 N	*Head.* In sphenoid sinus, 4 mm beyond anterior inferior margin of sella. (On lateral surface, over temporal fossa on or near nasion-inion line.)
Head and neck: 52.9 N (7.9%)	*Head and neck.* On inferior surface of basioccipital bone or within bone 23 ± 5 mm from crest of dorsum sellae. (On lateral surface, 10 mm anterior to supratragal notch above head of mandible.)
Head, neck, and trunk: 395.3 N (59.0%)	*Head, neck, and trunk.* Anterior to eleventh thoracic vertebra.
	Upper Limb
	Upper limb. Just above elbow joint.
Arm: 18.1 N (2.7%)	*Arm.* In medial head of triceps, adjacent to radial groove; 5 mm proximal to distal end of deltoid insertion.
Forearm: 10.7 N (1.6%)	*Forearm.* 11 mm proximal to most distal part of pronator teres insertion; 9 mm anterior to interosseous membrane.
Hand: 4.0 N (0.6%) Upper limb: 32.8 N (4.9%) Forearm and hand: 14.7 N (2.2%)	*Hand* (in rest position). On axis of metacarpal III, usually 2 mm deep to volar skin surface; 2 mm proximal to transverse palmar skin crease, in angle between proximal transverse and radial longitudinal crease.
	Lower Limb
	Lower limb. Just above knee joint.
Thigh: 65.0 N (9.7%)	*Thigh.* In adductor brevis muscle (or magnus or vastus medialis) 13 mm medial to linea aspera, deep to adductor canal; 29 mm below apex of femoral triangle and 18 mm proximal to most distal fibers of adductor brevis.
Leg: 30.2 N (4.5%)	*Leg.* 35 mm below popliteus, at posterior part of posterior tibialis; 16 mm above proximal end of Achilles tendon; 8 mm posterior to interosseous membrane.
Foot: 9.4 N (1.4%) Lower limb: 104.5 N (15.6%) Leg and foot: 40.2 N (6.0%)	*Foot.* In plantar ligaments, or just superficial in adjacent deep foot muscles; below proximal halves of second and third cuneiform bones. On a line between ankle joint center and ball of foot in plane of metatarsal II.
	Entire body. Anterior to second sacral vertebra.

*Based on Dempster, 1955; value for head weight was computed from Braune and Fischer, 1889. Centers of mass loci are from Dempster except those for entire limbs and body.

within the femoral head, and the axis at the shoulder, within the humeral head. The humeral head moves downward as the arm is elevated. Both the elbow and knee axes are proximal to the respective articular surfaces. At the radiocarpal and tibiotalar joints, on the other hand, the axis is distal to the joint.

The central straight line, which extends between two axes of rotation, is termed a "link." Thus, the femur and humerus are longer than their respective links, and the tibia and radius are shorter. The bones form the rigid support required by the segment, but the bone itself is not the link. Link systems are interconnected by joints, which predetermine the particular type of motion permitted to the functional segments. In the case of the hands and feet, the terminal links are considered to extend from the wrist and ankle joint centers to the center of mass of these so-called end members.

In apportioning the overlying soft tissue to the respective functional links, some arbitrary decisions must be made. In designating link dimensions. Dempster (1955) stated:

Such segments are most readily recognized in the limbs, where the segments have a changing angular relation to one another. Skin flexure lines may sug-

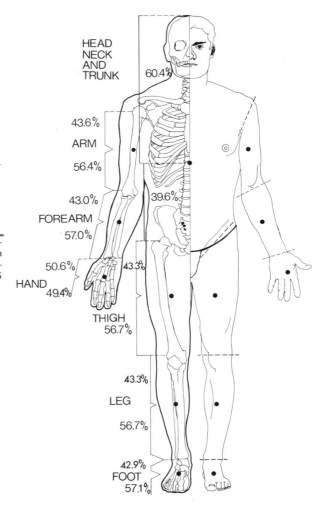

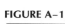

FIGURE A–1

Link boundaries (at the joint centers) and percentage distance of centers of gravity from link boundaries. (From Dempster WT: Space requirements of the seated operator. Wright-Patterson Air Force Base, Ohio, 1955 [WADCTR 55-159].)

gest boundaries in some instances; in others, the establishment of precise boundaries is not easy, since muscles and other structures cross from one region to the next, so that only the most arbitrary boundary lines can be drawn.

Another difficulty is that the joint axes shift about as the parts move in space. However, the instantaneous centers of motion plotted with the part in various positions are clustered in such a fashion that a mean position of the axis can be designated, which is adequate for our purposes. In certain positions, a link may be longer or shorter than the dimension based on a mean center.

In Dempster's view, the most satisfactory division of tissue in the experimental work involving sectioning of the body parts was obtained with the limb joints partially flexed. The following data on dimensions and mass of the functional body components have been obtained and reported with reference to the joint-and-link concept of body movement. Such quantitative data should have great importance for the study of biomechanics.

Table A–3 gives Dempster's estimates of link dimensions on living subjects (adult men). These represent the distances between joint centers at either end of the links, or between the

TABLE A–2. SURFACE LANDMARKS ASSOCIATED WITH JOINT CENTERS

Glenohumeral	Midregion of palpable bony mass of head and tuberosities of humerus.
Elbow	Midpoint of line between: (1) lowest palpable point of medial epicondyle of humerus, and (2) a point 8 mm above radiohumeral junction.
Wrist	Palmar surface: Distal skin crease at palmaris longus tendon; or midpoint of line between radial styloid and center of pisiform bone. Dorsal surface: Palpable groove between lunate and capitate bones, on a line with metacarpal III.
Hip	Lateral aspect: Tip of femoral trochanter 1.02 cm anterior to most laterally projecting part of femoral trochanter.
Knee	Midpoint of line between centers of posterior convexities of femoral condyles.
Ankle	At level of line between tip of lateral malleolus of fibula and a point 5 mm distal to tibial malleolus.
Link lengths (distances between the respective joint centers)	Hand link: Slightly oblique line from wrist joint center to center of mass of the hand. Foot link: Line between ankle joint center and center of mass of the foot.

joint center and center of mass in the case of the hand and foot. Thigh and leg, arm and forearm, and foot and hand links are nearly equal to each other. Another useful comparison among segments is the remarkably constant location of the center of mass of the arm, forearm, thigh, and leg when considered in terms of percentage distance from the proximal to distal axes of rotation. Deviations of loci in these segments were found to be less than 1 percent (Fig. A–1). Centers of mass of the limb segments lie along link lines (lines connecting adjacent joint axes).

On the basis of the various anthropometric measurements, joint range, and link dimensions, a drafting board manikin of a seated male figure was developed by Dempster's group for use in cockpit design. Three sizes were suggested, based on large, medium, and small body build. The pattern for a figure of average dimensions has been adapted for use in this test (Fig. A–2). Such a model should be helpful in diagramming and solving problems.

Dempster's report did not include percentage ratios of link or bone length to total body height. However, Trotter and Gleser's (1952) data were cited, based on measurements of 710 white Army men, in which the lengths of certain bones are plotted against stature. Extrapolating from these charts, we find that at the midrange of the distribution for the 50th percentile group (average height, 68.9 in, or 1750 mm) ratios were approximately as shown in Table A–4. These figures, together with the data in Table A–3, will be helpful in estimating segment and link lengths in setting up problems. Such estimates, which can be made on oneself, on another person, or from photographs and moving pictures, are admittedly rough approximations but can be of great practical value if careful attention is paid to anatomic landmarks.

SUMMARY OF BRAUNE AND FISCHER'S DATA

These data are based on measurements of three cadavers. The limb segments were divided at the joint axes. Total heights of the cadavers were 1.70 m, 1.69 m, and 1.67 m; mean height was 1.69 m. Weights were 736 N, 546 N, and 596 N, respectively; mean weight was 626 N. Landmarks were defined as follows:

1. Upper limb. Steel pins were inserted through the humeral head in the anteroposterior direction and through the head of the capitate bone. The elbow axis was marked medially and laterally on the skin.
2. Lower limb. The skin was marked over the anterosuperior iliac spine, upper prominence of the greater trochanter (considered to be at the level of the center of the femoral head), at the

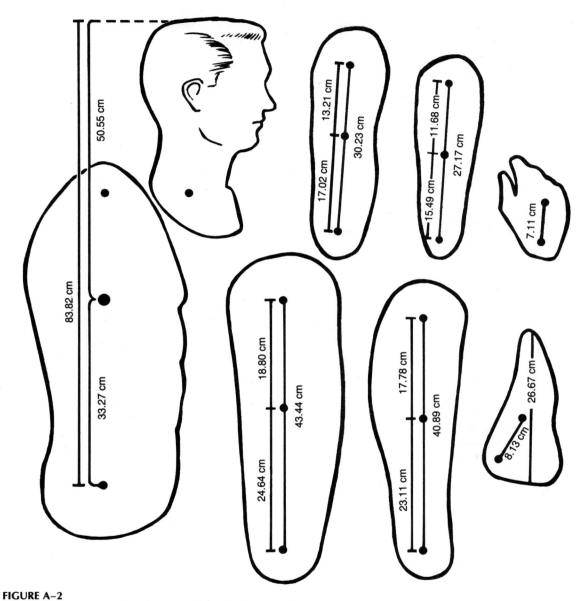

FIGURE A–2

Pattern for manikin. Dimensions are adapted from Dempster's drawing board model for a man of average build. (From Dempster WT: Space requirements of the seated operator. Wright-Patterson Air Force Base, Ohio, 1955 [WADCTR 55-159].)

TABLE A–3. ESTIMATES OF LINK DIMENSIONS*†

Segment	50th Percentile	Link-to-Length Ratio (Percent)	5th and 95th Percentiles	
Humerus link	11.9⎱	89.0	⎧11.3	12.6
Humerus length	13.3⎰		⎩12.6	14.1
Radius link	10.7⎱	107.0	⎧10.1	11.2
Radius length	10.0⎰		9.4	10.5
Hand link (wrist center to center of mass)	2.8⎱	20.6	⎧ 2.6	2.9
Hand length	7.5⎰		6.9	8.0
Femur link	17.1⎱	91.4	⎧15.9	18.1
Femur length	18.7⎰		⎩17.4	19.8
Tibial link	16.1⎱	110.0	⎧15.0	17.3
Tibial length	14.6⎰		⎩13.6	15.7
Foot link (talus center point to center of mass)	3.2⎱	30.6	⎧ 3.0	3.5
Foot length	10.5⎰		9.8	11.3
Vertical distance from midtalus to floor level	3.2			
Head, neck, and trunk	33.0			

*From Dempster, 1955.
†Young adult men, based on ratios from cadaver measurements (inches).

medial and lateral points of the knee axis, and at the medial and lateral points of the ankle axis.

The dimensions of the segments were measured from these landmarks. For center of mass determinations, the cadavers were frozen and segmented, and the parts were studied by balancing them over a knife-edge and suspending them by slender rods in such a fashion that they were free to oscillate until equilibrium was reached. The head and trunk were included in these investigations.

The location of centers of mass was given in terms of percentage of the distance from proximal to distal joint centers of the segments (the means of right and left sides of three subjects).

Additional centers of mass reported by Braune and Fischer were:

Head: Behind the sella turcica in the sagittal plane.

Trunk: In or anterior to the first lumbar vertebra.

Entire upper limb: In the area of the elbow axis.

Entire lower limb: A few centimeters (2 to 5 cm) above the knee axis in the substance of the femur.

DATA FROM CLAUSER, McCONVILLE, AND YOUNG

The purpose of a study by Clauser and associates (1969) was to transfer the findings of the interrelationships in cadavers to living persons.

TABLE A–4. RATIO OF BONE LENGTH TO BODY HEIGHT*

Ratio of stature to length of:			
femur	1750:477 mm	27.3%	47.75 cm (bone length)
tibia	1750:372 mm	21.2%	37.08 cm (bone length)
humerus	1750:338 mm	19.3%	33.78 cm (bone length)
radius	1750:252 mm	14.4%	22.15 cm (bone length)

*Data extrapolated from Trotter and Gleser, 1952.

From comparison of cadaver body dimensions to similar dimensions of Air Force studies on living subjects, even though the cadavers were smaller than the living subjects, these investigators found essentially the same type and degree of interrelation in the living as in the cadavers.

Thirteen male cadavers were each dissected into 14 segments. The weight, volume, and center of mass of each segment were determined, and sufficient anthropometry of the cadavers was taken to describe the length, circumference, and breadth or depth of each segment. The relationships between the size of the segment and its weight, volume, and the location of its center of mass formed the basis for estimating these parameters of living populations.

Regression equations were set up for prediction of segmental variables from anthropometric dimensions. Only three or fewer steps in the equations were used. For example, the weight of the arm could be predicted from linear measures of the arm or from total body weight (or both). From these equations, total body weight seemed to be the best, and most often used, predictor of weight and volume of segments. Circumferences were found to be better than lengths for predicting segment weight, whereas segment lengths most often were used in predicting the location of center of mass of segments. The prediction of segmental masses and mass centers on cadavers by the three-step regression equations were compared with prediction by simple ratios and by single step equations. The three-step equations provided the smallest average error for predicting the unknown variables on the cadavers. The simple ratios provided the poorest average estimate. When the single step equation used body weight as the predicting variable, the results were identical to those obtained using the simple ratio established by Dempster (1955).

Owing to problems involved in applying equations to the living from those formulated on a cadaver population, however, validation of these predictive equations was needed. To attempt this, Clauser and his associates took repeated observations on the major segments, such as arms or legs. These were found to have errors of from 3 to 5 percent of the total average volume. One major error was due to difficulties encountered in maintaining a subject's body segment relatively motionless in the overflow tank. Thus, they concluded that until new techniques of measuring segmental volumes accurately on the living can be developed, this approach to the validation of the predictive equations does not appear to be satisfactory. The authors suggested that the use of body circumferences of the living would tend to overestimate the segmental weight predicted by the cadaver-based equations, owing to reduction of the body circumferences of the cadavers from loss of fluid. They concluded from their study that this system of equations allows for the segmental parameters to be based more upon the individual variability in body size, which was not adequately considered in other cadaver studies.

Gross comparisons of (1) the segmental weights as a ratio of total body weight and (2) the location of the center of mass from the proximal end of the segment as a ratio of segment length from the preceding investigators (Braune and Fischer, 1889; Dempster, 1955), as presented by Clauser and associates (1969), are shown in Tables A–5 and A–6. The values presented in these comparisons were obtained using differences in techniques by the separate investigators. Therefore, only a general comparison of the similarities and/or differences in these parameters can be made.

MOMENTS OF INERTIA AND RADII OF GYRATION

For dynamic studies, the moment of inertia and radius of gyration must be known. In his cadaver study, Dempster (1955) used a pendulum system to determine the moments of inertia for the various body segments. The formula used was

$$I_o = \frac{WL}{4\pi^2 f^2}$$

TABLE A–5. SEGMENTAL WEIGHT/BODY WEIGHT RATIOS FROM SEVERAL CADAVER STUDIES*

Source	Braune and Fischer (1889)	Dempster (1955b)	Dempster[†] (1955b)	Clauser et al. (1969)
Sample Size	*3*	*8*	*8*	*13*
Head	7.0%	7.9%	(8.1)%	7.3%
Trunk	46.1	48.6	(49.7)	50.7
Upper arm	3.3	2.7	(2.8)	2.6
Forearm	2.1	1.6	(1.6)	1.6
Hand	0.8	0.6	(0.6)	0.7
Total arm	6.2	4.9	(5.0)	4.9
Forearm and hand	2.9	2.2	(2.2)	2.3
Thigh	10.7	9.7	(9.9)	10.3
Calf	4.8	4.5	(4.6)	4.3
Foot	1.7	1.4	(1.4)	1.5
Total leg	17.2	15.7	(16.1)	16.1
Calf and foot	6.5	6.0	(6.1)	5.8
Sum[‡]	99.9	97.7	100.0	100.0

*From Clauser et al., 1969.
[†]Adjusted values.
[‡]The sum is calculated as Head + Trunk + 2 (Total arm + Total leg).

where I_o is the moment of inertia from the proximal end of the segment, L is the distance from the center of mass to the point of suspension, and f is the frequency of oscillation. The moment of inertia at the center of mass was calculated by using the parallel axis theorem equation:

$$I_{CM} = I_o - \frac{w}{g} L^2$$

A summary of Dempster's results is shown in Table A–7.

Hanavan (1964) developed a computerized segment model of the human body from which body segment parameters could be obtained from 25 standard anthropometric measurements of the individual. His main objective was to determine the inertial properties of the body as a whole. From Hanavan's subroutines, however, Miller and Nelson (1973) generated the segmental moments of inertia of an adult male subject. Their results, determined from this computer model, are compared to the moment of inertia data found by Dempster. Some of the differences in their findings may be due to differences in body size and Hanavan's estimate of the segmental forms.

From Dempster's moment of inertia data, Plagenhoef (1966) calculated the segmental radii of gyration for the moments of inertia about an axis perpendicular to the long axis of the body segment. The radii of gyration were determined about the proximal and distal ends of the limbs by use of the parallel axis theorem. These proximal and distal radii of gyration are shown in Table A–8.

METHOD OF FINDING THE WEIGHT OF A SEGMENT

The following is the derivation of the formula for determining the weight of a body part. In Figure A–3 the upper subject lies prone on a board, one end of which rests on a scale. We take moments about the left support:

$$(SL) + (-WX) = 0$$
$$SL = WX \tag{1}$$
$$X = \frac{SL}{W}$$

TABLE A–6. CENTER OF MASS/SEGMENT LENGTH RATIOS TO PROXIMAL END FROM SEVERAL CADAVER STUDIES*

Source	Braune and Fischer (1889)	Dempster (1955b)	Clauser et al. (1969)
Total body	— %	— %	41.2%
Head	—	43.3	46.6
Trunk	—	—	38.0†
Arm	47.0	43.6	51.3
Forearm	42.1	43.0	39.0
Hand	—	49.4	48.0†
Total arm	—	—	41.3
Forearm and hand	47.2	67.7†	62.6†
Thigh	44.0	43.3	37.2†
Calf	42.0	43.3	37.1
Foot	44.4	42.9	44.9
Total leg	—	43.3	38.2†
Calf and foot	52.4	43.7	47.5

*Adapted from Clauser et al., 1969.
†These values are not directly comparable owing to variations in the definition of segment length used by the different investigators.

Then, taking moments about the same point, since the moments of the components must be equal to the moment of the resultant,

$$WX = W_1X_1 + W_2X_2 \qquad (2)$$

Now, applying the same equations to the lower figure,

$$(S'L) + (-WX') = 0$$
$$S'L = WX' \qquad (3)$$
$$X' = \frac{S'L}{W}$$

and

$$WX' = W_1X_1 + W_2X_2' \qquad (4)$$

Subtracting equation (4) from equation (2):

$$\begin{aligned} WX &= W_1X_1 + W_2X_2 \\ WX' &= W_1X_1 + W_2X_2' \\ \hline W(X - X') &= W_2(X_2 - X_2') \\ W_2 &= \frac{W(X - X')}{(X_2 - X_2')} \end{aligned} \qquad (5)$$

TABLE A–7. PRINCIPAL MOMENTS OF INERTIA ($Kg = m^2 \times 10^{-4}$)

Segment	From Dempster (1955) I_{cm} $\bar{x} \pm S$	From Dempster (1955) I_0 $\bar{x} \pm S$	From Miller and Nelson (1974) I_{cm} I_x	From Miller and Nelson (1974) I_{cm} I_y	From Miller and Nelson (1974) I_{cm} I_z
Head and neck	294 ± 62	1419 ± 268*			
Head			379	379	177
Thorax	1154 ± 56	3881 ± 1690†			
Upper trunk			602	360	664
Abdominal-pelvic region	4337 ± 3132	7265 ± 3666‡			
Lower trunk			5463	4546	2365
Arm	140 ± 45	408 ± 145	179	179	23
Forearm	56 ± 9	183 ± 47	71	71	8
Hand	47 ± 1.9	303 ± 8	3.8	3.8	3.8
Upper limb	1039 ± 264	3396 ± 1034			
Forearm and hand	190 ± 51	589 ± 152			
Thigh	1090 ± 864	2997 ± 1196	587	587	201
Leg	423 ± 144	1405 ± 602	465	465	39
Foot	30.1 ± 4.7	646 ± 26	58	58	5.6
Lower limb	6904 ± 1994	18176 ± 5901			
Leg and foot	1077 ± 377	3332 ± 1143			

*From hip joint.
†From T_{12} vertebra.
‡From C_7 vertebra.

TABLE A–8. RADIUS OF GYRATION AS PERCENTAGE OF SEGMENT LENGTH*

	Radius of Gyration	
Segment	From Proximal End	From Distal End
Head, neck, and trunk	49.7%	67.5%
Arm	54.2	64.5
Forearm	52.6	64.5
Hand	58.7	57.7
Upper limb†	64.5	59.6
Forearm and hand†	82.7	56.5
Thigh	54.0	65.3
Leg	52.8	64.3
Foot	69.0	69.0
Lower limb‡	56.0	65.0
Leg and foot‡	73.5	57.2

*Data from Plagenhoef, 1966.
†To the ulnar styloid.
‡To the medial malleolus.

Substituting equations (1) and (3) for X and X′,

$$W_2 = \frac{W\left(\dfrac{SL}{W} - \dfrac{S'L}{W}\right)}{(X_2 - X_2')}$$

$$W_2 = \frac{L(S - S')}{(X_2 - X_2')} \tag{6}$$

Then the weight of the leg and foot (W_2) is equal to the distance between the supports for the board, multiplied by the difference between scale readings with the leg horizontal and with it vertical, and divided by the distance the center of mass of the leg and foot moves horizontally as the limb moves from the first to the second position.

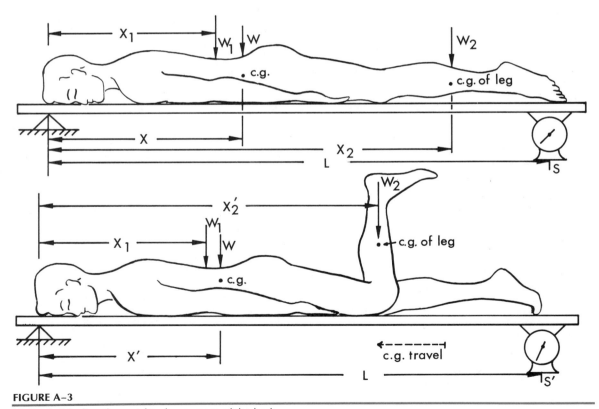

FIGURE A–3

Method of finding the weight of a segment of the body.

REFERENCES

Braune W, Fischer O: Über den Schwerpunkt des menschlichen Korpers mit Rucksicht auf die Austrustung des deutschen Infanteristen. Abh. d. Math.-Phys. cl. d. K. Sachs. Gersellsch. der Wiss. 26:561–672, 1889. *In* Krogman WM, Johnston FE (Eds): Human mechanics—four monographs abridged. Wright-Patterson Air Force Base, Ohio, 1963 (AMRL-TDR-63-123).

Brooks CB, Jacobs AM: The gamma mass scanning technique for inertial anthropometric measurement. Med Sci Sports 7:290–294, 1975.

Clauser CE, McConville JT, Young JW: Weight, volume, and center of mass of segments of the human body. Wright-Patterson Air Force Base, Ohio, 1969 (AMRL-TR-69-70).

Dempster WT: Space requirements of the seated operator. Wright-Patterson Air Force Base, Ohio, 1955 (WADCTR 55-159).

Dempster WT: Free-body diagrams as an approach to the mechanics of human posture and locomotion. *In* Evans FG (Ed): Biomechanical Studies of the Musculoskeletal System. Springfield, IL, Charles C Thomas, 1961.

Drillis R, Contini R: Body Segment Parameters. Tech. Report 1166.03. New York, New York University, 1966.

Drillis R, Contini R, Bluestein M: Body segment parameters: A survey of measurement techniques. Artif Limbs 8:44–68, 1964.

Hanavan EP: A mathematical model of the human body. Wright-Patterson Air Force Base, Ohio, 1964 (AMRL-TR-64-102).

Hay JG: The center of gravity of the human body. Kinesiology III. Washington, DC, American Association of Health, Physical Education, and Recreation, 1973.

Miller DI, Nelson RC: Biomechanics of Sport. Philadelphia, Lea & Febiger, 1973.

Plagenhoef SC: Methods for obtaining data to analyze human motion. Res Q Am Assoc Health Phys Educ 37:103–112, 1966.

Plagenhoef SC: Patterns of Human Motion: A Cinematographical Analysis. Englewood Cliffs, NJ, Prentice-Hall, 1971.

Trotter M, Gleser GC: Estimation of stature from long bones of American whites and Negroes. Am J Phys Anthrop 10:463–514, 1952.

Appendix B

Glossary

Acceleration—Time rate of change of velocity.

Anisotropic—A material that has directional structural orientation with its mechanical properties different in different directions.

Axis of rotation—Line about which all points in a rotating body describe circles.

Biomechanics—Branch of mechanics applied to biologic tissues.

Brittle—Property of a material in which only small amounts of energy are absorbed before failure. Dry bone and dry noodles are examples.

Center of gravity—Point in the body through which resultant force of gravity acts.

Center of mass—Point in the body, or body part, at which all the mass seems to be concentrated.

Centroid—Point in a two-dimensional figure at which area can be considered to be concentrated.

Colinear—Lying along the same line.

Composition of forces—Obtaining a resultant force from two or more forces.

Compression—Colinear forces acting in opposite directions to push together.

Concentric—Having the same center.

Concurrent—Meeting at a point.

Coplanar—Lying in the same plane.

Couple—Two equal but opposite parallel forces.

Creep—The increase of strain of a material that occurs during constant loading over a long time period.

Damping—Property of an object to resist speed of deformation.

Displacement—Distance and direction of movement.

Ductile—Ability of a material to absorb large amounts of energy before failure, e.g., wire.

Dynamics—Study of motions of bodies and forces acting to produce the motions.

Elasticity—Property of an object to return to its original size and shape after removal of loading.

Equations of motion—Equations based upon Newton's second law and expanded by Euler demonstrating that the resultant of the external forces and inertial forces acting on a body equals zero.

Equilibrant—A force that is equal in magnitude and opposite in direction to the resultant or a force that keeps the system in equilibrium.

Equilibrium—State in which a body is at rest with neither translatory nor rotatory motion (static equilibrium) or in which a body is in constant motion with no acceleration (dynamic equilibrium).

Fatigue—Failure of a structure following repetitive application of low-magnitude loads.

Force—A push or a pull produced by the action of one body on another.

Force systems:
  Linear (colinear)—Forces in one line.
  Parallel—Forces parallel to each other.
  Concurrent—All forces meeting at a common point.
  General—Any system of forces that cannot be classified as linear, parallel, or concurrent.

Free body diagram—Diagram of a body or portion thereof showing all forces acting on it.

Friction—Tangential force acting between two bodies in contact that opposes motion.

Gravity line (line of gravity)—Action line of force of gravity.

Hysteresis—Loss of energy during cycles of loading and unloading an object.

Inertia—That property of a body which makes it resist a change in motion.

Inverse dynamics—Evaluating values of forces based upon kinematic information.

Isotropic—A material that has no directional structural orientation with its mechanical properties the same in all directions.

Kinematics—Study of the relation between displacement, velocity, and acceleration.

Kinetics—Study of moving bodies, including forces producing motion.

Line diagram—Simple graphic portrayal of a body or part.

Link—Distance between joint centers of body segments.

Load—An externally applied force.

Mass—Resistance of change in linear velocity: the amount of matter equals weight divided by accleration of gravity ($m = W/g$).

Mechanics—Study of the action of forces on bodies.

Modulus of elasticity—Ratio of stress to strain during loading in the elastic range.

Moment of force—Product of force and distance (moment arm) from any point to the action line of force.

Moment of inertia—Resistance to change in angular velocity ($I = \Sigma mr^2$).

Momentum—Product of mass and its velocity (mv) or moment of inertia and its angular velocity (Iw).

Normal—Perpendicular to the surface.

Parallelogram law—Resultant of two concurrent forces is the diagonal of a parallelogram whose sides are the original forces.

Plane motion—Motion in a single plane.

Plasticity—Permanent deformation of a material following loading beyond the elastic limit.

Polygon—Multisided figure.

Power—Time rate of doing work, e.g., newton-meters per minute.

Pressure—Quantity of force per unit area.

Radian—Measure of angular displacement. One radian equals 57.3°.

Radius of gyration—Distance from the axis of rotation to a point on a rigid body at which if all the mass were concentrated, the mass times this radius squared would equal the moment of inertia of the body.

Rectangular components—Components of a force at right angles to each other.

Rectilinear motion—Motion in which all points in a body describe straight parallel lines.

Resilience—Ability of an object to vigorously rebound to its original size and shape.

Resolution of forces—Forming two or more forces from one force, usually forming rectangular components from a single force.

Resultant—Simplest equivalent force system that will replace any given system.

Reverse effect—Inertial forces that oppose change in motion.

Rigid body—An object in which the distance between every pair of points on the object remains the same.

Rotatory—Motion in which all particles of the body move in concentric circles.

Scalar quantity—Quantity having magnitude only.

Shear—Forces that are coplanar and opposite in direction, but not colinear; a force that causes one surface of a body to slide past an adjacent surface.

Statics—Study of forces acting on bodies at rest.

Stiffness—Resistance offered by a structure to external loads.

Strain—Deformation (lengthening or shortening) of any body or member.

Strength (mechanical)—Stress at which an object fails.

Strength (muscular)—Amount of force produced by a muscle.

Stress—Internal force between molecules.

Stress relaxation—Decrease of stress within a material following the loading and maintenance of constant strain.

Tension—Colinear forces acting in opposite directions to pull an object apart.

Torque—Moment of force (term generally applied to rotation of shaft).

Translatory (translational) motion—Motion in which all points in a body describe parallel lines, either straight or curved.

Vector quantity—Quantity having both magnitude and direction.

Velocity—Time rate of change of displacement.

Viscoelasticity—Behavior of a material that combines the properties of viscosity and elasticity.

Work—Product of force and displacement.

Appendix C

Answers to Selected Questions

CHAPTER 4

7. Swing 336 N, or 75 lb. Hammock at 20° angle with horizontal 982 N, or 220 lb.
8. Vertical = 22.24 N, or 5 lb. Horizontal = 38.5 N, or 8.66 lb.
9. Angle with river bank is 32°. She will travel 195 m or 640 feet downstream.
10. Sin 25° = 0.4226, or 42.26 percent.
    Cos 25° = 0.9563, or 95.63 percent.
    Sin 73° = 0.9063, or 90.63 percent.
    Cos 73° = 0.2924, or 29.24 percent.
11. Resultant decreases. The maximum resultant will be 0° between the two concurrent forces.
12. (a) The Rx component of the muscles is −25.7 N, or −5.78 lb. The Ry component of the muscles is 611.5 N, or 137.48 lb. The resultant magnitude is 611.6 N, or 137.6 lb. The resultant direction is 2.5° with the vertical up and left.
    (b) If tendon force equals 611.6 N (137.6 lb) then resultant of patella is −25.7 N (−5.78 lb) at an angle of 1.19° with the horizontal to the left and down.
    (c) The resulting magnitude of force on the patella is 17 N, or 3.82 lb, at an angle of 3.22° with the horizontal up and to the right.
    (d) The muscle resultant would be 628.6 N, or 141.33 lb, at an angle of 1.04° with the vertical up and to the left. The resultant on the patella would be 11.43 N, or 2.57 lb, at less than 1° with the horizontal.

CHAPTER 5

5. Table A–1 gives a force of gravity on the arm of 32.5 N (7.3 lb). The total tension force would be 57.5 N (12.9 lb).
6. (a) 605 N (136 lb).
   (b) 302.5 N (68 lb).
   (c) Compression.
7. (a) 120 N (27 lb).
   (b) Tension
   (c) 135 N (30.35 lb).
8. 300 N (67.45 lb).
9. Head weight from Table A–5 is 7.3 percent of the body weight.
   (a) Tension on tissues of the neck is 34.4 N (7.7 lb).
   (b) Tension on tissues of the neck is 234.3 N (52.7 lb).
10. (a) Force on each hand is 300 N (67.4 lb).
    (b) Force on each hand is 235 N (52.8 lb).
11. (a) 1200 N (270 lb).
    (b) 250 N (56 lb).
12. Table A–5 shows the total force of gravity of the lower limb as 16.1 percent of body weight and of the leg and foot as 5.8 percent of body weight.
    (a) 183.8 N (41.32 lb).
    (b) 101.4 N (22.8 lb).
13. (a) 117 N (26.3 lb).
    (b) 47.9 N (10.8 lb).
    (c) Less.
14. 52 N (11.7 lb).
15. (a) F = 50 N.
    (b) T = 90 N.
    (c) B = 150 N and H = 450 N.
    (d) C = 173.2 N.
    (e) B = 150 N and G = 450 N.
    (f) M = 725 N and J = 575 N.

(g) M = 725 N, J = 66.3 N, and θ = 18.7°
with the horizontal.

(h) F = 200 N.

18. (a) 16.5 N (3.7 lb).
(b) 31.9 N (71.7 lb).

19. 69.15 N (15.5 lb).

29. (a) 144 m.
(b) 0.96 m.

30. Tables A–1 and A–5 show that the forearm and hand equal 2.2 percent body weight and that the center of mass is 62.6 percent of the entire forearm and hand length.
(a) Varies about 4.42 Nm.
(b) 88 N.

32. (a) For a 670 N (68.4 kg) person, the resultant moment is 2680 Nm.
(b) 3.2 m.

34. 2.67 times more force at 15 cm.

37. (a) 164.7 N.
(b) 535.3 N.

38. (a) 200 Nm at 0°.
173 Nm at 30°.
141 Nm at 45°.
100 Nm at 60°.
0 Nm at 90°.

CHAPTER 6

2. μ = 0.3.

3. 24.4 N (5.5 lb).

4. 24.2°.

5. (a) 150 N (33.7 lb).
(b) 254.9 N (57.3 lb).
(c) More to slide 266.4 N (60 lb).
(d) 19.8° if μ = 0.36.

6. (a) 60 N (13.5 lb).
(b) It will tip over.
(c) 1 m or below.

9. 16.7°.

CHAPTER 7

2. 6.67 minutes.

3. (a) 0.25 m/sec.

(b) 5.5 m/sec.

(c) 22 m.

4. (a) 50°/sec, or 0.87 rad/sec.
(b) −4.0 rad/sec.
(c) 52.36 rad/sec.

5. (a) 7.85 rad/sec.^{2}
(b) 2 rad/sec.^{2}
(c) −20 rad/sec.^{2}

6. (a_1) 1.047 m/sec.
(a_2) 1.047 rad/sec.
(b_1) 1.047 m/sec.
(b_2) 0.346 m/sec.

7. (a) 3.14 rad/sec.
(b) 188.4 cm/sec.
(c) 47.1 cm/sec.

16. 45.36 N (10.2 lb).

24. Moment equals 55.02 Nm
Muscle force equals 1556.2 N (349.86 lb).
F_T = 353.6 N (79.5 lb), F_R = 1166.5 N (262.26 lb), and F = 1219 N (274 lb).

CHAPTER 8

5.

Joint Angle	Muscle Force	Tibial-femoral Joint Force
Degrees	N (lb)	N (lb)
90	0	27 (6.1)
60	608 (136.7)	562 (126.3)
45	860 (193.3)	808 (181.7)
30	1053 (236.7)	1024 (230.2)
0	1216 (273.4)	1168 (262.6)

8. (b) 53.3 N (12 lb).
(c) 1040 N (233.8 lb).

9. 8.7 N.

12. (a) 45 N (10.1 lb).
(b) 1298 N (291.8 lb).

13. (a) 144.2 Nm (106.3 ft-lb).
(b) 183.8 Nm (135.6 ft-lb).

14. Approximately 70 N (15.7 lb) at 34.5 cm (13.58 inches) from the proximal end of the limb. The moment equals 24.15 Nm (17.8 ft-lb).

22. (a) 300 N (67.4 lb).
(b) 360 N (80.8 lb).

27. (a) 50 N (11.2 lb), 50 N, and 0 N.
    (b) 800 N (179.9) lb).
    (c)

Forearm Angle	Muscle Angle	Muscle Force	Rotatory Force	Nonrotatory Force	Joint Force
Degrees	*Degrees*	*N (lb)*	*N (lb)*	*N (lb)*	*N (lb)*
0	90	923.8 (184.75)	800 (179.8)	461.9 (103.8)	680 (152.9)
0	15	3091 (694.9)	800 (179.8)	2985.6 (671.2)	3061 (688.2)
30	45	980 (220.3)	692.8 (155.8)	692.8 (155.8)	864.4 (194.3)
30	45	980 (220.3)	692.8 (155.8)	692.8 (155.8)	955.8 (214.9)

INDEX

Note: Page numbers in *italic* type indicate illustrations; those followed by a (t) refer to tables.

A

Abdominal muscles, strengthening of, gravitational force in, 276–277, *278*

Abductor muscles, of hip, weakness of, walking method in, 262–263, *264*

Acceleration, angular, average, calculation of, *157*, 157–158
   components of, 159, *160*, 161
      of forearm motion, in unloaded and loaded elbow flexion, 165, 166(t)
         unloaded, graph of, 165, *167*
   components of, correlation of, 163–166, 164(t), *165*, 166(t)
   definition of, 308
   in walking, 24–25
   instantaneous, analysis of, acceleration approach to, 166
   kinematic parameters of, recording and measuring techniques for, 163–164
   linear (translational), calculation of, 154, *155*
      definition of, 153
      instantaneous, 154
      magnitude and direction of, in exercise systems, 169–170, *170*
      negative, 153
      relationship between angular acceleration and, 158–159, 161, *161*
      relationship to force and mass of, 167–168, *168*
   Newton's law of, 24
   of runner, 154, *155*
      maximum, resultant force necessary for, 169, *169*
   radial, components of, relation to rectangular components of, *160*, 163
      equations for, 159
      of rigid body, 162–163
      relation to Newton's first law of, 159, 161
   rectangular components of, equations for, 163
      in determining reaction force, 185, 187

Acceleration *(Continued)*
   tangential, components of, relation to rectangular components of, *160*, 163

Achilles tendon, upward force on, 70–71, *71*

Aluminum, for orthotics and prosthetics, mechanical properties of, 48
   for surgical implants, mechanical properties of, 47, 48(t)

Amputation, center of mass after, 245–246
   kinematic and kinetic study of, 218–219
   mechanical energy changes after, 217
   muscle and joint forces after, 217–218

Anisotropic, definition of, 308

Ankle, forces at, following heel strike, 193–195, *195*
      in joint disease, 218
   moments at, following heel strike, 193–195, *195*
      in joint disease, 218
   surface landmarks associated with, 300(t)

Aorta, mechanical properties of, 43(t), 44

Arms, function of, during walking, 222–223

Arthritis, gait analysis in, 219
   hand deformity from, force resolution in, 86

Athletics, application of force in, 196
   conservation of angular momentum in, 201
   protective equipment for, biomechanical principles of, 6

Autograft, fresh, mechanical properties of, 55

B

Back, injuries to, unsafe lifting techniques and, 237
   low, forward trunk flexion of, forces on, 257, *258*
      strain from, 255, *256*
      while lifting, magnitude of forces during, 258–260, *259*
   posture of, mechanics of, 255–260, *256–259*
   stress to, during lifting, 225

313

ISBN 0-7216-5743-5

90016